Advanced Practice in Critical Care

Advanced Practice in Critical Care

A Case Study Approach

Edited by

Sarah McGloin, RN, BSc, MA

Senior Lecturer in Acute Care
Anglia Ruskin University, Chelmsford, UK

Anne McLeod RN, BSc, MSc

Senior Lecturer in Critical Care
School of Community and Health Sciences
City University, London, UK

WILEY-BLACKWELL

A John Wiley & Sons, Ltd., Publication

Library of Congress Cataloging-in-Publication Data

McGloin, Sarah, RN.
    Advanced practice in critical care : a case study approach / Sarah McGloin, Anne McLeod (eds.).
        p. ; cm.
    Includes bibliographical references and index.
    ISBN 978-1-4051-8565-3 (pbk. : alk. paper) 1. Intensive care nursing – Case studies.
I. McLeod, Anne, RN. II. Title.
    [DNLM: 1. Critical Illness – nursing. 2. Critical Care – methods. WY 154 M478a 2010]
    RT120.I5M38 2010
    616.02'8 – dc22
                                                                    2009037543

A catalogue record for this book is available from the British Library.

Typeset in 9.5/10.5pt Sabon by Laserwords Private Limited, Chennai, India.
Printed and bound in Malaysia by KHL Printing Co Sdn Bhd.

1   2010

Contents

Preface

Nursing interventions and medical management of the critically ill patient have evolved considerably as clinical advancements and technological developments are introduced into everyday practice. This has required experienced critical care nurses to extend their knowledge so that they can provide care that is grounded in evidence.

The aim of this book is to provide in-depth rationale for contemporary critical care practice in an effort to increase the depth of knowledge of nurses who care for the critically ill patient, so that they can truly evaluate their care interventions in view of underlying pathophysiology and evidence. Critically ill patients often experience multiple system dysfunctions within their critical illness trajectory; therefore, this book is written with an emphasis on holistic care rather than compartmentalising patients by their primary illness or organ dysfunction. Through this, the impact of critical illness and the development of multi-organ involvement will be explored.

As nurses become more assertive and partners in health-care decision-making, a knowledge base that reflects contemporary practice is required to enable active participation. This book, therefore, will provide experienced critical care practitioners with the depth of knowledge that he or she needs to be confident in leading and negotiating care whilst offering the critically ill patients and their family the support they require.

It is anticipated that this book will act as an essential resource to experienced practitioners, including critical care outreach, who primarily care for patients requiring high dependency or intensive care.

All of the scenarios are fictitious and are not based on real patients. Any similarities to real situations are coincidental. Nursing and Midwifery Council (NMC) regulations on confidentiality have been maintained throughout.

Sarah McGloin
Anne McLeod

Contributors

Elaine Cole, RN, BSc, MSc
Senior Lecturer–Practitioner in Trauma/Emergency Care, School of Community and Health Sciences, City University, London, UK

Glenda Esmond, RN, BSc, MSc
Respiratory Nurse Consultant, Barnet Primary Care Trust, London, UK

Tracey Bowden, RN, BSc, MSc
Lecturer in Cardiac Nursing, School of Community and Health Sciences, City University, London, UK

Sarah McGloin, RN, BSc, MA
Senior Lecturer in Acute Care, Anglia Ruskin University, Chelmsford, UK

Anne McLeod, RN, BSc, MSc
Senior Lecturer in Critical Care, School of Community and Health Sciences, City University, London, UK

Mark Ranson, RN, BSc
Senior Lecturer in Acute and Critical Care, University Campus Suffolk, Ipswich, UK

Phillipa Tredant, RN, BSc
Sister, Intensive Care Unit, St Bartholomew's Hospital, Barts and the London NHS Trust, London, UK

Acknowledgements

We would like to thank our families and friends for the patience and support. We would also like to thank previous clinical colleagues who have shared their knowledge with us.

Chapter 1

Challenges in contemporary critical care

Sarah McGloin

Introduction

The long-held traditional view that critical care nursing is regarded to be a 'speciality within nursing that deals specifically with human responses to life threatening problems' (American Association of Critical Care Nurses, 2009) is being increasingly challenged. The concept of the traditional intensive care unit (ICU), where patients, staff and equipment are geographically co-located is being increasingly challenged by the concept of 'critical care without walls'.

This chapter examines contemporary aspects relating to critical care nursing, with practices at both national and international levels being explored. Implications regarding new roles and new ways of working for the critical care nurse are also considered.

Critical care without walls

The philosophy of 'critical care without walls' has gained increasing momentum over the past decade, especially with support from policy documents such as *Critical to Success* (Audit Commission, 1999) and *Comprehensive Critical Care* (DH, 2000). Brilli *et al.* (2001) translate this contemporary view of critical care as being the appropriate medical care given to any physiologically compromised patient. Consequently, the underpinning philosophy to 'critical care without walls' is that any patient whose physiological condition deteriorates should receive both the appropriate medical and nursing care to which their condition dictates, no matter where they are physically located within the primary or tertiary care setting.

Importantly, Endacott *et al.* (2008) argue that this new approach to the delivery of critical care will aim to address Safar's long-held concerns from as far back as 1974 that critical care is no more than an increasingly unnecessary and expensive form of terminal care in a lot of cases (Safar, 1974). Similarly, Rosenberg *et al.* (2001) suggest that mortality rates and lengths of stay are also enhanced through a more effective and coordinated approach to the discharge and follow-up of patients from the critical care unit.

To facilitate this shift in the approach to the delivery of critical care, Endacott *et al.* (2008) argue that there is now an emphasis on empowering both the medical and nursing staff, who work within the acute care settings such as acute medical and surgical wards, with the knowledge, skills and attitude to recognise and effectively manage the deteriorating patient before they become severely and critically ill. Endacott *et al.* (2008) believe that it is the critical care nurse consultant who is ideally placed to support the empowerment of nurses working on general wards, particularly with regard to the development and assessment of decision-making skills.

Coombs *et al.* (2007) also support the empowerment of nurses with regard to clinical decision-making skills. They found that the nurses have become proficient at managing patients with long-term conditions such as chronic renal failure and respiratory failure. They argue that by pushing the boundaries of the traditional nursing role, the nursing contribution to the delivery of care has been enhanced.

Advanced practice

The expansion in the role of the nurse has not been confined to the United Kingdom. Kleinpell-Nowell (1999) and Kleinpell (2005) studied the steady growth of the acute care nurse practitioner (ACNP) role within the United States. Coombs *et al.* (2007) now see such opportunities developing within the United Kingdom. Such roles tend to come under the umbrella term of 'advanced practice'.

The concept of advanced practice is gaining increasing momentum within contemporary health-care practice. The notion of advanced practice is being driven by such factors as the demographic changes associated with an increasingly elderly population, budgetary constraints and workforce considerations, such as the European Working Time Directives, and the impact these have had on junior doctors' working hours and the General Medical Council (GMC) contract. Such factors demand a more streamlined and efficient health service. As a consequence, inter-professional groups within health care are developing additional knowledge, skills and practice, which were formerly the domain of other health professional groups. Within current health-care practice, some members of inter-professional groups such as nurses, paramedics, pharmacists and health scientists are developing advanced roles within their scope of practice. However, such advanced roles do not simply revolve around the ability to develop invasive procedures such as line insertions or intubation.

Despite its proliferation, there is much ongoing debate around the definition of 'advanced practice' (Furlong and Smith, 2005) along with acknowledgement of advanced skills being practiced in a huge variety of clinical settings. On the whole, many agree that 'autonomy' is the central ethos for advanced practice and the freedom to make informed treatment decisions based on acquired expertise within the individual's area of clinical practice.

Skills for Health (2009) does provide a useful definition of advanced practitioners as:

> *Experienced clinical professionals*
> *who have developed their skills and*
> *theoretical knowledge to a very high*
> *standard. They are empowered to make*
> *high level decisions and will often have*
> *their own caseloads.*

(Skills for Health, 2009)

The Skills for Health (2009) definition provides a generic definition for a range of inter-professional health-care practitioner's roles. For a nursing-profession-specific definition of advanced practice, the International Council for Nurses' (ICN, 2001) definition is widely considered:

> *A registered nurse who has acquired the expert knowledge base, complex*
> *decision making skills and clinical competencies for expanded practice, the*
> *characteristics of which are shaped by the context and for the country*
> *in which s/he is credentialed to practice. A masters degree is*
> *recommended for entry level.*

(ICN, 2001)

Advanced practice – an international perspective

The United States has developed a variety of advanced practice roles; however, within critical care, it is the nurse practitioner and the clinical nurse specialist (CNS) roles that dominate. Ackerman (1997) argued that these two roles could be blended together, based on the finding of Forbes *et al.* (1990) that educational programmes for both roles shared the same basic curriculum; however, the nurse practitioner programme included history taking, physical assessment techniques and pharmacology. There are, however, intrinsic differences to both roles. Hravnak *et al.* (1996) found that the CNS facilitates the care of the critically sick, and consequently, Mick and Ackerman (2000) argued that such facilitation means the CNS actually provides indirect care; their overall influence on patient outcome is difficult to quantify. Hravnak *et al.* (1996) believe it is the nurse practitioner who is directly involved with the delivery of care. As mid-level practitioners in the United States, the role of the advanced practitioner is far more quantifiable in terms of patient outcome and financial savings than that of the CNS (Rudy *et al.*, 1998).

The development of the advanced practitioner within the critical care arena in the United Kingdom is to some extent being driven by a reduced number of senior medical staff within the acute care setting. This mirrors the development of such roles within the United States, with rural areas experiencing difficulty recruiting medical staff, thus necessitating the need for nurses to develop their role to address such shortfalls in care (Dunn, 1997).

Within the United States, there is now an emerging role – that of the acute care nurse practitioner (ACNP). This role was initially developed within the tertiary care setting where the need arose for an advanced practitioner with the ability to directly manage the care of acute and critically ill patients within ICUs and high-acuity settings. The role remains supported by a national educational programme, which is delivered at masters' or post-masters' level of study (National Panel for Acute Care Nurse Practitioner Competencies, 2004). The ACNP receives credentials to practice and the role is highly regulated.

Kleinpell-Nowell (1999) and Becker *et al.* (2006) examined the role of the ACNP and found that the main focus was on direct patient care. This was in the form of liaising with families regarding plans of care, discharge planning and evaluating laboratory results to enhance the management of individual patients. In contrast to a common misconception regarding the role, Kleinpell-Nowell (1999) found that the degree to which the ACNP became involved with invasive procedures depended on the local patient population and local health-care policies. Importantly, back in 1999, Kleinpell-Nowell found that the ACNP also became involved in teaching, research, project work and quality assurance, which at that time resulted in the potential to fragmentate the role.

In 2005, Kleinpell published the results of a 5-year longitudinal study into the ACNP's role, where subjects had been questioned on an annual basis to collect data. The results found that most ACNPs were practising within a variety of intensive care settings. Some ACNPs were also practising in emergency care, oncology, multi-practice clinics and paediatric settings. Similarly, Becker *et al.* (2006) found that ACNPs were practising in areas outside the normal critical care domains such as cardiac catheterisation laboratories, burns units, outpatient clinics and private practice. Interestingly, Becker *et al.* (2006) also found the ACNP focused attention on those who had experienced cerebral vascular accidents, hypoglycaemia and gastro-oesophageal reflux. Such conditions are associated more with chronic conditions and so this again indicates that the role of the ACNP is far less easily confined to the care of just those experiencing acute illness. The expansion of the role to areas outside the usual boundaries of traditional critical care settings reflects the 'critical care without walls' philosophy now being practised.

Such an expansion of the scope of critical care within the United States found that by 2005 the ACNP's role had expanded to include history taking, physical assessment and diagnosis, conducting autonomous ward rounds, managing care through formulating written plans of care, interpreting results, performing procedures, education, consultancy and discharge planning (Kleinpell, 2005). Interestingly, there still remains a common misconception that the main function of the ACNP's role is to undertake invasive procedures. In fact,

Kleinpell (2005) still found that the opportunity for the ACNP to undertake invasive procedures remained restricted by local policies, with Becker *et al.* (2006) finding invasive procedures, such as insertion of central venous lines and arterial lines, by the majority of ACNPs occurring less than once a month.

In particular, Kleinpell (2005) found that not only did ACNPs find the role interesting but also the additional benefits, such as their own continuing professional development opportunities, conference attendance and journal subscriptions, enhanced their job satisfaction and contributed to good retention rates for the role. Strong collaboration with medical colleagues was also cited as a positive aspect of the role. However, Kleinpell (2005) found that some ACNPs were still citing a lack of recognition for the role and the perception by some other health-care professionals that ACNPs were not an equivalent professional peer.

Despite this, Kleinpell's (2005) longitudinal study found that the ACNP's role did have a significant impact on health-care outcomes. Such influences included decreased cost of care due to reduced lengths of stay and readmission rates (Russell *et al.*, 2002; Miers and Meyer, 2005), enhanced quality through increased compliance with clinical guidelines (Garcias *et al.*, 2003), effective medical management and enhanced continuity of care (Hoffman *et al.*, 2004; Vazirani *et al.*, 2005). Kleinpell (2005) also identified appropriate resource management, patient satisfaction and overall education associated with the role.

Similar to the evolution of the ACNP within the United States, Australia too has adopted similar roles in critical care. Again, the reason for the emergence of such roles includes such factors as a large proportion of rural health-care settings and lack of recruitment of medical staff to such areas. However, unlike the United States where there are clear education and credentials for the ACNP, such a role in Australia is far less defined or regulated.

Despite this, there is now the emergence of the ICU liaison nurse. This role is still in its infancy; however, it appears to display similarities to the role of the critical care outreach team within the United Kingdom. The ICU liaison nurse aims to enhance the discharge of the patient from the ICU to the general ward setting. An important feature to this role is also the responsibility the ICU liaison nurse has for educating the ward team as well (Chaboyer *et al.*, 2004).

Advanced practice in the United Kingdom

Within the United Kingdom critical care services, Coombs *et al.* (2007) identified two main advanced roles: the critical care outreach nurse and the consultant nurse. The consultant nurse's role was formally introduced into the National Health Service (NHS) in 1999 (Health Service Circular, 1999). The nurse consultant in critical care often has responsibility for developing the individual Trust's critical care outreach services (Coombs *et al.*, 2007).

Within critical care, these roles were developed as an integral component of the changes to critical care services driven by *Comprehensive Critical Care* (DH, 2000). Similar to the Australian ICU liaison nurse model, the critical care outreach team aims to bridge the gap between critical care settings and the acute care settings, thereby facilitating a seamless delivery of care for the patients on their discharge from the critical care unit and reducing the risks of readmission. Such teams also aim to help identify and stabilise the deteriorating patient in an attempt to prevent admission in the first instance to the critical care unit (Coombs *et al.*, 2007). The outreach nurse is expected to work across both professional and structural boundaries to enhance the care of the critically ill in a variety of settings. To facilitate these aims, a major role of the team is to act as an educator to both medical and nursing staff regarding the care of the deteriorating patient. Because development of such teams is relatively new, the effectiveness of the critical care outreach team is the focus of much of the research currently being undertaken (Coombs *et al.*, 2007).

An example of the potential career progression of an individual nurse in the field of critical care within the United Kingdom can be found in Box 1.1.

Box 1.1 Example of career progression for a critical care nurse

Carol qualified as an enrolled nurse (EN) in 1988. She worked on a medical ward for 18 months before she moved into critical care nursing. Initially, she gained a post as a D grade staff nurse on a general intensive care unit. Carol remained at this grade for 4 years whilst she developed her knowledge and competence for nursing the critically sick individual.

Between 1994 and 1996, Carol undertook her conversion course to registered nurse (RN) and following successful completion of this she gained an E grade staff nurse post. As an E grade nurse in critical care, Carol undertook teaching and assessing in clinical practice and became a mentor and assessor for pre-registration nursing students who were on placement within the intensive care unit.

In 1998, Carol commenced her BSc (Hons) Nursing Practice, which included the intensive care nursing pathway, providing her with the opportunity to rotate around a variety of intensive care units to gain experience in specialities such as neurosurgical intensive care nursing, burns and plastics intensive care and cardiac intensive care practice. In 2000, Carol not only successfully gained a first class Honours degree but also became the senior staff nurse in a large inner city intensive care unit with 14 critical care beds.

By 2002, having completed a leadership programme, she gained the position of Sister Critical Care and commenced an MSc in Critical Care. Carol successfully completed her MSc in 2005. As part of her MSc, Carol had studied the effectiveness of the Critical Care Outreach Team, which did not exist in her Trust at that time. In 2005, she successfully put together a bid for funding to set-up and manage a Critical Care Outreach Team in her Trust.

Carol is now a consultant nurse in acute and critical care and is responsible for the management of the Critical Care Outreach team within the Trust. She is also a teaching fellow at the local university and is undertaking a research study into critical care nursing.

Interprofessional roles within critical care

Physician assistant

The physician assistant (PA) is a role that has been evolving within the US health-care system since the early 1960s. The first PA training programme was developed by Stead in 1965, with the role initially being developed to serve the shortfall in primary care provision for rural communities as well as to provide a role for ex-military personnel returning from the Vietnam conflict, who had delivered medical care during the war, though in an unqualified capacity.

The vision was for the PA to be a fully trained health-care professional with the ability to adopt the role of the junior doctor, that is, to take on the more routine and less complex areas of health care for the entirety of their career (Hutchinson *et al.*, 2001). Throughout the 1980s and 1990s, barriers fell and the scope of practice for the PA expanded, particularly in respect to the ability for such practitioners to prescribe. Indeed in 1991, Dubaybo and Carlson found that the role of the PA had shifted and that many were now being trained to care for the acutely ill patients within acute care settings, some of whom were experiencing multi-organ dysfunction. To support such role expansion, Dubaybo and Carlson (1991) found that new curricula were being developed to support the emerging role of the PA within the critical care setting.

The typical training programme for a PA takes on average 24 months and follows very much the medical model (American Association of Physician Assistant Programmes, 2000). Entry requirements vary from school leavers to those already with a degree, with prior experience of health care also varying; however, the PA in critical care has some previous health-care experience and is often already a graduate (Dubaybo and Carlson, 1991). Awards given are generally to degree level; however, there is currently a move for the training to be increased to Masters level. Larson and Hart (2007) argue that this will restrict the entry gate and that recruitment into the role could be severely compromised, particularly in rural areas within the United States.

> **Box 1.2 Role of physician assistant in critical care**
>
> (1) Documenting plans of care in the notes
> (2) Physical assessment of the critically sick
> (3) Initiation of therapy including antibiotic therapy, blood transfusion and medication
> (4) Cardiopulmonary resuscitation
> (5) Haemodynamic management
> (6) Management of the patient in shock
> (7) Cardioversion
> (8) Weaning respiratory support
> (9) Invasive procedures
> (10) Liaising with next of kin
> (11) Record keeping
>
> All this occurs under the direct supervision of the certified intensivist.

The role of the PA within critical care remains highly regulated (Dubaybo and Carlson, 1991). The PA will graduate with a degree. However, to be licensed and certified they also have to complete a certifying examination from the American Board of Physician Assistants.

On graduation, the PA then spends a 3-month period of consolidation, rotating with colleagues under the supervision of the certified intensivist. Following this, the PA will be formally certified. Despite this, they remain under direct supervision especially when performing invasive procedures. A summary of the role of the PA within critical care can be found in Box 1.2

In the United Kingdom, there remains an ongoing debate into the appropriateness of the PA's role within the NHS. Certainly, the PA would fill a gap at the middle level of practice, especially with the reduction of junior doctors' working hours (Hutchinson *et al.*, 2001). Indeed, Hutchinson *et al.* (2001) argue that it could be a way of attracting graduates with life science degrees, who rarely move into the current health-care system. It may also be seen as a way to retain staff from other health-care professions; however, the emergence of the critical care consultant nurse addresses this within nursing (Hutchinson *et al.*, 2001).

Advanced critical care practitioners

Latterly, the Department of Health has developed a *National Education and Competence Framework for Advanced Critical Care Practitioners* (DH, 2008). This role is seen by the Department of Health as a new way of working within critical care functioning, at a level similar to the specialist registrar, a role which, like the PA, is based on the medical model. The role would be fully accredited and regulated, much as that of the PA is in the United States.

A further role that is also envisaged is that of the assistant critical care practitioner. This practitioner will work with nursing staff and allied health professionals to support the work of the doctor.

After undertaking a formal training programme, the advanced critical care practitioner will work under the supervision of the medical team to undertake physical assessment: undertake or order diagnostic studies, prescribe medication and fluids, develop and manage plans of care, undertake invasive procedures, educate staff and patients alike and undertake patient transfers (DH, 2008). This role is in its infancy within the United Kingdom, with eight sites currently piloting the role; however, the benefits are purported to include reduced waiting times for procedures, appropriate investigations and treatment, expert delivery of patient care, enhancing the 'critical care without walls' philosophy, enhanced continuity of care, reduced length of stay and overall improved patient experience.

Conclusion

There has been an explosion of different roles within critical care over the past few years. It is widely agreed that such a plethora of roles has developed in response to factors such as reduced recruitment and retention of health-care staff as well as directives such as a reduction in the junior doctors' working hours. In particular, the influence of practices from the United States has been seen to have a direct effect on the delivery of health care in other countries such as Australia and the United Kingdom as well. The consequence of this is that there is now a blurring of the traditional professional boundaries, ensuring that the patient remains the focus of critical care no matter where they are located within the health-care setting.

References

Ackerman MH (1997) The acute care nurse practitioner: evolution of the clinical nurse specialist? *Heart and Lung* 26 (2) 85–86.

American Association of Critical Care Nurses (2009) Definition of Critical Care Nursing [online]. Available from: http://www.aacn.org/WD/PressRoom/Content/AboutCriticalCareNursing.pcms?pid=1... [Accessed 14th May 2009].

American Association of Physician Assistant Programmes (2000) *Physician Assistant Incomes, Results from the 1999 AAPA Physician Assistant Census*, American Association of Physician Assistants, Alexandria.

Audit Commission (1999) *Critical to Success - the Place of Efficient and Effective Critical Care Services Within the Acute Hospital*, Audit Commission, London.

Becker D, Kaplow R, Muenzen PM and Hartigan C (2006) Activities performed by acute and critical care advanced practice nurses: American Association of Critical-Care Nurses Study of Practice. *American Journal of Critical Care* 15 (2) 130–148.

Brilli R, Spevetz A, Branson RD, *et al.* (2001) Critical care delivery in the intensive care unit: defining clinical roles and the best practice model. *Critical Care Medicine* 29 2007–2019.

Chaboyer W, Foster MM, Foster M and Kendall E (2004) The intensive care unit liaison nurse: towards a clear role description. *Intensive and Critical Care Nursing* 20 (2) 77–86.

Coombs M, Chaboyer W and Sole ML (2007) Advanced nursing roles in critical care – a natural or forced evolution? *Journal of Professional Nursing* 23 (2) 83–90.

Department of Health (DH) (2000) *Comprehensive Critical Care*, The Stationery Office, London.

Department of Health (2008) *National Education and Competence Framework for Advanced Critical Care Practitioners*, The Stationery Office, London.

Dubaybo BA and Carlson RW (1991) The role of the physician assistants in critical care units. *Chest* 99 (1) 89–91.

Dunn L (1997) A literature review of advanced clinical nursing practice in the United States of America. *Journal of Advanced Nursing* 25 (4) 814–819.

Endacott R, Boulanger C, Chamberlain W, Hendry J, Ryan H and Chaboyer W (2008) Stability in shifting sands: contemporary leadership roles in critical care. *Journal of Nursing Management* 16 (7) 837–845.

Forbes KE, Rafson J, Spross J and Kozlowski D (1990) The clinical nurse specialist and nurse practitioner: core curriculum survey results. *Clinical Nurse Specialist* 4 (2) 63–66.

Furlong E and Smith R (2005) Advanced nursing practice: policy, education and role development. *Journal of Clinical Nursing* 14 (9) 1059–1066.

Garcias VH, Sicoutris CP and Meredith DM (2003) Critical care nurse practitioners improve compliance with clinical practice guidelines in the surgical intensive care unit. *Critical Care Medicine* 31 12 Abstract 93.

Health Service Circular (1999) *HSC 1999/217 Nurse, Midwife and Health Visitor Consultant*. National Health Service Executive, London.

Hoffman LA, Happ MB, Scharfenberg C, DiVirglio-Thomas D and Tasota F (2004) Perceptions of physicians, nurses and respiratory therapists about the role of acute care nurse practitioners. *American Journal of Critical Care* 13 (6) 480–488.

Hravnak M, Rosenzweig MQ and Baldisseri M (1996) Current questions with regard to acute care nurse practitioner preparation and role implementation. *American Association of Critical Care Nurses Clinical Issues* 7 (2) 289–299.

Hutchinson L, Marks T and Pittilo M (2001) The physician assistant; would the US model meet the needs of the NHS? *British Medical Journal* 323 (7323) 1244–1247.

International Council for Nurses (2001) *International Survey of Nurse Practitioner/Advanced Practice Nursing Roles [online]*. Available from: http://www.icn.ch/forms/networksurvey [Accessed 14 May 2009].

Kleinpell RM (2005) Acute care nurse practitioner practice: results of a 5-year longitudinal study. *American Journal of Critical Care* 14 (3) 211–221.

Kleinpell-Nowell R (1999) Longitudinal survey of acute care nurse practitioner practice: year 1. *American Association of Critical Care Nurses Clinical Issues* 10 (4) 515–520.

Larson EH and Hart GL (2007) Growth change in the physician assistant workforce in the United States 1967–2000. *Journal of Allied Health* 36 (3) 121–130.

Mick DJ and Ackerman MH (2000) Advanced practice nursing role delineation in acute and critical care: application of the strong model of advanced practice. *Heart and Lung* 29 (3) 210–221.

Miers S and Meyer L (2005) Effect of cardiovascular surgeon and advanced care nurse practitioner collaboration on post operative outcomes. *American Association of Critical Care Nurses Clinical Issues* 16 (2) 149–158.

National Panel for Acute Care Nurse Practitioner Competencies (2004) *Acute Care Nurse Practitioner Competencies*, National Organization of Nurse Practitioner Faculties, Washington.

Rosenberg AL, Hoffer TP, Hayward RA, Strachan C and Watts CM (2001) Who bounces back? Physiologic and other predictors of ICU readmission. *Critical Care Medicine* 29 (3) 511–518.

Rudy EB, Davidson LJ, Daly B, *et al.* (1998) Care activities and outcomes of patients cared for by acute care nurse practitioners, physician assistants and resident physicians: a comparison. *American Journal of Critical Care* 7 (4) 267–281.

Russell D, VordderBruegge M and Burns SM (2002) Effects of an outcomes-managed approach to care of neuroscience patients by acute care nurse practitioners. *American Journal of Critical Care* 11 (4) 353–364.

Safar P (1974) Critical care medicine – quo vadis? *Critical Care Medicine* 2 (1) 1–5.

Skills for Health (2009) Definition of Advanced Practice [online]. Available from: http://www.skillsforhealth.org.uk/page/careerframeworks [Accessed 17 May 2009].

Vazirani S, Hays RD, Shapiro MF and Cowan M (2005) Effect of a multidisciplinary intervention on communication and collaboration among doctors and nurses. *American Journal of Critical Care* 14 (1) 71–77.

Chapter 2

The physiological basis of critical illness

Mark Ranson

Introduction

Many of the physiological changes that occur in response to critical illness have a profound effect on the human body, particularly at a cellular level. Reynolds (2007) suggests that, in critical illness, there are many factors conspiring at the cellular level to inhibit the activity of mitochondria, damage them or reduce the production of new mitochondrial protein. This leads to the suggestion that cellular and mitochondrial pathology may lie at the root of the process of progressive organ failure. If this hypothesis is correct, then supportive therapy should be aimed at preserving and improving mitochondrial function to provide the necessary energy to enable normal metabolic processes. Whilst this represents one of many views held regarding the physiological basis of critical care, the notion of physiological changes at cellular level and the subsequent impact on the systemic progression of critical illness can serve as the foundation for further exploration of the mechanisms of cellular damage, the inflammatory response and haemostasis in the critically ill. The following scenario will be considered to establish a physiological basis of critical illness.

Patient scenario

Deborah was admitted to the critical care setting with multi-organ failure as a result of shock. Her assessment findings were:

HR	130 BPM SR
BP	80/35 mmHg (MAP 50)
CVP	3
RR	30 BPM
SaO$_2$	97% on a non-rebreathing system
Capillary refill	4 seconds
UOP	10 ml for last hour
AVPU	V
Temperature (core)	36.2°C

Peripheral oedema is evident

Blood gases:
pH   7.2
pO_2 12 kPa
pCO_2 4.0 kPa
HCO_3 16 mmol/l
BE   −6
Lactate 4

Blood results indicate that she had developed a coagulopathy and had altered liver function. Her C-reative protein (CRP) was elevated.

Key considerations

What are the key physiological changes that occur in critical illness?
How do these contribute to the findings of Deborah's clinical condition?

Mechanisms of cellular damage

In order to grow, function and reproduce, cells must harvest energy and convert the same into a useable form that can facilitate the work of the cell and synthesise new cell components to maintain the integrity of their structure and the ability to perform their particular functions. Within this section, the aim is to focus on the conversion of nutrients and raw materials to the energy stored in adenosine triphosphate (ATP) through the process of cellular respiration. By understanding this process, the impact of reduced perfusion in relation to energy production can be explored, leading to an evaluation of the concept of ischaemia: reperfusion injury.

Cellular respiration

Key consideration

What processes are used to provide cellular energy?

Cellular respiration refers to the processes used by cells to convert energy in the chemical bonds of nutrients to ATP energy. Depending on the organism, cellular respiration can be aerobic, anaerobic or both.

Aerobic respiration is an exergonic pathway which allows energy release out of the system but requires the presence of molecular oxygen for it to take place. Anaerobic respiration includes endergonic pathways where the system absorbs energy from the surroundings. These pathways do not require the presence of molecular oxygen and include anaerobic respiration and fermentation.

Aerobic respiration

Aerobic respiration is the aerobic catabolism of nutrients to form carbon dioxide, water and energy. Aerobic catabolism is the breakdown of molecules into smaller units, with the aim of releasing energy in the presence of molecular oxygen. This process involves an electron transport system, a mechanism by which electrons are passed along a series of carrier molecules, releasing energy for the synthesis of ATP in which oxygen is the final electron acceptor. The overall reaction of aerobic respiration is shown in Figure 2.1.

$$C_6H_{12}O_6 + 6O_2$$

Yields

$$6CO_2 + 6H_2O + \text{energy (as ATP)}$$

Figure 2.1   The overall reaction of aerobic respiration. Note that glucose ($C_6H_{12}O_6$) is oxidised to produce carbon dioxide (CO_2) and oxygen (O_2) is reduced to produce water (H_2O).

Aerobic respiration can be broken down into two main stages to aid further consideration:

(1) Glycolysis – a transition reaction that produces acetyl coenzyme A;
(2) The citric acid (Kreb's) cycle.

Glycolysis
Glycolysis is a metabolic pathway found in the cytoplasm of all cells in living organisms and does not require oxygen – it is an anaerobic process. This process converts one molecule of glucose into two molecules of pyruvate and makes energy in the form of two net molecules of ATP. Four molecules of ATP per molecule of glucose are actually produced; however, two of the ATP molecules are consumed in the preparation phase of glycolysis. During the payoff phase of glycolysis, four phosphate groups are transferred to adenosine diphosphate (ADP) and are used, through phosphorylation (the addition of phosphate), to produce four molecules of ATP. The overall reaction can be seen in Figure 2.2.

Through a transition reaction, glycolysis is linked to the citric acid (Kreb's) cycle. This transition reaction converts the two molecules of three-carbon pyruvate from glycolysis into two molecules of the two-carbon molecule acetyl coenzyme A (acetyl-CoA) and two molecules of carbon dioxide. The overall reaction for the transition stage is shown in Figure 2.3. The two molecules of acetyl-CoA can now enter the citric acid cycle.

The citric acid (Kreb's) cycle
This cycle takes the pyruvates from glycolysis and other pathways, such as the transition reaction mentioned earlier, and completely breaks them down into carbon dioxide and water, thus generating ATP molecules by oxidative phosphorylation. In addition to this role in ATP production, the citric acid cycle also plays an important role in the flow of carbon through the cell by supplying precursor metabolites. The overall reaction can be seen in Figure 2.4.

$$\text{Glucose} + 2\ NAD^+ + 2\ P_i + 2\ ADP$$

Yields

$$2\ \text{pyruvate} + 2\ NADH + 2\ ATP + 2H^+ + 2\ H_2O$$

Figure 2.2   The overall reaction of glycolysis. NAD^+, hydrogen carrier; P_i, phosphoglucose isomerase; ADP, adenosine diphosphate; NADH, nicotinamide adenine dinucleotide; H^+, hydrogen ion; ATP, adenosine triphosphate; H_2O, water; pyruvate, carboxylate anion of pyruvic acid.

$$2\ \text{pyruvate} + 2\ NAD^+ + 2\ \text{coenzyme A}$$

Yields

$$2\ \text{acetyl-CoA} + 2\ NADH + 2\ H^+ + 2\ CO^2$$

Figure 2.3   The overall reaction of the transition stage. Pyruvate, carboxylate anion of pyruvic acid; NAD^+, hydrogen carrier; acetyl-CoA, molecule of metabolism; NADH, nicotinamide adenine dinucleotide; H^+, hydrogen ion; CO_2, carbon dioxide.

$$2 \text{ acetyl groups} + 6 \text{ NAD}^+ + 2 \text{ FAD} + 2 \text{ ADP} + 2 \text{ P}_i$$

Yields

$$4 \text{ CO}_2 + 6 \text{ NADH} + 6 \text{ H}^+ + 2 \text{ FADH}_2 + 2 \text{ ATP}$$

Figure 2.4 The overall reaction of the citric acid (Kreb's) cycle. NAD^+, hydrogen carrier; FAD, flavin adenine dinucleotide; ADP, adenosine diphosphate; P_i, phosphoglucose isomerase; CO_2, carbon dioxide; NADH, nicotinamide adenine dinucleotide; H^+, hydrogen ion; $FADH_2$, energy carrying molecule; ATP, adenosine triphosphate.

The theoretical, maximum yield of ATP molecules during aerobic respiration is between 30 and 38 molecules of ATP per molecule of glucose. Although most energy (ATP) production by cells involves the use of oxygen, we have noted that some ATP production occurs during glycolysis in the absence of oxygen.

Anaerobic respiration

Anaerobic respiration is the process by which the normal pathway of glycolysis is routed to produce lactate. It occurs at times when energy is required in the absence of oxygen. It is, therefore, vital to tissues with high-energy requirements, insufficient oxygen supply or lack of oxidative enzymes. Anaerobic respiration is less efficient than aerobic metabolism in that it only generates approximately 8 ATP molecules from the potential 38 available per molecule of glucose. The ATP generated by anaerobic respiration is an important contribution, but it is insufficient on its own to sustain cell function for long periods of time. In addition to the low yield of ATP, anaerobic respiration produces lactic acid, which is highly toxic to cells and has to be removed or at least deactivated. Lactate may diffuse out of the cell and pass to the liver where it is transformed into glucose. The glucose is then capable of passing back to peripheral cells where it can re-enter the glycolysis pathway. This entire process is known as the *Cori cycle*. However, the ability of the liver to detoxify lactic acid and produce glucose as the end product is totally dependent on the presence of oxygen in sufficient quantities. The elevated lactate level seen in Deborah's scenario suggests that because of multi-organ failure as a complication of shock, the normal pathway for glycolysis has been routed to anaerobic respiration, resulting in the production of excess lactate.

Impact of reduced perfusion on energy production

Key consideration

What is the impact of reduced blood supply in the production of energy?

It has become clear that oxygen must be continually available to all cells in the body. Oxygen delivered to the cells is consumed by the mitochondria to provide the energy for metabolism (this energy is in the form of ATP), which is required for many chemical and mechanical processes within the body. Under normal circumstances, energy production is facilitated by oxygen – aerobically. If oxygen is unavailable anaerobic respiration (respiration in the absence of oxygen) will occur. This is an inefficient way for metabolism to occur and results in the production of lactic acid as an end product. Accumulation of lactic acid can result in metabolic acidosis. Therefore, if a defect occurs physiologically or mechanically in the oxygen delivery pathway, normal oxygenation can be reduced or impaired. This lack of oxygen delivery prompts the onset of anaerobic respiration as the cells attempt to maintain the energy supply needed for metabolic activity. The resulting accumulation of lactic acid and onset of acidosis will, ultimately, lead to cell death and tissue damage.

Hypoxic states, therefore, arise when the oxygen supply to a tissue cannot match the cellular requirements of that particular tissue group. Aerobic metabolism will decline and the production of lactic acid will increase as anaerobic respiration begins to dominate. The inefficient production of ATP by anaerobic respiration will soon become inadequate to maintain cell function, whilst the excessive production of lactic acid may also disrupt cell structures and their functions. It is worth noting here that there is a point at which the effects of the lack of oxygen are irreversible; from then on the cells will die, even if oxygenation is restored. In Deborah's case, the hypoxic state caused by the initial insult and onset of shock has allowed anaerobic respiration to become dominant, resulting in the excessive production of lactic acid, as evidenced by the raised serum lactate level and metabolic acidosis. It has also led to the respiratory system becoming involved, as indicated by her tachypnoea, to compensate for the metabolic acidosis. This important point can help to rationalise the need for prompt detection and early intervention in the critically ill patient.

Evaluation of ischaemia: reperfusion injury

Key consideration

What are the consequences of restoring perfusion to ischaemic tissues?

Ischaemia: reperfusion injury refers to the damage caused to tissues when the blood supply is returned to the tissue after a period of ischaemia. The absence of oxygen and nutrients in the blood during the hypoxic episode results in conditions in which the restoration of circulation and blood flow results in inflammation and oxidative damage through the induction of oxidative stress rather than the restoration of normal function (Polderman-Keys, 2004).

As already discussed, in aerobic organisms, the energy needed to fuel biological processes is produced in the mitochondria via the electron transport chain. In addition to energy, however, reactive oxygen species (ROS) are also produced and have the potential to cause cellular damage. ROS are produced as a normal product of cellular metabolism. Contained within the cell are catalase and superoxide dismutase, which serve to break down the potentially harmful components of ROS into oxygen and water. However, this conversion is not 100% efficient and residual components such as peroxide can be left in the cell. As such, whilst ROS are a product of normal cellular function, excessive amounts can lead to a deleterious effect (Muller *et al.*, 2007).

The damage of reperfusion injury is caused in part by the inflammatory response of damaged tissues. White blood cells carried to the site by the returning blood flow release a host of inflammatory mediators such as interleukins as well as free radicals in response to tissue damage. The restored blood flow reintroduces oxygen to the cell, which has the potential to damage cellular proteins, DNA and the plasma membrane. Damage to the cell's membrane may also, in turn, lead to the release of more free radicals. These reactive species are thought to contribute to redox signalling in that they take on a messenger role within the biological tissue that they inhabit. Through this process of redox signalling, cell apoptosis, a mechanism of programmed cell death, may be switched on. Returning leucocytes may also accumulate in small capillaries, obstructing them and leading to more ischaemia (Clark, 2007).

In prolonged ischaemia (60 minutes or more), hypoxanthine is formed as a breakdown product of ATP metabolism. When delivery of molecular oxygen is restored, the presence of this enzyme results in the conversion of the molecular oxygen into highly reactive superoxide and hydroxyl radicals. In Deborah's scenario, the refractory hypotension caused by the initial insult has led to end-organ hypoperfusion and the onset of multi-organ failure, as indicated by the reduction in urine output and alteration in liver function as well as her slightly reduced level of consciousness. It has also caused the shock state that Deborah was demonstrating.

In recent years, nitric oxide (NO), a diffusible short-lived product of arginine metabolism, has been found to be an important regulatory molecule in several areas of metabolism, including vascular tone control. In a healthy state, endothelial cells produce low levels of NO that regulates blood pressure by mediating adjacent smooth muscle relaxation. In a state of shock such as Deborah's, cytokines such as interleukin 1 and tumour necrosing factor induce a separate high-output form of the enzyme that synthesises NO in both endothelial and smooth muscle cells. The resulting high rates of NO formation result in extensive smooth muscle relaxation and pressor refractory vasodilatation, ultimately worsening the shocked state. Excessive NO produced during reperfusion reacts with superoxide to produce the potent reactive species, peroxynitrite. Such radicals and reactive oxygen species attack cell membrane, lipids and proteins, causing further cell damage (see Figure 2.5).

Hence, restoring blood flow after more than 10 minutes of ischaemia can become more damaging than the ischaemia itself because the stage is then set for oxygen to produce free radicals and ROS rather than to contribute to cellular energy production. Indeed, some medical approaches now suggest that the rapid reperfusion of ischaemic patients with oxygen actually causes cell death to occur through the above mechanisms. A more physiologically informed aim may be to reduce oxygen uptake, slow the metabolism and adjust the blood chemistry for gradual and safe reperfusion (Adler, 2007).

The inflammatory response and the role of mediators

Key consideration

What is the inflammatory response?

In 1992 (Bone *et al.*, 1992), the American College of Chest Physicians (ACCP) and the Society of Critical Care Medicine (SCCM) suggested definitions for systemic inflammatory response syndrome (SIRS), sepsis, severe sepsis, septic shock and multiple organ dysfunction syndrome (MODS). The rationale behind defining SIRS, now often called systemic inflammatory syndrome (SIS), was to define a clinical response to a non-specific insult of either infectious or non-infectious injury. Previous terminology had reflected the historical importance that infection has played in the development of sepsis; however, SIRS is not always related to infection. SIRS is non-specific and can be caused by ischaemia, inflammation, trauma, infection or a combination of several of these insults. Bone *et al.* (1992) published the consensus conference agreement of the definitions for SIRS and sepsis. These definitions emphasise the importance of the inflammatory response in these conditions, regardless of the presence of infection. The term *sepsis* is reserved for SIRS when infection is suspected or proved.

It therefore becomes clear that SIRS, independent of the aetiology, has the same pathophysiologic properties, with only minor differences in the inciting cascades. Inflammation is the body's response to non-specific insults that arise from chemical, traumatic or infectious stimuli. The inflammatory cascade is a complex process that involves humoral and cellular responses, complement and cytokine cascades. Bone (1996) summarises the relationships between these complex interactions and SIRS as a three-stage process:

- *Stage I:* Following an insult, cytokine is produced with the goal of initiating an inflammatory response, thereby promoting wound healing and recruiting the reticular endothelial system.

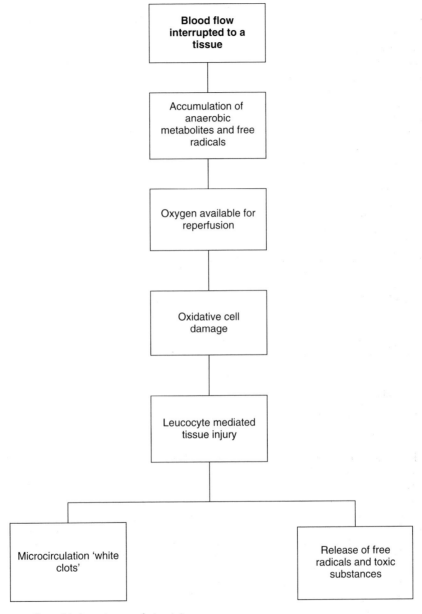

Figure 2.5   Effect of ischaemia: reperfusion injury.

- *Stage II:* Small quantities of local cytokines are released into the circulation to improve the local response. This leads to growth factor stimulation and recruitment of macrophages and platelets. This acute phase response is typically well controlled by a decrease in the proinflammatory mediators and by the release of endogenous antagonists.
- *Stage III:* If homeostasis is not restored, a significant systemic reaction occurs. The cytokine release leads to destruction rather than protection. A consequence of this is the activation of numerous humoral cascades and the activation of the reticular endothelial system, resulting in subsequent loss of circulatory integrity. This, ultimately, leads to end-organ failure.

The inflammatory response is, therefore, a protective response intended to eliminate the cause of an insult and any necrotic tissue present as a result of that insult. This response has three main stages:

(1) Vasodilatation – increased blood flow causing phagocytes, clotting factors, antibodies, etc. to be circulated to the area
(2) Increased permeability of blood vessels – allows plasma proteins to leave the circulation and access the site of insult
(3) Migration of leucocytes to the site of insult

In the critically ill, the processes caused by the immune response and resulting inflammation are disordered and out of control. A massive systemic reaction occurs and an excess of inflammatory mediators are released, causing an overwhelming physiological response, ultimately leading to tissue damage and organ dysfunction, as evidenced by the presentation scenario described for Deborah.

Within a very short period following the initial insult, blood vessels carrying the circulation away from the site of insult constrict, resulting in engorgement of the capillary network. The engorged capillaries produce the characteristic swelling and redness associated with inflammation. An increase in capillary permeability facilitates an influx of fluid and cells from the engorged capillaries into the surrounding tissues. The fluid that accumulates (exudate) contains much higher protein content than the fluid normally released from capillaries. The accumulation of this fluid around the site of insult gives rise to the characteristic swelling associated with inflammation due to the formation of oedema by the extra fluid volume within the tissue – hence the oedema that Deborah has. The increased capillary permeability, decreased flow velocity and the expression of adhesion molecules also facilitate the migration of various leucocytes from the capillaries into the tissues.

Phagocytic cells are the first type of leucocytes to migrate, neutrophils first followed by macrophages. Neutrophils are short-lived and die within the tissues, having exerted their effects. Macrophages are much longer lived and can provide longer term phagocytic activity at the site of insult. Later, lymphocytes (B and/or T) may also enter the site. Blood cells are able to leave the capillaries through a combination of the following processes:

• Margination – the adherence of the blood cells to the capillary walls
• Diapediesis/extravasation – emigration between the capillary endothelial cells and the tissues
• Chemotaxis – directed migration through the tissues to the site of the inflammatory response

Because phagocytic cells accumulate at the site, lytic enzymes are released, causing damage to nearby cells. This activity can lead to pus formation as dead cells, digested material and fluid accumulate.

Chemical mediators of inflammation

Key consideration

What mediators are involved in the inflammatory process?

The events in the inflammatory response are initiated by a complex series of interactions involving several chemical mediators whose interactions are still only partially understood. Some of these are derived from invading organisms, released by the damaged tissue, generated by several plasma enzyme systems or are the products of some of the white blood cells involved in the inflammatory response.

Histamine

Most histamine in the body is generated in the granules within mast cells or in basophils. The most important pathophysiologic mechanism of mast cell and basophil histamine is immunologic. These cells, if sensitised by immunoglobulin E antibodies attached to their membranes, degranulate when exposed to the appropriate antigen. Histamine release facilitates vasodilatation and increased capillary permeability.

Lipid-derived chemical mediators

Cell membrane phospholipids are hydrolysed by phospholipases at a reasonably high rate during inflammation. The arachidonic acid pathway leads to the production of leukotrienes and prostaglandins. Further evolving pathways result in the production of platelet-aggregating factors. The modes of action for the chemicals produced can be seen in Table 2.1.

Chemokines

Chemokines are small proteins produced by a wide variety of cells, of which 50 have currently been described. Chemokines are the major regulators of leucocyte traffic and help to attract the leucocytes to the site of inflammation. These proteins bind to proteoglycans on the cell surface and within the extracellular matrix and set up chemokine gradients for the migrating leucocytes to follow. An example of a well-characterised chemokine is interleukin 8 (IL-8).

Pro-inflammatory cytokines

Responding to the presence of chemokines, phagocytes enter the site of inflammation within a few hours. These cells release a variety of soluble factors, many of which have potent pro-inflammatory properties. Three of these cytokines, in particular, have very well-characterised activity – interleukin 6 (IL-6), interleukin 1 (IL-1) and tissue necrosis factor alpha (TNF-α). All three of these cytokines are known to be endogenous pyrogens because they induce fever by acting directly on the hypothalamus. They also induce production of acute phase proteins by the liver and trigger increased haematopoiesis (blood cell production) in the bone marrow, leading to leucocytosis.

Other mediators

The process of phagocytosis also results in the production of a variety of mediators of inflammation, including nitric oxide, peroxide and oxygen radicals. These oxygen and nitrogen intermediates have the potential to be toxic to the host micro-organism.

Table 2.1 Lipid-derived chemical mediators

Prostaglandins	Increase vasodilatation
	Increase vascular permeability
	Act as chemoattractants for neutrophils
Leukotrienes	Increase smooth muscle contraction
	Act as chemoattractants for neutrophils
Platelet-activating factors	Cause platelet aggregation
	Act as chemoattractants for neutrophils

Acute phase proteins

As mentioned earlier, the synthesis of acute phase proteins is triggered by the pro-inflammatory cytokines. Well-characterised examples include C-reactive protein (CRP) and mannose-binding protein. Therefore, in acute inflammatory situations, serum levels of these proteins become elevated as seen with Deborah's elevated CRP levels. CRP and mannose-binding protein are both capable of triggering complement fixation, leading to the formation of the membrane attack complex and the release of complement components, such as C3b, which function as opsonins, a binding enhancer in the process of phagocytosis.

Products of the four major plasma enzyme systems also serve as chemical mediators:

- Kinin system
- Complement system
- Coagulation system
- Fibrinolytic system

The four pathways are interconnected. These four enzyme systems generate factors that induce constriction of damaged blood vessels, general vasodilatation, increased capillary permeability, extravasation, chemotaxis and clearance of pathogens. Specifically, initial tissue damage triggers the activation of Hageman factor (one of the plasma clotting factors). Activated Hageman factor serves to trigger the kinin cascade and the clotting cascade. This in turn leads to fibrin deposition and clot formation. Fibrin clot serves to 'wall off' the insulted area from the rest of the body and serves to prevent the spread of infection. Ultimately, the fibrinolytic system leads to the synthesis of plasmin, which degrades/dissolves the fibrin clot when no longer needed and activates the complement system.

Kinins

Kinins are small peptides usually present in the blood in an inactive form. Tissue insult induces activation of these peptides, which serve to enhance the process of vasodilatation and increase capillary permeability. Specifically, bradykinin stimulates pain receptors. The presence of pain will usually prompt the individual to protect the insulted area from further insult.

It can, therefore, be seen that the inflammatory response is a complex interaction of a variety of processes and chemical activity designed to act as a protective mechanism following an insult to the tissues of the body. However, the progress of inflammation must be closely observed to avoid the potential for extensive tissue damage.

The inflammatory response in relation to tissue perfusion

Key consideration

How does the inflammatory response influence tissue perfusion?

It has been shown that the inflammatory response is a complex set of pathophysiological changes triggered by an insult to the tissues of the body. Activation of the inflammatory response in response to insult also results in the activation of the coagulation cascade and the temporary impairment of the fibrinolysis system. The immune system functions to initiate mediator responses that serve to increase the inflammatory and coagulatory activity. Cytokines released from white blood cells during phagocytosis and from the activated cell endothelium produce pro-inflammatory and pro-coagulation responses. The concurrent fibrinolysis impairment leads to decreased clot breakdown.

Kleinpell (2004) describes how an imbalance in the combination of inflammation, coagulation and fibrinolysis in the critically ill can result in widespread inflammation, microvascular thrombosis, endothelial injury and systemic coagulopathy. These are all conditions that have the potential to result in impaired tissue perfusion and organ system dysfunction. In Deborah's case, changes in vital signs and laboratory results, along with clinical signs of altered tissue perfusion, reflect acute organ system dysfunction.

As SIRS progresses, the potential for MODS increases and becomes one of the major causes of SIRS-related mortality. Whilst all organ systems are at risk from SIRS, cardio-vascular, pulmonary and renal system dysfunctions are commonly seen. As organ system failure leads to a cumulative risk of mortality from SIRS, the need for early recognition and treatment of the condition can be rationalised.

Mechanisms for haemostasis in relation to critical illness

Key considerations

What is haemostasis?
How does this normally occur?

Haemostasis, in simple terms, is the process designed to prevent excessive blood loss in the human body. In order for this mechanism to function efficiently, four main components need to be available:

(1) Vascular system – endothelial cell lining
(2) Platelets – number and function
(3) Plasma proteins – coagulation factors
(4) Fibrinolytic mechanisms

Damage to blood vessels leads to exposure of basement membranes and collagen. The initial response to this insult is vasoconstriction, which slows the blood flow to the damaged area. This reduction in flow velocity allows the platelets to come into contact with the damaged endothelium. When platelets become attached to the damaged endothelium, they are activated and undergo an initial change in shape as the pseudopodia (false feet) form around the damaged area, coupled with a shift of the granular content towards the centre of the platelet. The canalicular system allows release of the granular contents from the platelet. This granular content includes adenosine diphosphate in dense granules and fibrinogen in alpha granules. Release of these two main chemicals serves to both cause and aid platelet aggregation around the damaged epithelial site.

Endothelial cell lining

The endothelial cell lining consists of the basement membrane and matrices of collagen and muscle fibres. This lining, in normal function, can be described as anti-thrombogenic, that is, it does not promote blood clotting. However, when damaged, it has the potential to release a number of substances that can be considered as pro-thrombogenic, that is, aimed at promoting blood clotting. The anti- and pro-thrombogenic chemical potential of the endothelial lining is summarised in Table 2.2. The combination of these two potentials means that the endothelial cell lining can prevent thrombus formation during normal function but actively promote thrombus formation at times of insult and injury.

Platelets

Platelets are highly refractile, disc-shaped structures that have no nucleus, that is, they are not cells and have an average lifespan of about 10 days. These complex structures contain a number of structures, each with a specific role and function.

- Platelet membrane – consists of a bi-lipid (often referred to as *platelet factor 3*), which contains receptor sites for adenosine diphosphate, Von Willebrand factor and fibrinogen.

Table 2.2 Antithrombogenic and prothrombogenic potential of the endothelial cell lining

Antithrombogenic	Prothrombogenic
Protein S	Tissue factor
Thrombomodulin	Von Willebrand factor
Heparan	PAI : 1 and -2
Heparan sulphate-proteoglycans (HS-PG)	PAF
Antithrombin	Endothelins
t-PA	Adhesion molecules (E-CAM1; V-CAM1; I-CAM 1 + 2)
U-plasminogen activator	Fibronectin
Urokinase	Collagens
EDRF (NO)	Clotting factors V and VIII
13-HODE	Factor IX receptor; factor X receptor
PGI$_2$	
PGE$_2$	

PAI, plasminogen activator inhibitor; PAF, platelet activating factor; t-PA, tissue plasminogen activator; E-CAM, endothelial cell adhesion molecule; V-CAM, vascular cell adhesion molecule; I-CAM, intercellular cell adhesion molecule; EDRF, endothelium-derived relaxing factor; 13-HODE, 13-hydroxy octadecadienoic acid; PGI$_2$, prostacyclin; PGE$_2$, prostaglandin.

- Sol-gel zone – consists of microtubules allowing platelet contraction and microfilaments, allowing pseudopodia production.
- Organelle zone – contains alpha granules that house platelet-derived growth factors as well as clotting factors I, V and VIII and dense granules housing calcium, ADP/ATP and serotonin.
- Tubular system – an open canalicular system linking the interior of the platelet to the exterior. The system contains calcium and is a site for prostaglandin synthesis (e.g. Thromboxane A$_2$).

After adhesion and aggregation, as mentioned earlier, platelets disintegrate and liberate platelet factors 1, 5, 6, 8 and 9, which correspond to plasma clotting factors V, I, X, VIII and XIII, respectively. As a consequence of this factor release, the local concentration of clotting factors is elevated. In this way, the platelets actively support the plasma clotting mechanism. The formation of the platelet plug and the subsequent release of local clotting factors are termed as *primary haemostasis*.

Plasma proteins

During the process of primary haemostasis, a simultaneous, secondary haemostatic mechanism is activated. This secondary mechanism involves the proteins in plasma, also known as *coagulation factors*. A complex cascade of events is initiated with the ultimate goal of producing fibrin strands to strengthen the platelet plug formed in the primary haemostatic response.

The coagulation cascade, like the complement system, is a proteolytic cascade. Each enzyme of the pathway is present in the plasma as zymogen, in other words, as an inactive form, which, on activation, undergoes proteolytic cleavage to release the active factor from the precursor molecule. The coagulation cascade of secondary haemostasis has two main pathways, the contact activation pathway (intrinsic pathway) and the tissue factor pathway (extrinsic pathway). Whilst these pathways describe the initial onset of the coagulation cascade, it is known that both pathways eventually converge into a final common pathway that completes the coagulation cascade (see Figure 2.6).

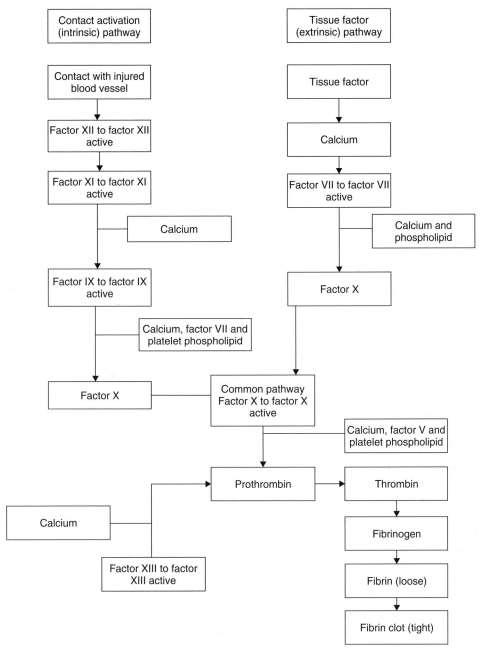

Figure 2.6   Clotting cascade.

Tissue factor (extrinsic) pathway

The overall aim of this pathway is to produce a thrombin burst. By this process, thrombin, as probably the most important constituent of the coagulation cascade in terms of its feedback and activation role, is released instantaneously. Factor VII actively circulates in higher amounts than any other clotting factor.

Contact activation (intrinsic) pathway

This pathway begins with the formation of the primary complex on collagen by high-molecular weight kininogen (HMWK), prekallikrein and factor XII (Hageman factor). This, in turn, leads to the cascade activation of clotting factors, as shown in Figure 2.6. The relatively minor role played in the coagulation cascade by this pathway can be rationalised by the fact that individuals with severe deficiencies of factor XII, HMWK and prekallikrein do not suffer from bleeding disorders.

Final common pathway

Thrombin has a large array of functions, with its primary role being the conversion of fibrinogen to fibrin, which forms the building block for the haemostatic plug. In addition, it activates factors VIII, V and XIII, which form covalent bonds that cross-link and strengthen the fibrin polymers.

Following activation by the tissue factor or contact activation pathways, the coagulation cascade is held in a pro-thrombotic state by the continued activation of factors VIII and IX to form the tenase complex. The tenase complex forms on a phospholipid surface in the presence of calcium and is responsible for the activation of factor X, which initiates the final common pathway.

Cofactors

To ensure that the coagulation cascade functions correctly, certain substances must be present in sufficient quantities. Calcium is required at various stages of the cascade but, most importantly, is essential to the function of the tenase and prothrombinase complexes. Vitamin K plays a crucial role in the ability of proteins to bind with calcium ions. Seven of the coagulation factors are completely dependent on vitamin K to bring about a physiological change in their structure, which facilitates the ability of these factors to bind with calcium and become active in the coagulation cascade.

Regulation

The body needs to keep platelet activation and the coagulation cascade under control to prevent the potential complications of prolonged thrombus formation. Five mechanisms are employed to keep the cascade in check:

(1) Protein C – a major physiological anticoagulant. It is a vitamin K-dependent enzyme that is activated by thrombin. The activated form, along with protein S and a phospholipid as cofactors, degrades the active forms of coagulation factors V and VIII.
(2) Antithrombin – a protease inhibitor that degrades thrombin and active coagulation factors IX, X, XI and XII. It is constantly active but the presence of heparin or the administration of heparins increases its affinity to thrombin and the coagulation factors.
(3) Tissue factor pathway inhibitor – limits the action of tissue factor as well as inhibits excessive activation of coagulation factors IX and X by tissue factor.
(4) Plasmin – created by the proteolytic cleavage of plasminogen; plasmin cleaves fibrin into fibrin degradation products that inhibit excessive fibrin formation.
(5) Prostacyclin – released by the endothelial lining, prostacyclin activates platelet G_s protein-linked receptors. This results in the activation of adenylyl cyclase, which synthesises cyclic adenosine monophosphate (cAMP). cAMP impedes platelet activation and, subsequently, inhibits the release of granular material that would lead to activation of additional platelets and the coagulation cascade as a whole.

Fibrinolysis

Fibrinolysis is the final process whereby the fibrin clot product of the coagulation cascade is broken down and redistributed or reabsorbed. Its main enzyme, plasmin, cuts the fibrin mesh in various places, leading to the production of circulating fragments or fibrin degradation products. Some elements of these degradation products are modified by other proteinases to allow the reusable components to be absorbed, whilst the remaining waste products are ultimately removed via the kidney or the liver.

Haemostasis in the critically ill

> **Key consideration**
>
> How does haemostasis alter during critical illness?

Deborah had developed a coagulopathy, which is often seen during critical illness (Levi and Opal, 2006). Altered coagulation parameters such as thrombocytopenia, prolonged coagulation times, reduced levels of coagulation inhibiting factors and high levels of fibrin split products are often measured in the critically ill patient. Indeed, Chakraverty *et al.* (2003), in a study of 235 patients admitted to an adult intensive care unit, found that clinical coagulopathy was found in 13.6% of patients. Laboratory evidence of coagulopathy was even more common with coagulopathy found in 38 to 66% of critically ill patients. In the vast majority of critically ill patients, coagulopathies are acquired mostly because of impaired synthesis, massive loss or increased turnover of coagulation factors and cofactors caused by the underlying condition. In Deborah's case, this would relate to the end-organ hypoperfusion associated initially with her shocked state leading to multi-organ failure.

In relation to the occurrence of a severe inflammatory response, as discussed earlier, it can be seen that pro-inflammatory cytokines lead to activation of mononuclear and endothelial cells, which, in turn, can also produce cytokines. Activated mononuclear and endothelial cells will express tissue factor, the main initiator of the coagulation cascade. At the same time, impairment of the physiological anticoagulant mechanism by the down-regulation of endothelial bound proteins and the alteration of biological function within endothelial cells can lead to an insufficient counterbalance in favour of intravascular fibrin formation, which may, ultimately, contribute to organ failure. Simultaneously, consumption of platelets and clotting factors by increased metabolic processes may lead to serious bleeding. The use of this example can help to illustrate the potential for coagulopathies in the critically ill.

Disseminated intravascular coagulation

Disseminated intravascular coagulation (DIC) is a syndrome caused by intravascular activation of coagulation that is seen to occur in a substantial proportion of intensive care patients (Bakhtiari *et al.*, 2004). Formation of microvascular emboli in conjunction with inflammatory activation may lead to failure of the microvasculature and contribute to organ failure. Ongoing and inadequately compensated platelet and coagulation factor consumption may be a risk factor for bleeding, especially in peri-operative patients. High circulating levels of plasminogen activator inhibitor type 1 can lead to impaired fibrin degradation, thus further enhancing intravascular deposits of fibrin (see Figure 2.7).

It becomes clear that abnormal tests of coagulation in the critically ill occur frequently and should never be considered to be inconsequential. Coagulopathies may significantly contribute to morbidity and mortality and require prompt detection to facilitate the initiation of prompt corrective and supportive treatment.

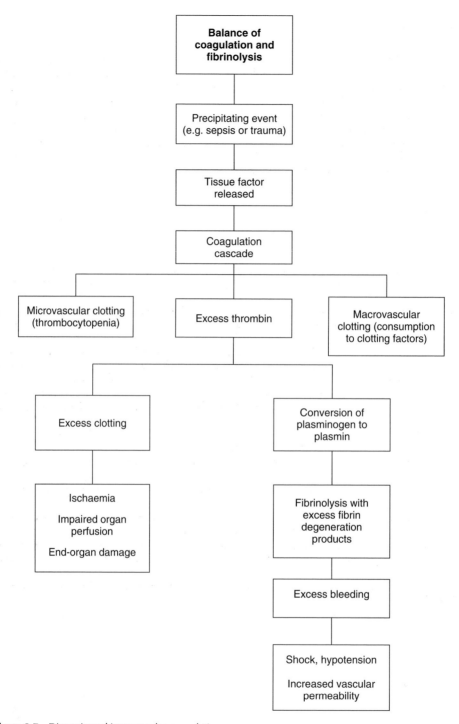

Figure 2.7   Disseminated intravascular coagulation.

Conclusion

By using Deborah's scenario of presentation in multi-organ failure due to shock, it becomes clear that a complex and multifaceted sequence of physiological events takes place in response to an initial insult and the onset of shock. It has been shown that these physiological responses have a profound effect on the human body, particularly at a cellular level. A better understanding of these physiological responses and the subsequent progress of critical illness can serve to underpin current and developing practices in the care of the critically ill individual. Ongoing studies in these important areas should allow practice in the care of the critically ill to remain dynamic and responsive to the complex care needs and challenges that these patients present.

References

Adler J (2007) To Treat the Dead [online]. Available from: http://www.newsweek.com/id/35045 [Accessed 8th August 2008].

Bakhtiari K, Meijers JC, de Jonge E and Levi M (2004) Prospective validation of the international society of thrombosis and haemostasis scoring system for disseminated intravascular coagulation. *Critical Care Medicine* 32 (12) 2416–2421.

Bone RC (1996) Toward a theory regarding the pathogenesis of the systemic inflammatory response syndrome: what we do and do not know about cytokine regulation. *Critical Care Medicine* 24 (1) 163–172.

Bone RC, Balk RA and Cerra FB (1992) Definitions for sepsis and organ failure and guidelines for the use of innovative therapies in sepsis. The ACCP/SCCM Consensus Conference Committee American College of Chest Physicians/Society of Critical Care Medicine. *Chest* 101 (6) 1644–1655.

Chakraverty R, Davidson S, Peggs K, Stross P, Garrard G and Littlewood TJ (2003) The incidence and cause of coagulopathies in an intensive care population. *British Journal of Haematology* 93 (2) 460–463.

Clark WM (2007) Reperfusion Injury in Stroke [online]. Available from: http://www.emedicine.com/neuro/topic602.htm [Accessed 7th August 2008].

Kleinpell RM (2004) Working out the complexities of severe sepsis [critical care]. *Nursing Management* 35 (5) 48A–48H.

Levi M and Opal SM (2006) Coagulation abnormalities in critically ill patients. *Critical Care* 10 (4) 222.

Muller FL, Lustgarten MS, Jang Y, Richardson A and Van-Remmen H (2007) Trends in oxidative ageing theories. *Free Radical Biological Medicine* 43 (4) 477–503.

Polderman-Keys H (2004) Application of therapeutic hypothermia in ICU: opportunities and pitfalls of a promising treatment modality. Part 1: indications and evidence. *Intensive Care Medicine* 30 (12) 556–575.

Reynolds T (2007) From small things: mitochondrial research. *British Medical Journal* 335 (7623) 747–748.

Chapter 3

The patient with haemodynamic compromise leading to renal dysfunction

Tracey Bowden and Anne McLeod

Introduction

A myocardial infarction (MI) is a common medical emergency; there are an estimated 146,000 episodes of acute MI in the United Kingdom each year (Allender *et al.*, 2008). It is one of the most frequent causes of hospital and intensive care unit admissions (Edwards, 2002). Approximately one-third of the deaths resulting from MI occur within the first hour following the onset of symptoms (NICE, 2002); therefore, the effects of MI on a patient within the first hour can be life threatening. The medical and nursing intervention given to patients is closely linked to the physiological processes occurring in the body. An understanding of the association between physiology and practice is essential for nurses if they are to care for MI patients effectively and to reduce mortality during this vital period (Edwards, 2002). Through the application of a scenario, this chapter initially explores the current evidence base that informs the assessment, clinical decision-making and selection of nursing interventions in the first 12 hours of holistic care of a patient with an MI.

As the effects of cardiogenic shock progress, the systemic effects of the altered cardiac physiology will be demonstrated through the development of acute renal failure (ARF). ARF is also referred to as *acute kidney injury* (AKI). Koreny *et al.* (2002) found that a third of patients who had an MI developed ARF within 24 hours and this significantly increased their mortality to 87% (as compared to 53% of patients who did not develop ARF). Therefore, the pathophysiology, assessment and management of ARF will be explored as part of the developing patient scenario. In conjunction with this, in-depth cardiovascular assessment will be explored.

Patient scenario

Robert, a 65-year-old man, presented to the emergency department with central crushing chest pain that was radiating to his jaw, back and down his left arm. He had a history of stable angina; however, he had been experiencing this more frequently over the last few weeks. It is usually relieved with glyceryl trinitrate (GTN); however, more recently GTN has not relieved the angina and sometimes the angina occurred at rest. The pain awakened Robert from sleep and commenced approximately 2 hours prior to admission to the emergency department. A 12-lead electrocardiogram (ECG) revealed ST segment elevation in leads V_1–V_4 and a diagnosis of an acute anterior ST segment elevation myocardial infarction (STEMI) was made. Observing the indications and contraindications to thrombolysis, 45 mg tenecteplase (based on Roberts's weight of 80 kg) and adjunctive therapy were administered with his consent within 20 minutes of his arrival at the emergency department.

Initial assessment in the emergency department found the following:

HR   120 BPM SR
BP   150/90 mmHg (MAP = 110)
RR   28 BPM
Temp   37.2°C
Blood sugars 9 mmol/l

He had shortness of breath and was diaphoretic. Crackles were heard in the basal lung fields.

Following the administration of thrombolytic therapy and analgesia, his pain had been relieved. Robert was then transferred to cardiac care unit (CCU) where an urgent echocardiogram demonstrated an ejection fraction of 30% and dyskinesia of the septum, apex and anterior wall.

Ongoing assessment found the following:

HR   105 BPM SR, with some PVCs
BP   140/95 mmHg (MAP = 110)
RR   30 BPM
JVP   6 cm

He was commenced on a GTN infusion.

Robert was demonstrating signs of cardiac compromise during and following his MI. It is important that critical care practitioners have an understanding of the rationales for interventions in relation to the underlying physiological changes and assessment findings.

Underlying physiology and pathophysiology

Key consideration

What are the underlying physiological changes in myocardial infarction?

The vast majority of MIs result from the formation of an acute thrombus that obstructs an atherosclerotic coronary artery. The thrombus transforms a region of plaque narrowing into one of total occlusion. The thrombus is generated by interactions between the atherosclerotic plaque, the coronary endothelium, circulating platelets and the dynamic vasomotor tone of the vessel wall, all of which overwhelm the body's natural protective mechanisms (Naik *et al.*, 2006).

Thrombus formation

Under normal circumstances when a blood vessel is damaged or ruptured, the body initiates a number of responses to induce haemostasis: vascular spasm, platelet plug formation and blood clotting (Tortora and Derrickson, 2009). There is little difference between this physiologic response and the pathological process of coronary thrombosis triggered by the disruption of an atherosclerotic plaque. To prevent spontaneous thrombosis and occlusion of normal blood vessels, several homeostatic control mechanisms exist.

- Anticoagulants such as antithrombin and heparin are naturally present in the blood; these delay, suppress or prevent blood clotting.
- Endothelial cells produce natural fibrinolytic substances (tissue-plasminogen activator [tPA] and thrombin) to dissolve small and inappropriate clots.
- Prostacyclin and endothelium-derived relaxing factor (EDRF) are secreted by endothelial cells. Both substances inhibit platelet activation and induce vasodilation.

(Naik *et al.*, 2006; Tortora and Derrickson, 2009)

Despite these natural homeostatic mechanisms, a thrombus can develop in the cardiovascular system. Atherosclerosis contributes to thrombus formation in two ways: (1) when the plaque ruptures, thrombogenic substances within the atherosclerotic core are exposed to circulating platelets and (2) the plaque itself disrupts the endothelial lining, thereby reducing the release of the protective antithrombotic and vasodilatory substances (Naik *et al.*, 2006).

The innermost arterial layer (tunica intima) is thickened by the development of fibrous tissue and the accumulation of lipid-forming plaques, which continue to grow over a number of years, resulting in a narrowed lumen. Blood flow through the narrowed coronary arteries is lessened and some patients, such as Robert, may begin to experience angina (Gardner and Altman, 2005). Rupture or fissuring of the atherosclerotic plaque exposes the circulating platelets to thrombogenic substances contained within the core of the plaque, resulting in thrombus formation at that site (Young and Libby, 2006). Factors such as stress from blood flow or inflammation can cause the plaque to rupture (Tough, 2006). Platelets migrate quickly to the site of rupture, resulting in platelet adhesion, activation and aggregation. Activation of the clotting cascade results in the formation of fibrin which binds with the platelets and leads to clot formation (Gardner and Altman, 2005; Tough, 2006).

There are three different potential outcomes of plaque disruption:

(1) Acute coronary thrombosis and occlusion leading to an acute coronary syndrome (ACS)
(2) Plaque growth and expansion causing new onset or deteriorating angina
(3) Complete resolution and healing with little or no symptoms

(Newby and Grubb, 2005)

Acute coronary syndrome

The extent to which these events reduce the flow of blood to the myocardium largely determines the nature of the clinical ACS that ensues. ACS is an umbrella term for a group of conditions that shares the same underlying pathophysiological process and includes unstable angina, non-ST segment elevation myocardial infarction (NSTEMI) and STEMI (Gardner and Altman, 2005). Unstable angina and NSTEMI are closely linked as both represent the formation of a thrombus that does not result in a sustained complete occlusion of the coronary artery. The differentiating factor is that a NSTEMI will result in myocardial cell necrosis. STEMI is characterised by the formation of a fixed and persistent clot that causes a complete sustained occlusion of the affected coronary artery (Gregory, 2005). The prolonged unrelieved ischaemia results in hypoxia, and as the amount of oxygen to the cardiac cells diminishes, cellular death or necrosis ensues (Edwards, 2002). The definition of, and distinction between, these syndromes is based on the patient's clinical presentation, serial ECGs and biochemical markers of necrosis (Newby and Grubb, 2005).

Myocardial infarction

The wall of the heart consists of three layers: the epicardium (external layer), the myocardium (the middle layer/cardiac muscle) and the endocardium (innermost layer) (Tortora and Derrickson, 2009). The inner layer is particularly susceptible to ischaemia because it is subjected to higher pressures from the ventricular chamber and is perfused by vessels that must pass through layers of the contracting myocardium (Naik *et al.*, 2006). The extent of damage is determined by the size of the obstructed vessel and the capacity of the collateral circulation bringing additional blood to the areas deprived of oxygen (Edwards, 2002). Antman *et al.* (2000) state that infarctions are usually classified by size.

- Microscopic – focal necrosis
- Small – less than 10% of the myocardium
- Medium – 10–30% of the myocardium
- Large – more than 30% of the myocardium

After the onset of ischaemia, cellular changes in the myocardium begin immediately. If the ischaemic condition is severe or prolonged, the area of ischaemia becomes more and more injured, cell function ceases and irreversible cell death ensues producing a mass of necrotic tissue (Conover, 2002). Irreversible ischaemia develops within 15 (Antman *et al.*, 2000) to 30 minutes (Gardner and Altman, 2005) of coronary artery occlusion. There are three zones of tissue damage following the occlusion of a coronary artery: ischaemia, injury and infarction. Ischaemia occurs almost immediately and results in a delay in depolarisation and repolarisation of the cardiac cells. If blood flow is restored, this area may recover. If, however, blood flow is not restored, myocardial injury occurs. At this stage cardiac cells begin to lose their ability to conduct impulses and contract. The myocardial cells may survive if adequate circulation to this area is restored; but if ischaemia persists, progression to necrosis is inevitable.

Another consequence of anaerobic metabolism and reduced adenosine triphosphate (ATP) levels is cellular membrane disruption leading to electrolyte imbalances. The plasma membrane can no longer maintain normal ionic gradients across the membranes and the sodium/potassium pump can no longer function (Edwards, 2002). The levels of intracellular sodium $[Na^+]$ and calcium $[Ca^+]$ increase, causing cellular oedema. There is also an increase in the level of extracellular potassium $[K^+]$. This electrolyte imbalance predisposes the myocardium to arrhythmias (Kelly, 2004; Naik *et al.*, 2006). Cardiac monitoring is essential for assessment of arrhythmias and ST segment monitoring. Robert has experienced some premature ventricular contractions (PVCs). PVCs may be aggravated by ischaemia, increased sympathetic activity and increased heart rate. The presence of PVCs following MI identifies patients at greater risk for sudden cardiac death (Conover, 2002).

Necrotic myocardial tissue has been irreversibly destroyed; cardiac cells in this area are electrically inert and unable to contract (Edwards, 2002; Gregory, 2005). Loss of functional myocardium results in reduced left ventricular (LV) function, affecting the patient's quality of life and mortality (Gardner and Altman, 2005). The priority, therefore, when patients present with a STEMI is to commence treatment as early as possible to restore the blood flow to the myocardium in an attempt to salvage any viable cardiac muscle (Gregory, 2005). Key phrases such as 'time is muscle' or 'minutes equals myocardium' have been used to encourage clinicians to act quickly (Tough, 2004). Robert was assessed and diagnosed with a STEMI and treatment was commenced within 20 minutes of arriving at the hospital.

MI classification

Classification of MI is based on the location of the infarction and the layers of the heart involved. The location or site of infarction depends on which coronary artery is blocked, and can be identified on the 12-lead ECG. Robert's ECG demonstrated ST segment elevation in leads V_1–V_4. It is generally accepted that these leads relate to the anterior wall of the left ventricle (Morris and Brady, 2002; Leahy, 2006). An anterior MI results from the occlusion of the left anterior descending (LAD) artery, which usually supplies the anterior wall of the left ventricle and part of the intraventricular septum. This is a large portion of the left ventricle and occlusion of this artery can cause severe left ventricular dysfunction, resulting in congestive heart failure or cardiogenic shock (Del Bene and Vaughn, 2005). Ischaemia or infarction of the intraventricular septum can result in varying degrees of heart block. Frequent observation and monitoring will allow early recognition of any complications or signs of deterioration in Robert.

Cardiac output

Key considerations

Upon what physiological principles is cardiac output based?
What are the physiological responses to reduced cardiac output (shock)?

The coronary circulation perfuses the myocardium, which in turn is responsible for producing adequate output and blood flow to perfuse all of the body's organs including the heart itself. The heart requires an oxygen-rich supply of blood as the myocardium of the left ventricle extracts approximately 75% of the oxygen supplied by the coronary arteries at rest (Green and Tagney, 2007). Hypoxia induces a rapid shift from aerobic to anaerobic metabolism. Although anaerobic metabolism produces some energy (in the form of ATP), it is insufficient to maintain homeostasis of the myocardial cells. This shift results in increased intracellular hydrogen ions and accumulation of lactic acid. Myocardial compliance and contractility is reduced as a consequence of the reduced pH (Gardner and Altman, 2005; Naik *et al.*, 2006). The affected area of the myocardium becomes depressed or hypokinetic. Echocardiography is a useful tool to evaluate the location and extent of damage caused by the MI. It allows identification of regions of abnormal wall motion (Del Bene and Vaughn, 2005).

The performance of the heart as a pump is measured as cardiac output (CO), which is the volume of blood ejected from the left ventricle into the aorta each minute. CO is the product of stroke volume (SV) and heart rate (HR) (CO = SV × HR) and is usually altered by changes in both factors (Levick, 2003). A healthy heart will pump out the blood that entered its chambers during the previous diastole. Three factors regulate the stroke volume and ensure that the left and right ventricles pump equal amounts of blood: preload, contractility and afterload (Tortora and Derrickson, 2009). Stroke volume may fall if the ventricular myocardium is damaged, for example, following MI. In order to fully understand the consequences of MI related to ventricular function, and subsequent treatment options, it is important to consider the factors that affect the regulation of stroke volume.

Preload

Preload is the degree of stretch on the heart before it contracts. A greater preload (stretch) on cardiac muscle fibres prior to contraction increases their force of contraction. The Frank–Starling law of the heart states that the preload is proportional to the end-diastolic volume (EDV). Under normal circumstances the greater the EDV, the more forceful the subsequent contraction. The duration of ventricular diastole and venous return determines EDV and therefore the impact upon the preload. For example, in a tachycardic patient such as Robert, diastole is reduced, resulting in a reduced filling time. The ventricles will contract before they are adequately filled. The most important effect of the Frank–Starling law is to balance the outputs of the right and left ventricles to ensure that the same volume

Table 3.1   Clinical spectrum of haemodynamic states in MI

Haemodynamic state	Clinical spectrum
Normal	Normal blood pressure, heart rate and respiratory rate; good peripheral circulation
Hypovolaemia	Venoconstriction, low JVP, poor tissue perfusion; responds well to fluid infusion
Pump failure	Tachycardia, tachypnoea, reduced pulse pressure, poor tissue perfusion, hypoxia, pulmonary oedema
Cardiogenic shock	Very poor tissue perfusion, oliguria, severe hypotension, reduced pulse pressure, tachycardia, pulmonary oedema

(Adapted from Van de Werf *et al.*, 2003)

of blood is flowing to both the systemic and pulmonary circulations (Levick, 2003; Tortora and Derrickson, 2009).

Contractility

Contractility relates to the forcefulness of contraction of individual ventricular muscle fibres. Substances that decrease contractility are known as *negative inotropic agents*. Acidosis and increased $[K^+]$ levels in the interstitial fluid have negative inotropic effects, which explains the reduction in myocardial contraction and compliance (Levick, 2003; Tortora and Derrickson, 2009).

Afterload

Afterload is the pressure that must be exceeded before ejection of blood from the ventricles can occur. The vascular resistance primarily contributes to afterload (Levick, 2003; Tortora and Derrickson, 2009).

Robert's echocardiogram has demonstrated that there is a significant loss of pumping efficiency of his heart. As the pump becomes less effective, more blood remains in the ventricles at the end of each cycle, and gradually the EDV (preload) increases. The Frank–Starling mechanism increases preload to improve the force of contraction; however, as the preload continues to increase, the heart is overstretched and contractility is reduced. The anterior segment of Robert's left ventricle is significantly damaged and, therefore, cannot pump out all the blood it receives. Consequently, blood backs up in the lungs and causes pulmonary oedema. Left ventricular failure ranges from mild decreases in left ventricular ejection fraction to cardiogenic shock. The degree of haemodynamic compromise parallels the degree of LV dysfunction as do the clinical manifestations (Table 3.1) (Del Bene and Vaughan, 2005). At present, Robert is demonstrating clear signs of pump failure.

Assessment and diagnosis

Key consideration

What is the significance of the assessment findings?

The diagnosis of ACS can be challenging. Rapid diagnosis and early risk stratification of patients presenting with acute chest pain are important to identify those in whom early interventions can improve outcome (Van de Werf *et al.*, 2003). Initial assessment should be as rapid as possible and treatment should be started immediately to provide prompt relief of symptoms, limit myocardial damage and risk of cardiac arrest (Tough, 2004). On arrival in the emergency department, Robert would have been assessed using an ABCDE process.

Airway: Robert was able to respond verbally to questions, indicating that his airway was patent.

Breathing and ventilation: Robert was tachypnoeic and appeared to have shortness of breath. He could only answer questions with short sentences because of his shortness of breath. An increase in respiratory rate is usually observed following an MI as the acidic myocardium, secondary to anaerobic metabolism, results in an increase in rate and depth of breathing in an attempt to remove excess acid. Left ventricular dysfunction will also result in increased respiratory rate. On auscultation, fine crackles were heard, indicating the development of pulmonary oedema. Therefore, a chest X-ray would be useful to assess for pulmonary oedema as well as heart size.

Circulation: Significant arterial occlusion and pain will stimulate the sympathetic nervous system. Evidence of autonomic nervous system activation includes diaphoresis, tachycardia and cool and clammy skin due to vasoconstriction. Robert was tachycardic. This is common in the patient with an anterior MI because of excess sympathetic stimulation. He appeared to be normotensive; however, it would be important to find out whether he was normally hypertensive. His jugular venous pressure (JVP) was slightly elevated in view of the fact that he was self-ventilating: this could indicate that he has pulmonary hypertension. Peripheral oedema should be assessed for in case Robert has developed right ventricular failure. Fingernail clubbing could indicate cardiovascular disease and any xanthelasma is also an indicator of hypercholesterolaemia. Auscultation of the heart should be undertaken as in situations of ACS a third (S_3) or fourth (S_4) heart sound indicates left ventricular failure or decreased left ventricular compliance, respectively.

Disability: Robert was alert. However, his blood sugars were slightly elevated. Elevated blood sugars levels are associated with elevated free fatty acids levels and these are considered to have an adverse effect on myocardial function, increasing the size of the infarction. The Diabetes and Insulin-Glucose Infusion in Acute Myocardial Infarction (DIGAMI) study (Malmberg, 1997) found that mortality was significantly reduced when intensive insulin therapy was used. Therefore, Robert's blood sugars will need to be closely monitored and an insulin infusion commenced if his blood sugars are over 11 mmol/l.

Exposure: Robert should be assessed for any other clinical signs of disease. Robert had a low-grade pyrexia. Following an MI, an inflammatory response is initiated, leading to the release of mediators by the damaged endothelium to protect the body from invading microorganisms, to limit the extent of blood loss from injury and to promote rapid healing of the tissues involved. This leads to swelling, oedema, redness and heat around the injured myocardium, resulting in a mild fever. This is usually observed within the first 24–48 hours. In addition, patients experience nausea, vomiting and weakness due to a vagal response. Therefore, Robert should be asked whether he is nauseated or needs to vomit (Edwards, 2002; Van de Werf *et al.*, 2003; Naik *et al.*, 2006; Green and Tagney, 2007).

Following this rapid assessment, a more detailed assessment of Robert's cardiac history and presentation would be required.

Clinical presentation

MI should be suspected if the patient describes the following:

- History of severe chest pain lasting for 20 minutes or more, which has not responded to nitrate therapy. Common descriptions of pain associated with MI include crushing,

---

Box 3.1 PQRST pain assessment for chest pain

P   *Precipitating and palliative factors*
       What brought on the chest pain? What were you doing when the chest pain started?
       What measures have helped relieve the pain (position, medication, relaxation)?
Q   *Quality*
       Can you describe your pain in your own words? What does it feel like?
R   *Region and radiation*
       Can you show me where the pain is? Do you have pain anywhere else?
S   *Severity*
       On a scale of 0 (no pain) to 10 (worst pain ever experienced), how would you rate your pain?
T   *Timing*
       How long did it last?

(Adapted from Kelly, 2004; Albarran, 2002)

---

heaviness, tightness or a dull ache. Radiation of the pain to the neck, lower jaw or left arm is common.
• Discomfort in the chest described as indigestion but associated with other symptoms of ACS.

Green (2007)

Chest pain assessment is a priority because continued pain is a symptom of ongoing MI, which places viable ischaemic and injured tissue at risk of necrosis. The pain experienced during an MI is caused by insufficient oxygen supply to the myocardium, the presence of lactic acid in the myocardial tissues and inflammation exerting pressure on the nerve endings (Edwards, 2002). The PQRST approach is a common tool used to assess chest pain (Box 3.1).

Robert has a previous history of coronary artery disease; therefore, the likelihood of this episode of chest pain having a cardiac origin is increased. If the patient history is consistent with ACS, ECG changes and elevated biochemical markers will determine the diagnosis (Tough, 2004).

ECG changes associated with myocardial infarction

Key consideration

What is the significance of the ECG changes in relation to the location of the infarction?

The ECG is central to the diagnosis of acute MI and should be obtained as quickly as possible. An ECG provides evidence of the location of ischaemia, injury and infarction. If ST segment elevation is present, a rapid decision on reperfusion therapy is required. Patients with an appropriate clinical history and any of the following criteria should be treated as STEMI.

• ST segment elevation of >1 mm in at least two adjacent limb leads
• ST segment elevation of >2 mm in at least two adjacent chest leads
• New or presumed new left bundle branch block (LBBB)
• True posterior MI

(Myerson *et al.*, 2006; Green, 2007)

ST segment elevation is one of the earliest recognised signs of acute myocardial infarction (AMI); however, less than half of patients will fulfil the criteria for revascularisation on the first ECG. It is therefore important to undertake serial ECGs on patients who are suspected

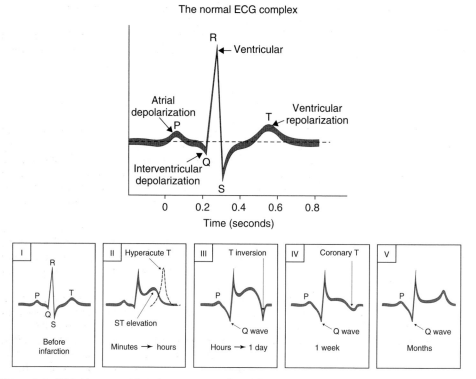

Figure 3.1   ECG changes with ischaemia. Reproduced from Gregory J (2005) Using the 12-lead ECG to assess acute coronary patients. *British Journal of Nursing* 14 (21) 1135–1140, by permission of MA Healthcare Limited.

of experiencing an AMI (Potts, 2006). As the MI evolves, specific changes may be observed on the ECG (Figure 3.1). Changes to the QRS complex include loss of R wave height (poor R wave progression), and the development of pathological Q waves may be observed in an evolving MI. Abnormal Q waves are identified when there is an increase in duration and depth of normal Q waves or the appearance of new Q waves and these indicate the loss of viable myocardium beneath the recording electrode. They have a depth of at least 25% of the succeeding R wave. Pathological Q waves are a permanent feature on the ECG and indicate an old MI (Conover, 2002; Morris and Brady, 2002; Gregory, 2005).

It is possible to identify the location of infarction through the 12-lead ECG. The anatomical relationship of leads on the ECG is as follows:

Standard leads

Inferior wall	Leads II, III and aVF
Anterior wall	Leads V_1–V_4
Lateral wall	Leads I, aVL, V_5 and V_6

Non-standard leads

| Right ventricular | Right-sided chest leads V_1R–V_6R, particularly V_4R. |
| Posterior wall | V_7–V_9. If using standard leads ST segment depression and tall R waves in leads V_1–V_3 |

Green (2007)

Robert has a previous history of ischaemic heart disease; his angina symptoms have been increasing in frequency and duration over the past few weeks. The most recent episode of chest pain is typical of pain associated with an ACS. A rapid ECG revealed ST segment elevation in leads V_1–V_4, indicating an anterior STEMI.

The final diagnosis of myocardial necrosis depends on the detection of elevated levels of biochemical markers as ST segment elevation may resolve following therapy (Antman *et al.*, 2000).

Biochemical markers of necrosis

Myocardial necrosis results in, and can be recognised by, the appearance in the blood of different proteins released into the circulation because of damaged myoctes including cardiac troponin T (cTnT), cardiac troponin I (cTnI), creatine kinase (CK) and lactate dehydrogenase (LDH) (Antman *et al.*, 2000). Cardiac troponins are now considered to be the gold standard biochemical marker for myocardial necrosis; troponin measurement has largely superseded measurement of CK and LDH (Myerson *et al.*, 2006). They are components of the cardiac contractile apparatus where they act as a calcium-sensitive molecular switch to regulate muscular contraction. As they are only found in cardiac tissue, raised levels occur only where there is cardiac damage (Collinson, 2006). Levels are detectable in the bloodstream within 4 hours of ischaemic injury, peak at around 24 hours and remain elevated for up to 14 days (Myerson *et al.*, 2006; Green and Tagney, 2007).

It is important to recognise that the initial diagnosis of STEMI is based on clinical diagnosis and the 12-lead ECG; management is aimed at re-establishing patency of the acutely occluded vessel by primary percutaneous coronary intervention (PPCI) or thrombolytic therapy. There is no role for cardiac troponin measurement in the initial management of these patients (Collinson, 2006). It does, however, play an important role in risk stratification as a raised cardiac troponin value at first presentation identifies a high-risk subgroup. There is a direct proportional relationship to the risk of mortality; as the level of troponin rises, so does the risk of death and re-infarction (Green and Tagney, 2007). The role of cardiac troponin measurement in STEMI is to confirm the final diagnosis (Collinson, 2006).

Other conditions such as myocarditis, pericarditis, pulmonary embolism, sepsis and renal failure can lead to troponin elevation; therefore, it is important to observe caution when interpreting elevated troponin results in the absence of a typical history and ECG (Myerson *et al.*, 2006).

Evidence-based care

Key consideration

What interventions are required for patients presenting with ACS?

Initial treatment for ACS

Initial treatment for patients presenting with any ACS can be memorised using the pneumonic MONA (Tough, 2004) and comprises the following:

- Morphine
- Oxygen
- Nitrate (sublingual GTN)
- Aspirin (antiplatelet)

Morphine

Pain is associated with sympathetic activation, which causes vasoconstriction and increases the workload of the heart. Anxiety is a natural response to pain (Van de Werf *et al.*, 2003). The administration of morphine or diamorphine relieves pain as well as anxiety and may lead to a lowered threshold for cardiac arrhythmias (Kelly, 2004). Diamorphine depresses the exaggerated respiratory effort caused by myocardial ischaemia, reduces distress and helps redistribute some of the increased pulmonary blood to the peripheries (Edwards, 2002). An anti-emetic should also be given; cyclizine should be avoided in patients with signs of left ventricular failure.

Oxygen

It is particularly important to administer high-flow oxygen to patients who are dyspnoeic or those who are displaying signs of heart failure or shock as the lungs will not be able to adequately respond to the body's increased demand for oxygen to remove excess acid.

Nitrate

Sublingual GTN should be administered if the systolic blood pressure (SBP) is greater than 90 mmHg. Nitrates are not only useful in the treatment of pain associated with ACS but also in the treatment of left ventricular failure. Nitrates release nitric oxide (NO) in vascular smooth muscle resulting in vasodilation. They act predominantly on the venous system causing venodilation, which reduces venous return to the heart, preload and myocardial oxygen demand. In addition, there is some arterial dilation resulting in an increased blood supply to the myocardium (Filer, 2007). Peripheral arterial vasodilation reduces the afterload, which is beneficial in patients with signs of left ventricular failure. For these reasons, Robert was commenced on a GTN infusion.

Aspirin

The main function of aspirin is the inhibition of thromboxane in individual platelets. This prevents platelets from adhering to each other and to the atheromatous plaques, thereby preventing formation or extension of thrombus (Gibson, 2007). An initial dose of 300 mg is given, followed by low-dose aspirin to prevent further cardiovascular events. The concurrent use of aspirin with a thrombolytic drug reduces mortality far more than either drug alone (Lip *et al.*, 2002). Clopidogrel is a thienopyridine antiplatelet drug that inhibits platelet aggregation by irreversibly modifying the platelet adenosine diphosphate. This should be administered in combination with low-dose aspirin. This combination is recommended to be continued for 1 month.

Reperfusion

After Robert's being diagnosed with STEMI, the main aim of his treatment is to restore the blood flow to the myocardium in an attempt to salvage any viable cardiac muscle. The probability of a successful outcome is maximised if prompt and complete reperfusion of the infarcting myocardium can be achieved (Pollack, 2008). Reperfusion can be attempted

- pharmacologically by the administration of an intravenous thrombolytic drug, such as tenecteplase, which is administered in an attempt to dissolve the clot, or
- mechanically by PPCI.

Regardless of the reperfusion strategy employed, the most important factor is to start treatment as early as possible (Tough, 2006). Extensive research has shown that the

Table 3.2   Thrombolysis in Myocardial Infarction (TIMI) flow grading system

Grade	Definition
0	Complete occlusion, no perfusion
1	Minimal perfusion
2	Partial perfusion
3	Normal flow, brisk perfusion

prognosis for patients following an MI is closely related to the length of time the coronary artery remains blocked; the longer the duration of the blockage, the higher the mortality and morbidity results (Stenestrand *et al.*, 2006; DH, 2008).

The Thrombolysis in Myocardial Infarction (TIMI) flow grading system is used to evaluate the flow of blood before and after treatment with PPCI (Leahy, 2006) (Table 3.2). TIMI grade 3 flow is associated with improved left ventricular function and improvement in early and late mortality (Sutton *et al.*, 2000; Leahy, 2006).

Thrombolysis

Key consideration

Rationalise the use of tenecteplase in this situation.

The formation of an occlusive thrombus on an atherosclerotic plaque is responsible for an acute STEMI. Thrombolytic therapy can be administered to dissolve the thrombus in an attempt to restore the blood flow to the myocardium and limit necrosis. This is achieved by the activation of plasminogen into plasmin. Plasmin is a protease enzyme that breaks down the fibrin matrix of the clot (Filer, 2007). A number of landmark clinical trials carried out in the 1980s demonstrated that thrombolytic therapy resulted in preserved left ventricular function and decreased mortality in patients with an MI (NICE, 2002; Keeley *et al.*, 2003; Van de Werf *et al.*, 2003). Subsequently, thrombolytic therapy was introduced as routine clinical practice for the treatment of MI (Quinn, 2005). There are four thrombolytic agents available:

- *Non-fibrin specific*
  - Streptokinase which is administered as an infusion over 30–60 minutes.
- *Tissue plasminogen activator agents (fibrin-specific)*
  - Alteplase (tPA) is administered as a bolus followed by an infusion.
  - Reteplase (R-PA) requires two boluses which are administered 30 minutes apart.
  - Tenecteplase (TNK-tPA) is a single bolus dose.

The European Guidelines on the Management of STEMI (Van de Werf *et al.*, 2003) have provided a comparison of these drugs and summarise that accelerated tPA (when administered with concomitant IV heparin) resulted in fewer deaths and a higher incidence of stroke than streptokinase. A review of the three fibrin-specific fibrinolytics (Tsikouris and Tsikouris, 2002) demonstrates that although patency rates differ, overall mortality benefit is similar. Reteplase and tenecteplase offer ease of administration with bolus dosing (Potts, 2006). Increased fibrin specificity appears to play a significant role in differentiating between them. Tenecteplase, the most highly fibrin-specific fibrinolytic is associated with decreased risk of noncerebral bleeding and reduced need for blood transfusions in all patients, as well as longer survival in those with late presentation AMI (Tsikouris and Tsikouris, 2002; Myerson *et al.*, 2006). Evidence suggests that tenecteplase restores patency to the artery more quickly and effectively than other fibrinolytic drugs (Potts, 2006).

National guidelines recommend that eligible patients receive thrombolysis within 60 minutes of calling for help (call-to-needle time) and within 20 minutes of arriving in hospital (door-to-needle time) (DH, 2000). In order to meet the recommended door-to-needle time, prompt assessment of patients presenting with chest pain is required. The greatest improvements in mortality can be gained from patients receiving thrombolysis within 1 hour of calling for help. In order to achieve this, ambulance services are working with National Health Service (NHS) Trusts to ensure that patients receive thrombolysis before they reach hospital (pre-hospital thrombolysis) (Tough, 2004). MINAP (2008) data indicate an increase in the number of patients receiving pre-hospital thrombolysis.

Thrombolytic therapy has some important limitations:

- TIMI flow 3 (normal flow) is only achieved in 55% of patients treated with streptokinase or up to 60% of patients treated with accelerated tPA or equivalent.
- There is a risk of ischaemia or re-infarction.
- There is a 1–2% risk of significant haemorrhage, which increases with age.
- Optimum results are achieved if thrombolysis is administered within 1 hour of symptom onset.
- Up to 20% of patients presenting with STEMI have contraindications to thrombolysis (Box 3.2).

(Grech and Ramsdale, 2003; Leahy, 2006)

Primary percutaneous coronary intervention (PPCI)

PPCI is defined as intervention on the infarction-related artery within 12 hours after the onset of chest pain or other symptoms, without prior thrombolytic therapy (Silber *et al.*, 2005). This can be achieved with or without a stent, which is a small tubular structure

---

Box 3.2 Contraindications to thrombolysis

Absolute contraindications

- History or stroke (haemorrhagic stroke or stroke of unknown origin at any time, ischaemic stroke within 6 months)
- Recent head trauma or intra-cranial neoplasms
- Recent major trauma or surgery including dental extraction
- Gastrointestinal bleeding within the last month
- Known bleeding disorder
- Aortic dissection
- Previous allergic reaction to streptokinase

Relative contraindications

- Transient ischaemic attack within 6 months
- Oral anticoagulant therapy
- Pregnancy or within 1 week post-partum
- Non-compressible punctures
- Traumatic resuscitation
- Severe uncontrolled hypertension
- Advanced liver disease
- Infective endocarditis
- Active peptic ulcer
- Pain for more than 24 hours

(Van de Werf *et al.*, 2003; Myerson *et al.*, 2006; Green, 2007)

left in place after the balloon inflation to help keep the artery open. A specially designed catheter carrying either a balloon or a stent is inserted into the coronary artery under X-ray guidance, to a position inside the atherosclerotic narrowing. The balloon is then inflated and it squeezes the plaque against the vessel wall (Muggenthaler *et al.*, 2008).

Evidence suggests that PPCI is superior to thrombolytic therapy (Keeley *et al.*, 2003; Stenestrand *et al.*, 2006; DH, 2008). It is associated with early patency rates exceeding 90% and low rates of serious bleeding, recurrent ischaemia and death. In contrast, patency rates following thrombolytic therapy indicating full reperfusion can be as low as 50% (Leahy, 2006). Unfortunately, PPCI is associated with a number of logistical disadvantages. Most notably, delays are almost universally greater for PPCI than for thrombolytic therapy, which may be associated with a lessening of the relative advantage of mechanical reperfusion. In addition, there are a limited number of centres able to perform PPCI but this may not be a 24-hour service (Pollack, 2008).

Current guidelines recommend that the delivery of PPCI should occur within 90 minutes after the first medical contact or within 60 minutes of arrival at the hospital (door-to-balloon time). It is argued that if PPCI is unachievable within these time frames then thrombolysis is preferred (Van de Werf *et al.*, 2003; Silber *et al.*, 2005). Evidence does suggest that within the first 3 hours after the onset of chest pain, both reperfusion strategies seem equally effective in reducing the size of the infarct and mortality rates (Silber *et al.*, 2005). For these reasons, thrombolytic therapy is the chosen reperfusion strategy for many patients (Tough, 2006; Pollack, 2008). Encouragingly, there has been an increase in the number of PPCIs performed in the United Kingdom from 8% in 2006 to 22% in 2007 (DH, 2008).

Rationales for Robert's treatment

Reperfusion

Robert presented to the emergency department 2 hours after the onset of chest pain; therefore, either reperfusion strategy is viable. Rapid coronary perfusion is the main objective of Robert's treatment. PPCI may lose some of its advantage over thrombolysis if the additional delay incurred in waiting for PPCI is 60 to 90 minutes more than the time when thrombolysis could have been given (DH, 2008). As Robert did not have any contraindications to thrombolysis, weight-related tenecteplase and adjunctive therapy were administered within 20 minutes of his arrival at the emergency department. This is consistent with the national guidance (DH, 2000, 2008).

Treatment of pump failure

Left ventricular failure during the acute phase of an MI is associated with a poor short- and long-term prognosis (Van de Werf *et al.*, 2003). Robert is receiving oxygen therapy and a GTN infusion, both of which are beneficial in the treatment of left ventricular failure. Robert would also benefit from the administration of a loop diuretic such as frusemide to inhibit sodium and chloride reabsorption, resulting in an increased urine volume (Filer, 2007). This will help to offload his heart, which should improve his contractility and reduce his risk of developing significant pulmonary oedema.

Following the administration of thrombolysis, Robert was transferred to CCU where specialist staff can monitor him, provide expertise in rhythm recognition and facilitate rapid defibrillation and resuscitation in the event of a cardiac arrest (Quinn, 2005).

Ongoing patient scenario

Robert has been in CCU for 12 hours and it is becoming increasingly difficult to maintain his cardiovascular status. Dobutamine has been commenced and is currently infusing at 5 mcg/kg/min. His urine output has also reduced and he is now oliguric.

On assessment, the following are found:

HR   130 BPM SR
BP   86/45 mmHg (MAP = 58)
RR   35 BPM
CVP   12 mmHg
UOP   20 ml/hr for the last 2 hours

His capillary refill time is 4 seconds. His peripheries are cool. Blood results are as follows:

Troponin T   5.2 μg/L
K^+ 5.5 mmol/l
Na^+ 134 mmol/l
Mg^+ 0.7 mmol/l
PO_4 0.75 mmol/l
Urea   11 mmol/l
Creatinine   160 mmol/l

A 12-lead ECG shows that the ST segment elevation has resolved. However, he still has some intermittent chest pain. He has fine crackles on lung auscultation.

During the ward round, the following decisions are made:

(1) To commence Milrinone to aim for an MAP of >70 mmHg
(2) To consider the use of an intra-aortic balloon pump (IABP) if his MAP is not maintained
(3) To assess his cardiac output studies and determine variables
(4) To commence first-line renal management
(5) To consider the use of continuous renal replacement therapy (CRRT), if his urine output does not increase to >0.5 ml/kg

Robert is showing signs of continued cardiac compromise and reduced cardiac output, despite inotropic support. His renal function is becoming compromised as a consequence. He may need to be transferred from the CCU setting to the intensive care setting if his renal function does not improve and renal replacement is required. He may also need more invasive haemodynamic monitoring and cardiovascular support. It is important to consider why his renal function has reduced and therefore to have a clear understanding of the ongoing shock mechanisms, which can occur following an MI.

Progressing pathophysiology

Cardiovascular

Key consideration

What is the pathophysiology of cardiogenic shock?

Under normal circumstances, cardiovascular homeostasis is maintained by four essential components: blood/interstitial fluid volume, blood flow, vascular resistance and myocardial contractility. Following his MI, Robert demonstrated signs of reduced stroke volume, cardiac output and myocardial contractility. This resulted in the release of catecholamines in an attempt to compensate for the reduced myocardial contractility and to improve cardiac output. Compensatory mechanisms only improve blood flow temporarily and soon become counterproductive as they all increase the workload of the heart and therefore myocardial oxygen demand (Edwards, 2001; Shipgood, 2006; Migliozzi, 2009). As the myocardium is not able to function effectively, compensatory mechanisms are hindered, leading to a more rapid progression through the stages of shock.

Cardiogenic shock

Bench (2004) summarises the three stages of shock:

- Compensated shock – body mechanisms are triggered to maintain adequate BP and tissue perfusion.
- Progressive shock – compensatory mechanisms begin to fail and signs of inadequate organ perfusion become apparent.
- Decompensated or irreversible shock – there is no response to treatment, with death being imminent.

Shock is a severe, life-threatening clinical syndrome that results in inadequate tissue perfusion and impaired cellular metabolism. Shock is generally classified according to its aetiology (Foxall, 2009; Migliozzi, 2009). Cardiogenic shock is a progressive state of hypotension (SBP <90 mmHg or a MAP <60 mmHg) lasting more than 30 minutes, despite adequate preload and heart rate, which leads to systemic hypoperfusion (Ducas and Grech, 2003; Myerson *et al.*, 2006). Van de Werf *et al.* (2003) also indicate that cardiogenic shock should be considered if inotropes and/or mechanical support are required to maintain an SBP of >90 mmHg. At present Robert is receiving inotropic support (dobutamine), which is unable to maintain an adequate blood pressure. Robert is also demonstrating signs of hypoperfusion – cool, clammy peripheries, decreased urine output and decreased level of consciousness (Aymong *et al.*, 2007). Thus, Robert fulfils the diagnostic criteria of cardiogenic shock.

Cardiogenic shock (pump failure) occurs when the heart is unable to maintain a cardiac output sufficient to meet the metabolic needs of major organ systems. The organ dysfunction that results causes more damaging physiological effects, and a rapid, progressive, downward clinical course ensues (Darovic, 2002). Figure 3.2 demonstrates the cycle of clinical deterioration of patients who develop cardiogenic shock. The essential feature of cardiogenic shock is that decreased coronary blood flow results in a decrease in cardiac output. This leads to hypotension and progressively more ischaemia and dysfunction (Aymong *et al.*, 2007). If this vicious cycle of increased oxygen demand in the presence of inadequate perfusion is not interrupted, death becomes inevitable (Shipgood, 2006).

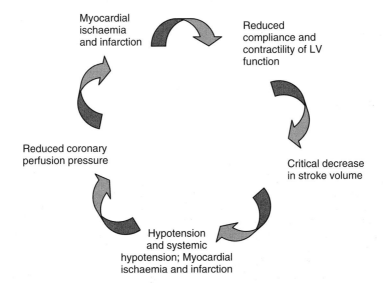

Figure 3.2   Vicious cycle of reduced LV function.

Cardiogenic shock occurs in approximately 8% of patients with MI of the left ventricle and is most often associated with STEMI (Ducas and Grech, 2003) and infarction of the anterior wall (Laurent and Shinn, 2005). This is consistent with Robert's presentation and diagnosis. Mortality rates remain high at 50–80% despite intervention (Bench, 2004; Myerson *et al.*, 2006).

Renal effects

Key considerations

What is the pathophysiology of acute renal failure?
What is the effect of ischaemia on renal structure and function?

Robert is now showing signs of renal compromise, secondary to his low cardiac output. ARF is characterised by an abrupt and reversible decline in renal function and can have a mortality of 80% in critically ill patients. There is an incidence rate of ARF in critical illness of 10–25%, with 3–5% requiring renal replacement (Tillyard *et al.*, 2005; Uchino, 2006). However, despite many definitions for ARF no consensus exists about what functions of the kidneys should be assessed, what variables are used to define ARF and how different degrees of renal dysfunction should be differentiated (Venkataraman and Kellum, 2007).

There is a broad range of factors that can cause ARF and these can lead to vascular, glomerular and tubular dysfunction. ARF can be caused by pre-renal, intra-renal and post-renal alterations.

Pre-renal renal failure

Pre-renal (sometimes referred to as *volume responsive acute kidney injury*) causes make up approximately one half of ARF cases and occur proximal to the kidney. A reduction in renovascular blood flow is a key characteristic of pre-renal renal failure and therefore is largely caused by situations of reduced renal perfusion. These situations include, for example, hypovolaemia, severe cardiac dysfunction and loss of vascular tone. Drugs, such as non-steroidal anti-inflammatory drugs, through their renal vasoconstrictor effects, can cause pre-renal renal failure as can angiotensin-converting enzyme inhibitor drugs as they reduce glomerular filtration pressure.

Normal renal function is dependent on the maintenance of renal blood flow as well as glomerular pressure for filtration.

Renal blood flow

The blood flow to the kidneys is about 22% of the cardiac output, and the renal circulation is unique in that there are two capillary beds: the glomerular and peritubular capillaries, which are separated by the efferent arteriole. Renal blood flow is determined by the pressure gradient across the renal vasculature, that is, the difference between arterial and venous hydrostatic pressure. The kidneys can autoregulate, thereby maintaining a steady blood flow despite changes in systemic blood pressure. The hydrostatic pressure in the glomerulus is one of the major determinants of glomerular filtration rate (GFR) and is influenced by the sympathetic nervous system, hormones and autacoids, which are substances that are released by the kidneys and that act locally. There are also feedback control systems that are intrinsic to the kidneys.

Sympathetic nervous system
Activation of the sympathetic nervous system decreases GFR. This is due to constriction of the blood vessels, which will therefore reduce blood flow and therefore GFR.

Hormonal and autacoid control

Noradrenaline, adrenaline and endothelin all constrict renal blood vessels and therefore reduce GFR. Endothelin is a peptide released by damaged vascular endothelial cells and is a powerful vasoconstrictor.

Angiotensin II preferentially constricts efferent arterioles as well as the systemic blood vessels. Increased angiotensin II levels will increase glomerular hydrostatic pressure while reducing renal blood flow. The efferent arteriole constricting effect of angiotensin II, in situations of shock, helps to maintain GFR by preventing a reduction in glomerular hydrostatic pressure.

NO decreases renal vascular resistance and therefore will increase GFR. NO is released from the vascular endothelium and will act locally to maintain hydrostatic pressure.

Prostaglandins and bradykinins both increase GFR through vasodilation. This may help prevent excessive reduction in blood flow and GFR, by dampening the effects of the sympathetic nervous system and angiotensin II.

Autoregulation of renal blood flow

Autoregulation helps maintain renal blood flow irrespective of changes in systemic blood pressure. This allows for the continued delivery of oxygen and nutrients to the tissues as well as the maintenance of a relatively constant GFR for homeostasis. There are several mechanisms that allow this to happen.

Tubuloglomerular feedback

The tubuloglomerular feedback mechanism has two components that help control GFR: the afferent arteriolar feedback system and the efferent arteriolar feedback system. Both of these depend on the juxtaglomerular apparatus, which consists of the macula densa of the distal tubule and the juxtaglomerular cells in the arterioles.

The macula densa senses changes in volume as well as concentration of sodium chloride of the filtrate as it flows past. A decreased GFR will reduce the flow of filtrate, which will give more time for sodium and chloride to be reabsorbed. The decrease in sodium chloride concentration will stimulate the macula densa, which in turn will lead to a decrease in resistance of the afferent arteriole. This will increase the hydrostatic pressure. Also, renin will be released from the juxtaglomerular cells of the afferent and efferent arterioles, thereby stimulating the renin–angiotensin–aldosterone system (RAAS). Angiotensin II will constrict the efferent arteriole and increase the glomerular hydrostatic pressure.

Myogenic autoregulation

Individual blood vessels have an ability to resist stretching because of increased arterial blood pressure; this ability is known as the *myogenic mechanism*. It has been shown that stretching of a blood vessel causes the muscle in the blood vessel wall to contract because of increased movement of calcium ions from the extracellular fluid. This prevents the blood vessel from becoming overdistended and also increases vascular resistance. This, in turn, prevents excessive rises in renal blood flow and GFR when arterial pressure increases.

Glomerular filtration

Urine formation begins with the filtration of large amounts of fluid through the glomerular capillaries within the Bowman's capsule of the nephron. The glomerular capillaries are relatively impermeable to protein. The concentrations of the solutes are similar to the concentrations within the blood: the exceptions to this include calcium and other protein-bound substances such as fatty acids. The GFR is dependent on several aspects.

The balance of hydrostatic and colloid oncotic pressures across the capillary membrane

If the pressures that favour filtration are greater than those that oppose it, filtration will occur:

Forces favouring filtration (mmHg):
Glomerular hydrostatic pressure: 60
Bowman's capsule colloid oncotic pressure: 0

Forces opposing filtration (mmHg):
Bowman's capsule hydrostatic pressure: 18
Glomerular colloid oncotic pressure: 32

Therefore the net filtration pressure = 60 – 18 – 32 = +10 mmHg

The capillary filtration coefficient (K_f)

The glomerular capillaries have a much higher rate of filtration than other capillaries because of the higher hydrostatic pressure and high K_f. In fact, the glomerular K_f is about 400 times higher than other capillaries. Because of this, the GFR is about 125 ml/min or 180 l/day. The fraction of the renal blood flow that is filtered averages about 0.2 or 20%.

The glomerular filtration membrane

The glomerular filtration membrane, unlike other capillaries, has three layers and has special characteristics that allow it to have such a high filtration rate.

The endothelium

The capillary endothelium is perforated by thousands of fenestrations. Although these fenestrations are relatively large, the endothelial cells have a negative charge, which restricts plasma proteins from passing through the fenestrations.

The basement membrane

The basement membrane surrounds the endothelium and consists of a meshwork of collagen and proteoglycan fibrillae. These have large spaces through which water and small solutes can pass. Plasma proteins cannot be filtered through the basement membrane because of the strong negative charge of the proteoglycans.

Layer of epithelial cells (podocytes)

There is a layer of epithelial cells that lines the outer surface of the glomerulus. These cells are not continuous but have large podocytes (foot-like projections) that encircle the outer surface of the capillaries. Slit pores separate the podocytes and it is through these that the filtrate passes. Again, the epithelial cells have a negative charge, which provides additional resistance to the movement of proteins through the filtration membrane.

Although the filtration membrane is thicker than other capillaries, it is much more porous. This allows for the high levels of filtration required. Despite the high filtration rates, the membrane is selective in which molecules can pass through it as this depends on their size and electrical charge. Electrolytes such as sodium are freely filtered as are organic compounds such as glucose. However, substances with a high molecular weight, such as myoglobin, have a much reduced capability of being filtered. In conjunction, those molecules that are negatively charged are filtered less easily than positively charged molecules.

Robert's blood pressure is low and therefore this will reduce the blood flow to his kidneys. The hydrostatic pressure within the Bowman's capsules of his nephrons will be lower than desired to maintain a normal GFR. Mechanisms to promote the maintenance of GFR and perfusion will have been activated. Even so, he has oliguria, and his blood chemistry indicates ARF as his urea and creatinine are rising.

Intra-renal renal failure

Intra-renal (or intrinsic) renal failure involves the renal parenchyma and is characterised by impaired glomerular filtration, renal tubular dysfunction or both. The disorders that are associated with intra-renal renal failure are usually described as three different syndromes: acute glomerulonephritis, acute tubular necrosis (ATN) and acute interstitial nephritis (AIN). In ARF, ATN is the most common cause of intra-renal renal failure. Situations that can lead to intra-renal renal failure include ischaemia episodes such as sepsis, shock or anything that can lead to prolonged pre-renal renal failure. There are also nephrotoxic causes such as a radiocontrast dye, drugs (such as aminoglycosides) and pigments (such as myoglobin). Robert could be developing intra-renal renal failure as he has been hypotensive for a sustained period of time and therefore his pre-renal renal failure has become prolonged.

In view of the lack of necrosis seen on biopsy, ATN perhaps more correctly should be termed as *acute tubular dysfunction* or *acute tubular injury* (Schrier *et al.*, 2004). During ischaemia, the reduction in blood flow to the outer medulla region of the kidneys is key in the pathogenesis of ATN. It has been found that during ischaemic injury there is a loss of renal autoregulation, and it appears that vasoconstriction, rather than vasodilation, occurs (Schrier *et al.*, 2004). This may be associated with an increase in renal nerve stimulation as well as an increase in responsiveness to noradrenaline and endothelin (Conger and Falk, 1993). Raised cytosolic calcium levels have been found in afferent arterioles and this could be related to the vasoconstriction observed in acute ischaemia.

Congestion within the outer medullary region of the kidney is a characteristic of acute renal ischaemia. This worsens the relative hypoxia in this region and, therefore, the hypoxic injury to the proximal convoluted tubule and Loop of Henle. Endothelial dysfunction is associated with ischaemic injury, which is likely to be due to increased oxidative injury. Increased oxidative injury may also lead to a decrease in NO and prostaglandin production with subsequent reduction in their vasodilatory properties (Schrier *et al.*, 2004). Additionally, the increased levels of endothelin may also be due to increase in oxidative injury.

Tubular dysfunction

Tubular dysfunction occurs in ARF. Sodium and water reabsorption becomes impaired and there is shedding of the brush border and epithelial tubule cells into the filtrate. Experiments have shown that there are changes in the tubular cells cytoskeleton during hypoxia/anoxia, primarily involving $Na^+/K^+/ATPase$, which has been shown to translocate from the basolateral membrane to the apical membrane. The translocation of $Na^+/K^+/ATPase$ could explain the decrease in tubular reabsorption of sodium that occurs in ARF (Schrier *et al.*, 2004). Actin-binding proteins are also found in higher concentrations within the cytoplasm of anoxic tubular cells, which could account for the increase in calcium concentration within the cells during ischaemia. This may then lead to tubular injury as demonstrated by an increase in lactic dehydrogenase release (Schrier *et al.*, 2004). The increase in calcium may also activate phospholipase A, which again may contribute to renal tubular injury during episodes of ischaemia (Choi *et al.*, 1995).

The shedding of the brush border and epithelial cells leads to the obstruction of the tubular lumen. This leads to dilation of the proximal tubules and will also increase the hydrostatic pressure within the tubules. This, in turn, will reduce the glomerular filtration pressure and, thus, GFR. The swollen tubules will also compress the vasa recta/peritubular capillaries, worsening the perfusion of the tubules further.

Tubuloglomerular feedback mechanisms involvement

Tubuloglomerular feedback mechanisms become involved in ischaemic ARF. The decrease in proximal tubular sodium reabsorption will increase the amount of sodium within the filtrate, which will be sensed by the macula densa. This will activate the tubuloglomerular feedback mechanism and decrease GFR. Even so, the degree to which GFR is reduced does not correlate with the clinical signs of ARF. However, this, in combination with the increased sensitivity of the afferent/efferent arterioles to vasoconstriction and the formation of casts within the tubules by the cells which are sloughed off into the tubule lumen, could offer an explanation to the decline in GFR seen in clinical practice.

Inflammatory involvement

Inflammation may also be partly responsible for the decline in GFR seen during ARF. Inducible nitric oxide synthase (iNOS) may contribute to the tubular injury, with an increase in NO occurring in hypoxia. Additionally, the scavenging of NO by oxygen radicals produces peroxynitrite, which also damages tubules (Wangsiripaisan *et al.*, 1999; Noiri *et al.*, 2001). However, endothelial nitric oxide synthase (eNOS) is inhibited, leading to a reduction in the vasodilatory effect of NO (Bonventre and Weinberg, 2003). Leucocytes are activated by a number of local factors such as cytokines, free radicals and eicosanoids and their accumulation contributes to the reduction in medullary blood flow seen in ARF. Other white blood cells such as neutrophils and macrophages may also infiltrate the renal cells, again contributing to the reduction in blood flow. Renal tumour necrosis factor (TNF) levels are elevated during ischaemia, upgrading the inflammatory response seen. Complement may also have a role in the potentiation of leucocyte–endothelial interactions, with the up-regulation of adhesion molecules leading to neutrophil aggregation within the renal vasculature (Bonventre and Weinberg, 2003). However, it is also thought that the primary effect of complement during renal ischaemia could be due to the direct membrane attack of complement as inhibition of C5 has been shown to protect against renal dysfunction (De Vries *et al.*, 2003).

Renal cell death

Renal cell death during ischaemia can either be due to necrosis or apoptosis.

Necrosis

Necrosis occurs as a consequence of severe ATP depletion due to poor perfusion. The lack of ATP will disrupt cellular Na^+, K^+, Ca^{2+} and volume homeostasis. Phospholipid metabolites will accumulate and protein dephosphorylation will occur, leading to cell membrane breakdown and cell death. Necrosis is seen predominately in the proximal tubule.

Apoptosis

Apoptosis, or programmed cell death, is less evident than necrotic cell death initially. This could be that apoptotic cells and their fragments are smaller and more easily cleared and therefore are less evident during pathological examination (Bonegio and Lieberthal, 2002). Another reason could be that ATP is required for the full apoptosis pathway. However, ATP is limited during ischaemia. Finally, there are two pro-apoptotic proteins that are required for initiating apoptosis. These proteins are down-regulated, however, before injury.

   However, following the initiating insult, apoptosis becomes more important. The expression of the pro-apoptotic proteins becomes more evident as do other components of the apoptosis pathway. These pro-apoptotic factors are initiated because of the primary insult and consequential DNA damage and production of free radicals. This leads to apoptosis in both the proximal and distal tubules.

Post-renal renal failure

Post-renal renal failure is characterised by occlusion of urine flow. Therefore, common causes include, for example, tumours (both intra- and extra-renal), kidney stones and urethral obstructions such as blocked catheters or an enlarged prostate gland.

Ongoing assessment

As Robert's condition is deteriorating rather than stabilising and improving, ongoing assessment is required. In any changing situation, the ABCDE assessment approach can be used to ensure that care remains prioritised. It is also clear that he requires a more in-depth assessment of his cardiovascular system as well as assessment of his renal function.

Cardiovascular function

> **Key consideration**
>
> Rationalise the use of different methods to assess cardiac output.

Robert has cardiovascular compromise following his cardiac event. He requires increasing doses of vasoactive support to try to restore and maintain tissue perfusion. Currently, his cardiovascular monitoring is limited to central venous pressure (CVP) and blood pressure monitoring. If an arterial line is not in situ, one should be inserted as Robert requires inotropic support; therefore, close observation of his response to the infusion is required (Marino, 1998).

Even so, more advanced assessment of his haemodynamics would assist the critical care team to accurately assess his response to interventions and to manipulate ongoing management.

Measurement of cardiac output

The Fick equation is the gold standard for assessment of cardiac output:

$$CO = VO_2/(C_aO_2 - C_vO_2)$$

VO_2 is whole body oxygen consumption and C_aO_2 and C_vO_2 are arterial and mixed venous oxygen content, respectively. VO_2 can be measured by indirect calorimetry. However, this assessment as a critical care tool can be difficult to implement in practice. Indirect calorimetry calculates heat production from carbon dioxide production and nitrogen waste, or oxygen consumption in a steady state. Critically ill patients do not meet the preconditions required for indirect calorimetry. Additionally, error is introduced by elevated oxygen consumption by inflamed lungs.

However, there are several options that can be used in critical care for direct assessment of Robert's haemodynamics.

Pulmonary artery catheter (PAC)

Pulmonary artery catheters (PACs) continue to be used despite the development of technology and concerns that the use of PACs increased mortality (Connors *et al.*, 1996). Further studies, however, have demonstrated that PACs do not appear to influence mortality (Murdoch *et al.*, 2000; Harvey *et al.*, 2005; Shah *et al.*, 2005). Even so, PACs are highly invasive and the critical care team needs to have adequate education in their usage and interpretation of waveforms/data.

Indications for PAC include the following:

(1) To differentiate between different shocks;
(2) To distinguish between cardiogenic and non-cardiogenic pulmonary oedema;
(3) To guide manipulation of drugs/fluid and diuretics.

A number of directly measured and derived measurements can be obtained with a PAC.

Pulmonary artery occlusion pressure

Assessment of preload can be made through measurement of pulmonary artery occlusion pressure (or wedge pressure) (PAoP). It is also a key determinant of pulmonary capillary pressure and therefore extravascular lung water (EVLW) (Morgan, 2003). This should be measured during end-expiration and ideally at end-diastole. There are, though, a number of situations in which PAoP does not accurately reflect left ventricular end-diastolic pressure (or preload). These include the following:

(1) Positive end-expiratory pressure (PEEP) (extrinsic and intrinsic)
    It can be difficult to assess how PEEP influences cardiac pressures. During temporary disconnection from mechanical ventilation, the lowest PAoP can be assessed as the effect of PEEP will have been eliminated, but this will also alter pre- and after-load as well as reduce alveoli recruitment. It could cause hypoxaemia. Generally, if lung and chest wall compliances are normal, about half of the total PEEP (intrinsic and extrinsic) is transmitted. If chest wall compliance is reduced, PEEP will have more of an influence, and when chest wall compliance is increased, it will have less of an effect (Morgan, 2003).
(2) Cardiac tamponade
(3) Pneumothorax
(4) Myocardial ischaemia
(5) Left ventricular hypertrophy

Pulmonary capillary hydrostatic pressure

In addition, pulmonary capillary hydrostatic pressure (PCP) can be assessed. PCP is an important determinant of EVLW and therefore pulmonary oedema. The simplified Garr equation can be used to assess this:

$$PCP = PAoP + 0.4 \text{ (pulmonary MAP} - PAoP)$$

In the equation, 0.4 represents the contribution of post-capillary resistance to total pulmonary vascular resistance.

Normally, PCP is only slightly greater than PAoP but in situations of increased pulmonary vascular resistance, PAoP may under-estimate PCP, depending on the pre:post capillary resistance ratio. If the ratio is low, PAoP and PCP may be fairly similar; however, if the ratio is high, there will be a significant hydrostatic influence on increase in lung water, which is not reflected without assessing the PCP.

Pulmonary artery diastolic pressure

One of the drawbacks of using a PAC is that with repeated measurement of wedge pressure, there is a risk of the balloon at the tip of the PAC bursting. Pulmonary arterial diastolic pressure (PADP) can be used to estimate PAoP as the normal PADP–PAoP gradient is <5 mmHg. Certain situations such as a tachycardia >120 BPM and increased pulmonary vascular resistance (e.g. in acute respiratory distress syndrome [ARDS] or chronic obstructive pulmonary disease [COPD]) will increase this gradient. However, once the gradient is known and if it is stable, then PADP can be used to track the PAoP without repeated inflation of the balloon.

Cardiac output measurement

Measurement of cardiac output with a PAC can be achieved through several methods:

Cold thermodilution
When a bolus of cold fluid is injected into the right atrium, there is a transient decrease in blood temperature in the pulmonary artery. The mean drop in temperature is inversely

proportional to the cardiac output as determined by the modified Stewart–Hamilton equation.

$$Q = \frac{V \times (Tb - Ti)\,K1 \times K2}{Tb\,(t)\,dt}$$

where Q is the cardiac output, V is the volume injected, Tb is the blood temperature, Ti is the injectate temperature, $K1$ and $K2$ are the corrections for specific heat and density of injectate and for blood and for dead space volumes and $Tb(t)dt$ is the change in body temperature as a function of time.

Too much or too little injectate will under- or overestimate cardiac output. Care does need to be taken if using cold injectate (0–4°C) as this can cause bradycardia; so an injectate temperature up to 12°C is usually acceptable. Measurements are only obtained when the thermodilution procedure is carried out.

Warm thermodilution

This method uses the same principle as cold thermodilution but allows for semi- continuous measurements. A thermal filament transmits low power pulses of heat, which are detected by a distal thermistor and they are cross correlated with the input sequence and power. From this, measurements of cardiac output can be made. Although semi-continuous, the measured cardiac output is an average over the preceding 3–6 minutes, which means that more than 10 minutes need to elapse before any acute changes can be accurately assessed. Therefore, real time beat-by-beat changes are not obtained.

Pulse contour analysis

Pulse contour analysis is based on the method of Wesseling *et al.* (1993), which uses a three-element model incorporating aortic impedance, arterial compliance and systemic vascular resistance. Stroke volume is ascertained by analysis of the arterial waveform systolic area with corrections for age and heart rate.

Peripheral arterial waveforms can be used following calibration via several methods.

Transpulmonary indicator dilution

This technique uses thermal and other indicators (such as dye), which are injected into a central vein. As the indicator substance passes through the heart and pulmonary circulation, additional information other than cardiac output is obtained. For example, central blood volumes and lung water determinants can be measured.

Transpulmonary thermodilution

PiCCO™ uses transpulmonary thermodilution to assess cardiac output and variables such as global end-diastolic volume (GEDV), intrathoracic blood volume (ITBV) and extravascular lung water index (EVLWI). During transpulmonary thermodilution with this device, cardiac output is measured by injecting a bolus of cold injectate into a central vein and an arterial line, which has a thermistor within it, is inserted. The thermistor detects the change in blood temperature and the Stewart–Hamilton equation is applied. During calibration, the following variables are obtained:

Global end-diastolic volume (GEDV)

GEDV represents the volume of blood in all the chambers of the heart at end-diastole.

Intrathoracic blood volume (ITBV)

ITBV assesses preload as a volume rather than CVP or PAoP, which assesses preload as a pressure. Therefore, ITBV is independent of intrathoracic pressures or myocardial compliance.

Extravascular lung water index (EVLWI)

Extravascular lung water index (EVLWI) gives an indication of the pulmonary capillary permeability and is a marker of severity of illness. A normal EVLWI is 3–10 ml/kg; an EVLWI >14 ml/kg has a higher risk of mortality.

Along with the usual haemodynamic variables (stroke volume, systematic vascular resistance, cardiac output), the stroke volume variation (SVV) can be obtained. This offers information about the effect of positive intrathoracic pressures on stroke volume and an SVV >10% indicates that the patient is preload responsive: if fluid is given, the stroke volume should improve.

Lithium

Lithium can also be used as a transpulmonary indicator for pulse contour analysis. With this method, corrections for packed cell volume are required as lithium is distributed only in plasma. Also, electrode drift occurs with patients receiving muscle relaxants. LiDCO™ uses lithium as its indicator and this system allows for continuous assessment of haemodynamic variables. It is unlicensed for patients <40 kg/88 lb. As with PiCCO, SVV can be assessed and used to guide fluid management if the patient is deemed to be preload responsive (Perry Jones and Pittman, 2003).

No calibration required

The recently developed Flo-Trac/Vigileo™ system calculates continuous cardiac output measurements by interpretation of the arterial waveform but does not require calibration. Arterial compliance is estimated by patient demographic data and real arterial pressure waveform interpretation. McGee *et al.* (2007) compared the use of this system for assessment of cardiac output against intermittent thermodilution via PAC and found that the arterial pressure based cardiac output was comparable to cardiac output via PAC. However, Mayer *et al.* (2007) found only moderate correlation between this device and PAC cardiac output measurement when used in patients undergoing cardiac surgery. Similar to the LiDCO, the Flo-Trac/Vigileo system can assess SVV, and Hofer *et al.* (2008) found that it could predict fluid responsiveness.

Pulse contour analysis allows beat-by-beat, real-time assessment of haemodynamics, such as blood pressure, stroke volume and systemic vascular resistance. The arterial waveform, however, needs to be accurate. There are some limitations to pulse contour analysis including the following:

- Aortic aneurysms/aortic valve regurgitation
- Alterations in abdominal pressure that can alter aortic compliance

Transoesophageal Doppler

Transoesophageal Dopplers can assess blood flow down the aorta, offering useful information about haemodynamics. At the tip of the probe is a crystal that emits an ultrasound beam. This beam is reflected off red blood cells and the differences in frequency between the emitted and reflected ultrasound beams are translated into information about speed of the movement of the red blood cells and the distance they travel during systole. The obtained waveform can be interpreted along with the variables obtained, which include the following:

Flow time corrected (FTc)

Flow time corrected (FTc) is an indication of preload and is corrected to the heart rate.

Peak velocity (PV)

Peak velocity (PV) is an indication of contractility.

Stroke volume

Stroke volume is calculated as the product of the mean systolic red cell velocity and the aortic cross-sectional area. This assumes that the descending aorta carries 70% of the cardiac output.

Systemic vascular resistance

This can be calculated when external pressures (CVP and MAP) are taken into consideration. However, changes in afterload are indicated when both the FTc and PV are altered.

Advantages include ease of use and interpretation of data. However, the probe is not easily tolerated unless sedation is used. Contraindications include aortic coarctation, pharyngo-oesphageal pathology and aortic balloon counterpulsation.

Fluid management

Fluid management can be guided using the Doppler. A patient is fluid responsive if the stroke volume and FTc increase by >10% following administration of fluid bolus. This can be nurse-led if protocols are in place, and this approach has been shown to reduce patient stay in post-operative cardiac patients (McKendry *et al.*, 2004). Gan (2000) compared the Doppler with the PAC, finding that the Doppler could be used to direct fluid administration, resulting in improvements in outcome and shortened hospital stay.

A range of variables can be obtained from contemporary cardiovascular assessment technologies, and these can offer guidance on the influences on haemodynamics (Table 3.3).

To enable the critical care team to have a more in-depth assessment of Robert's haemodynamic status, either a PAC or a pulse contour analysis would offer useful information on the variables that influence cardiac output as well as his left ventricular function. These devices would also enable the critical care nurse to assess the effectiveness of interventions and to guide manipulation of vasoactive drugs and fluid replacement.

Renal function

> **Key consideration**
>
> How is renal function assessed?

Changes in GFR and renal function are reflected within changes in serum creatinine levels from baseline. In critical care, blood urea nitrogen (BUN) and creatinine levels are usually used for assessment of renal function in conjunction with urine output and creatinine clearance. Therefore, indirect estimations of GFR (serum creatinine), solute clearance (BUN) and urine output offer guidance to clinicians of ARF and renal function (Venkataraman and Kellum, 2007).

Assessment of GFR

GFR is normally assessed through creatinine clearance. However, the accuracy of creatinine clearance is limited because as GFR decreases, creatinine secretion is increased with the subsequent rise in serum creatinine being less (Bellomo *et al.*, 2004). Therefore, creatinine excretion is greater than the filtered load, which leads to an overestimation of GFR. Also, GFR varies widely and baseline GFR does not necessarily correspond to the extent of

Table 3.3 Normal flow monitoring parameters

Parameter	Definition	Method used	Value
CI	Cardiac output related to body size	PAC/pulse contour/ transoesophageal Doppler	$2.5-4.2$ l/min/m^2
CO	Volume of blood ejected from left ventricle each minute	PAC/pulse contour/ transoesophageal Doppler	$4-8$ l/min
CVP (self-ventilating)	Pressure recorded within the vein near the heart	CVP	$0-8$ mmHg
DO$_2$	Delivery of oxygen to the tissues	Blood gas analysis	$900-1100$ l/min
EVLW	Presence of pulmonary oedema	Pulse contour analysis (PiCCO)	$5-7$ ml/kg
LCWI	Left cardiac work index	PAC	$3.4-4.2$ kg-m/m^2
LVSWI	Left ventricular stroke work index	PAC	$50-60$ g-m/m^2
PAP	Pulmonary artery pressure	PAC	$10-20$ mmHg
PVR	Pulmonary vascular resistance	PAC	<250 dynes/sec/cm^5
PVRI	Pulmonary vascular resistance related to body size	PAC	$255-285$ dynes/sec/ cm^5/cm^2
RVSWI	Right-sided cardiac values indicating right-sided cardiac function	PAC	$7.9-9.7$ g-m/m^2
SV	Volume of blood ejected from left ventricle per beat	PAC/pulse contour/ transoesophageal Doppler	About 70 ml at rest
SVI	Volume of blood ejected from left ventricle per beat related to body size	PAC/pulse contour/ transoesophageal Doppler	$35-70$ ml/beat/m^2
SVV	Stroke volume variation	Pulse contour analysis	$<10\%$
SvO$_2$	Venous saturation	Blood gas analysis	75%
SVR	Resistance to the left ventricle	PAC/pulse contour/ transoesophageal Doppler	$800-1200$ dynes/ sec/cm^5
SVRI	Resistance to the left ventricle in relation to body size	PAC/pulse contour/ transoesophageal Doppler	$2000-24,000$ dynes/ sec/cm^5/m^2
VO$_2$	Oxygen consumption at the tissues	Fick equation	$200-290$ l/min
VO$_2$I	Oxygen consumption at the tissues related to body size	Fick equation	$100-180$ ml/min/m^2
FTc	Preload	Transoesophageal Doppler	$330-360$ ms
PV	Contractility	Transoesophageal Doppler	20 years $90-120$ cm/sec 50 years $70-100$ cm/sec 70 years $50-80$ cm/sec

Many are indexed to height and weight.

functioning nephrons. If the renal reserve of a patient is not known, measurements of GFR will not offer an accurate estimate of global renal function. Even so, estimation of GFR is a useful strategy for assessing renal function, with, for example, a GFR of <30 ml/min denoting severe renal dysfunction in most patients (Venkataraman and Kellum, 2007).

Assessment of BUN and serum creatinine

BUN is a non-specific measurement of renal function and can vary widely. For example, gastrointestinal bleeding, nutritional status, dehydration and steroid administration can all influence BUN.

Creatinine, however, is more specific in assessing renal function. Studies have found an inverse relationship between serum creatinine levels and patient outcome (Brivet *et al.*, 1996; Mehta *et al.*, 2002) – this may be explained by other extra-renal factors, such as muscle mass and liver function, which can alter serum creatinine. Additionally, as previously indicated, using serum creatinine as an indicator of GFR can be inaccurate. Even so, serum creatinine is useful for assessing whether renal function is stable or improving/worsening (Venkataraman and Kellum, 2007).

Urine output

Urine output is a routine parameter in the assessment of renal function. Urine output is sensitive to renal blood flow, and changes in urine output are often seen prior to biochemical changes; however, severe renal failure can be present despite adequate urine output (nonoliguric renal failure). Venkataraman and Kellum (2007) identify the following to be of importance when considering the critically ill patient:

(1) Decreased urine output may indicate renal dysfunction in an adequately resuscitated patient; the degree of oliguria does not necessarily correlate with the severity of the renal dysfunction.
(2) Urine output may continue to be satisfactory despite ongoing renal dysfunction.
(3) Critical care interventions can lead to a disproportionately higher urine output when compared with severity of renal disease.
(4) Nonoliguric renal failure has a better prognosis than oliguric renal failure.

RIFLE criteria

As there are a number of abnormalities seen in ARF, the Acute Dialysis Quality Initiative (ADQI) group proposed that 'acute renal dysfunction' (ARD) better described an abrupt decline in renal function (or ARF). The term *acute kidney injury* has since been proposed by the Acute Kidney Injury Network (AKIN). The ADQI group has formulated a multilevel classification that defines three grades of increasing severity of ARD (Risk [R], Injury [I] and Failure [F]) as well as the two outcome variables of loss (L) and end-stage kidney disease (E) (Figure 3.3).

The RIFLE classification is unique in that it provides three grades of severity based on urine output or changes in serum creatinine value from baseline. A drawback to this classification is that it does not differentiate between different pathophysiologies, which could have a marked influence on patient outcome. For example, a patient with low urine output and increased creatinine due to urinary obstruction will have a better outcome than a septic patient with similar urine output and creatinine levels, even if they both have a similar RIFLE classification. Even so, Bell *et al.* (2005) have demonstrated that patients with a more severe RIFLE score have a higher mortality than patients with a lower score, indicating that the RIFLE criteria is a useful prognostic tool.

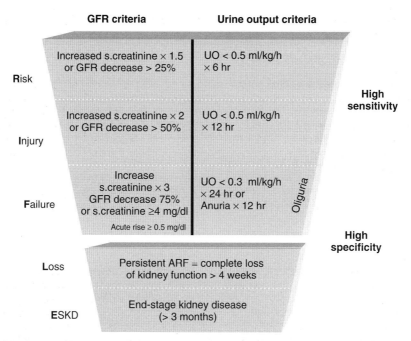

GFR criteria   **Urine output criteria**

Figure 3.3 RIFLE criteria. GFR, glomerular filtration rate; ARF, acute renal failure. Reproduced with permission from Bellomo R, Ronco C, Kellum J, Mehta R, Palevsky P and the ADQI workgroup (2004) Acute renal failure: definition, outcome measures, animal models, fluid therapy and information technology needs: the Second International Consensus Conference of Acute Dialysis Quality Initiative (ADQI). *Group Critical Care* 8 (4) R204–R212.

Evidence-based care

In view of Robert's continued hypotension and signs of reduced organ perfusion, several key changes have been decided upon in Robert's care. These, at the moment, are focused on improving his cardiovascular function and his renal function.

Cardiovascular function

In relation to improving his cardiovascular function, management strategies are aimed at

(1) improving myocardial oxygen supply by increasing aortic diastolic pressure and coronary blood flow as well as ensuring adequate arterial oxygenation;
(2) decreasing myocardial oxygen requirements by decreasing the workload of the heart;
(3) optimising cardiac output and systemic perfusion.

Darovic (2002)

Key consideration

Why is the team considering using milrinone and an intra-aortic balloon pump to improve Robert's cardiac output?

Inotropic support

A MAP of 60 mmHg is generally required for tissue perfusion (Iakobishvili and Hasdai, 2007). The use of inotropes stimulates cardiac function and increases vascular tone, which will optimise blood flow and oxygen delivery, thereby maintaining perfusion of vital organs (Ducas and Grech, 2003).

Dobutamine

Dobutamine is usually the first-line pharmacological management of cardiogenic shock. Dobutamine acts directly on beta 1 (β1) adrenergic receptors that are located in the myocardium and results in increased cardiac contractility, increased cardiac output and possibly a slight increase in heart rate (Foxall, 2009). In addition, dobutamine can lead to a more severe hypotension (Shipgood, 2006). A consequence of drugs that improve contractility is that they may have the undesirable effect of increasing automaticity and myocardial oxygen demand (Darovic, 2002).

At present, Robert is prescribed a continuous infusion of 5 mcg/kg/min of dobutamine. This has resulted in a slight increase in heart rate and it has been insufficient to maintain his blood pressure; therefore, a decision was made to commence milrinone as opposed to increasing the dobutamine infusion.

Milrinone

Milrinone is a phosphodiasterase inhibitor and is a positive inotrope and vasodilator but has little chronotropic effect. Phosphodiasterase is an intracellular enzyme that inactivates cyclic adenosine monophosphate (cAMP). cAMP is a secondary messenger which, when activated, increases intracellular calcium. The increase in calcium will enhance the contractile state of the myocyte, thereby improving contraction of the myocardium. As milrinone inhibits phosphodiasterase, intracellular levels of calcium are subsequently increased. Milrinone is clinically indicated for Robert as the dobutamine is having little effect, he has signs of pulmonary hypertension and an increase in his heart rate should be avoided.

Intra-aortic balloon pump (IABP) therapy

IABP therapy involves the use of a helium-filled balloon, which is inserted retrogradely via the femoral artery into the descending thoracic aorta, to a position just below the left subclavian artery (Kumar and Roberts, 2001). The underlying principle of IABP therapy is that inflation and deflation of the IABP causes the central aortic pressure to rapidly fall with systole and rapidly rise with diastole (Darovic, 2002). This assists the heart by

- increasing aortic diastolic pressure and coronary blood flow, and
- decreasing aortic systolic pressure to reduce the workload of the heart.

(Kumar and Roberts, 2001)

The majority of coronary artery perfusion occurs during diastole. Inflation is usually timed in response to a biological signal (usually ECG) and occurs during diastole, immediately after the aortic valve closes (Quaal, 2001). When inflation occurs, there is an increase in central aortic pressure, resulting in a displacement of blood volume from the aorta, which augments coronary perfusion.

Deflation occurs at the end of diastole, immediately before contraction. Since balloon inflation reduces aortic blood volume, deflation results in a subnormal central aortic pressure just prior to ventricular contraction. Therefore, the left ventricle encounters less resistance to opening the valve and ejecting blood into the systemic circulation; the workload of the left ventricle is reduced (Darovic, 2002).

The primary effects of IABP therapy are increase in myocardial oxygen supply, increase in cardiac output, and decrease in myocardial oxygen demand (Kumar and Roberts, 2001). Secondary effects observed are decreased HR and system vascular resistance (SVR) and increased MAP, all of which lead to increased perfusion of all the organ systems.

Therefore, with IABP therapy myocardial oxygen supply and demand becomes more balanced (Ducas and Grech, 2003). Evidence suggests that the use of IABP therapy, in combination with a thrombolytic agent, results in reduction in mortality (Sanborn *et al.*, 2000); subsequently the European Guidelines for Percutaneous Coronary Intervention (Silber *et al.*, 2005) recommend its use.

> **Key consideration**
>
> What else could be considered to improve Robert's prognosis?

Percutaneous coronary intervention

Although inotropic agents and IABP increase BP, these measures are temporary and have no effect on long-term survival unless combined with myocardial reperfusion (Ducas and Grech, 2003). Evidence suggests that a strategy of early revascularisation results in an improvement in 6-year survival compared with initial medical management (Hochman *et al.*, 2006). The European Guidelines for Percutaneous Coronary Intervention (Silber *et al.*, 2005) recommend that in the setting of cardiogenic shock the usual time frame for considering PCI should be extended and that multi-vessel PCI should be attempted in patients with multiple critical narrowings. If Robert does not show signs of improvement, mechanical revascularisation should be considered.

Renal function

> **Key consideration**
>
> What is renal rescue/first-line renal management?

Management of oliguria

The early management of oliguria is to identify and treat any pre-renal causes. Robert has been hypotensive for at least 12 hours despite efforts to improve his blood pressure with fluids and inotropic support. Marino (1998) identifies the following as key steps in the management of acute oliguria:

Optimising haemodynamics
Robert's cardiac filling pressure and cardiac output need to be optimised. His CVP appears to be adequate but his blood pressure is not, despite the dobutamine infusion. Milrinone has been suggested, as has an intra-aortic balloon pump been, in view of the persistent hypotension.

Improving glomerulotubular flow
If oliguria persists despite resolution of pre-renal causes (hypovolaemia and/or hypotension), it is likely that intra-renal renal failure has developed. Often loop diuretics, such as frusemide, are used if the patient appears to be normovolaemic and normotensive. The goal of using loop diuretics is to increase tubular flow, thereby reducing the raised tubular hydrostatic pressure. Tubular sediment may also be removed by increasing flow. However, there is no research-based evidence that demonstrates that loop diuretics reduce the incidence of renal failure (Marino, 1998; Bellomo, 2003). Even so, loop diuretics may protect the Loop of Henle from the effects of reduced perfusion by reducing the energy-dependent workload of the nephron. Loop diuretics may also reduce the requirement for renal replacement therapy (RRT) by inducing polyuria, which helps to reduce any fluid overload, acidosis and hyperkalaemia. These are the main triggers for RRT in critical care (Bellomo and Ronco, 2002a).

Low-dose dopamine, as a renal vasodilator, continues to be used in some critical care units despite the lack of evidence to support its use (Marino, 1998; Bellomo, 2003). Low-dose dopamine acts as a tubular diuretic so any increase in urine output is not due to an increase in GFR and does not improve renal function (Marino, 1998). However, dopamine as a β_1 agonist may help improve cardiac output and therefore GFR, as would dobutamine or milrinone.

If Robert's urine output does not improve once his cardiac output has been optimised, CRRT may be required. He is hyperkalaemic and his urea and creatinine are both elevated. In addition, he has started showing signs of fluid overload, as indicated by his serum sodium levels and the fact that he has fine crackles on auscultation. An arterial blood gas would be useful determining whether he has a metabolic acidosis – which is likely in view of his respiratory rate. All of these clinical signs indicate a need for RRT should his renal function not improve.

Renal replacement therapy (RRT)

> **Key consideration**
>
> When should renal replacement be used?

Timing of RRT

RRT is usually commenced when there are clinical indications of renal failure such as the following:

(1) Uraemia complications
(2) Elevated creatinine levels
(3) Hyperkalaemia
(4) Fluid overload
(5) Uncontrolled/worsening metabolic acidosis

Page *et al.* (2005) found that early continuous veno-venous haemodiafiltration (CVVHDF) improved the prognosis of sepsis-related multiple organ failure: this was demonstrated by an improvement in metabolic acidosis during early RRT. However, there is no consensus about when RRT should be started (Bellomo and Ronco, 2002a). Many, though, believe that it is physiologically unsound and potentially clinically dangerous to delay commencing RRT whilst waiting for the clinical complications of uraemia to develop. To this end, a more aggressive approach to renal failure has been advocated, when maintenance of homeostasis and prevention of complications is the desired therapeutic goal (Bellomo and Ronco, 1996). Therefore it is largely advocated to start RTT early (Schrier *et al.*, 2004). If a 'prevention' approach is used, then criteria for initiating RRT in critical care include, for example, the following:

Oliguria
Anuria
Hyperkalaemia (K^+ >6.5 mmol/l and rising)
pH <7.1
Urea >30 mmol/l and/or creatinine >300 μmol/l
Pulmonary oedema
Uraemic encephalopathy
Drug overdose
Severe hypernatraemia (>160 mmol/l) or hyponatraemia (<115 mmol/l)
(Bellomo and Ronco, 2002a; Intensive Care Society, 2009)

Aims and methods of RRT

The aim of RRT is to maintain the urea level at <30 mmol/l and preferably <25 mmol/l, as well as to achieve normalisation of electrolytes, calcium and phosphate. There is debate and discussion about how this should be achieved, with some clinicians advocating CRRT whilst others prefer intermittent haemodialysis (IHD). In general, Australian and European intensivists have adopted CRRT whereas American clinicians support the use of IHD (Bellomo and Ronco, 2002a). Uehlinger *et al.* (2005) found that there was no significant difference in survival benefit of continuous vs. intermittent RRT in intensive care. However, IHD is associated with complications, which may limit its use in the critically ill patient, such as in significant systemic hypotension as well as fluctuations in both fluid and electrolyte balance. Any of these could have a significant negative impact on the critically unwell patient. For example, fluctuations in fluid balance will not be well tolerated by a patient with ARDS as their EVLW will also fluctuate, worsening their hypoxaemia. Therefore, in this situation, CRRT could be more beneficial than IHD, even though Hoste *et al.* (2002) found, in a small trial, that CRRT did not significantly improve the respiratory status of patients with acute lung injury who were in ARF when an even fluid balance was aimed for (This trial did not compare CRRT and IHD but investigated the effect of CRRT with zero fluid balance in patients with acute lung injury and ARF).

Clearance of solutes is more consistent when CRRT is used. CRRT has been shown to be superior in the cumulative clearance of urea and creatinine as compared to four times a week IHD. Indeed, IHD would need to be used six times a week to achieve the same uraemic control as CRRT (Bellomo and Ronco, 2002a). IHD is more likely to cause solute disequilibrium as there is faster solute diffusion. This removal rate may be substantially faster than solute movement from the intracellular and interstitial compartments into blood. This could cause cerebral oedema and raised intracranial pressure. Conversely, CRRT does not create such pronounced alterations in solute balance and therefore is less likely to create deleterious rises in intracranial pressure.

CRRT may also enhance the nutritional requirements of the patient as nutrition can be delivered without restriction. Maintaining nutritional requirements of the critically ill patient has been shown to improve patient outcome, and CRRT allows for urea to be controlled whilst adequate nutritional support can be delivered. CRRT also reduces energy requirements as heat is lost during CRRT, and this may be beneficial should a patient be febrile.

CRRT removes inflammatory mediators, and this will be useful for patients who have severe sepsis and multiorgan dysfunction. This may increase the survival rate of this group of patients (Bellomo *et al.*, 1995). Even so, the Surviving Sepsis Guidelines (Dellinger *et al.*, 2008) currently do not recommend the use of CRRT to treat sepsis independent of renal replacement requirements.

Principles of RRT

Key consideration

How does RRT purify blood?

RRT purifies blood via three mechanisms of fluid and solute transport across a semi-permeable membrane.

Diffusion

During diffusion, solutes move across a semi-permeable membrane in relation to a concentration gradient. Solutes move from an area of high concentration to an area of low concentration in an effort to equalise the distribution of the solute on each side of the membrane. This is in accordance to Brownian motion, which identifies that particles move randomly, colliding with each other and altering their direction of travel. This type of motion results in the equal distribution of the particles through the solvent solution. The driving force for diffusion is the concentration of particles: the denser the concentration, the more frequent the collisions will be, leading to the spreading out of particles. How quickly this occurs depends on the concentration gradient.

Hydrophilic membranes soak up water and therefore enhance diffusion. Hydrophobic membranes have less diffusive properties as they do not absorb water. Molecules or ions can diffuse at an equal rate through an unrestricted membrane. However, in RRT, the membrane has pores in it, which restricts the movement of solutes depending on their size. Small solutes can move unrestricted through the pores; however, larger molecules will diffuse more slowly.

As diffusion is reliant on a concentration gradient, to maximise diffusion the concentration gradient must also be maximised. To achieve this, high concentrations of uraemic blood must enter the dialyser and the dialysate fluid should not contain the solute that needs to be removed from the blood. To also enhance diffusion, flow rates of both blood and dialysate need to be maximised.

Ultrafiltration

Ultrafiltration is the movement of plasma water across a semi-permeable membrane due to a transmembrane pressure gradient (TMP). This process is governed by

$$Qf = \text{Km} \times TMP$$

Qf is the ultrafiltration rate (ml/min), Km signifies the membrane coefficient (or how easily fluid can move across it) and TMP relates to the transmembrane pressure gradient.

The pressure differences on either side of the membrane create the TMP: the hydrostatic pressure of the blood largely creates the pressure gradient and therefore the movement of plasma water across the membrane. The hydrostatic pressure, in turn, is largely dependent on the blood flow – the greater the blood flow rate is, the greater the TMP will be. Also, measures that increase the negative pressure on the ultrafiltrate side of the membrane will enhance ultrafiltration as will methods that decrease the oncotic pressure (e.g. using predilution replacement fluid) on the blood side of the membrane.

The relationship between the TMP and the oncotic pressure will determine the amount (or fraction) of plasma water that is removed because of ultrafiltration: this volume is the filtration fraction. If a patient has a haemocrit of 30%, the ideal filtration fraction is 20–25% (Bellomo and Ronco, 2002a). This avoids excessive haemoconcentration and reduces the risks of the filter clotting during RRT.

Convection

During convection, solutes move across a semi-permeable membrane in conjunction with ultrafiltration and water transfer. Therefore, solutes are 'carried' or 'dragged' across the membrane by water (or the solvent) as the solvent is pushed across the membrane due to TMP. The hydrodynamic flow across the membrane is determined by the TMP, the surface area of the membrane and the intrinsic permeability of the membrane. It is important that the membrane used for convective methods of clearance has a high flux, which means that it has a high permeability. Therefore, fluid and solutes can readily pass through it.

The size of the pores in the membrane is another major determinant of which solutes can move across the membrane. 'Fouling' of the membrane can occur as protein and cells are pushed by the hydrostatic pressure but cannot move through the pores, thereby blocking the pores. This limits the size of the molecules that can be transported through the pores: even so, using convection greatly exceeds the size of the molecules which can move through the membrane via diffusion. Thus middle and even larger molecular weight molecules can be transported through the membrane via convection including septic mediators. It is largely the convective methods of RRT that are useful for the removal of septic mediators: De Vriese *et al.* (1999) demonstrated that a combination of high ultrafiltration rate (and therefore convection rate) and frequent filter changes results in measurable decreases in systematic cytokine concentrations.

Sieving coefficient

The ability of a solute to move through a membrane via convection is known as the *sieving coefficient*. This is estimated by determining the ratio of the solute concentration in the filtrate divided by the concentration within plasma water. A value of 1.0 indicates complete permeability whereas a value of 0 would indicate rejection. Molecular weight only has a minor role in sieving but once the molecular weight of a solute is >12 kDa, then convective transport of the solute becomes affected. Albumin has a molecular weight of 69 kDa and has a sieving coefficient of nearly zero. Any solute or drug which is bound to albumin therefore also will not move by convection through the membrane: this is of significance if a drug, for example, is bound to albumin (Golper, 2002).

Concept of clearance

Solute clearance is the time for a volume of blood to be completely cleared of solute. During RRT, this can be misleading if the concentration of a solute is changing as is seen during intermittent RRT. During CRRT, the solute concentration is more stable and therefore the concept of clearance is more useful. For example, when there is a steady BUN concentration of 70 mg/dl, a clearance of 30 ml/min will lead to a removal of 2.1 mg/min. CRRT interventions are probably equivalent to four to five intermittent treatments per week for solute removal.

Filtration membrane

The filtration membrane used in RRT can be divided into two different types:

Cellulose-based membranes

These membranes are low-flux membranes, which means that they have a permeability coefficient (Km) <10 ml/hr × mmHg/m^2. The membranes are very thin and are strongly hydrophilic.

Synthetic membranes

These membranes are high-flux membranes with a Km >30 ml/hr × mmHg/m^2. The thickness of the membrane is greater than in cellulose-based membranes and these membranes have large pores and are hydrophobic. Solutes with a wide range of molecular size are able to pass through the membrane and these membranes are more suitable for convective modes of RRT.

Adsorption

Molecules adsorb to membranes and this contributes to their removal from blood. Convection enhances adsorption by increasing the surface area. The molecules may, in time, be released either back into the circulation or into the filtrate. Inflammatory cytokines and endotoxic peptides are both examples of molecules that adsorb to the filter membrane (Golper, 2002).

Vascular access

Two different approaches are used in extracorporeal circulation of blood:

Arterio-venous approach

In this system, an artery and a vein are cannulated and no blood pumps are used; instead, the patient's blood pressure is the driving force to move blood through the circuit. As the difference between the arterial and venous pressure is largely responsible for maintaining the blood flow through the circuit, resistance to flow must be minimised. Therefore, short blood lines and filters are used. Blood flow speeds range between 50 and 150 ml/min depending on the blood pressure. Arterio-venous systems are largely obsolete in critical care.

Veno-venous approach
A single central vein is cannulated with a double-lumen catheter, and pumps are incorporated into the system to maintain blood flow. One of the lumens acts as the arterial or access port whereas the other is the venous or return line. In this system, blood flow can be kept between 150 and 200 ml/min. Veno-venous systems are generally used in contemporary critical care.

Modes of RRT

> **Key consideration**
>
> Rationalise the use of different modes of RRT.

There are different modes of RRT, with the difference between them largely due to the principles of blood purification being used.

Peritoneal dialysis (PD)
Peritoneal dialysis (PD) is a diffusive method of RRT that uses the peritoneal membrane as a semi-permeable membrane. Dialysate fluid is passed into the peritoneum via a peritoneal catheter and solutes move from the blood in the capillaries of the peritoneal membrane into the fluid via diffusion. Water can also move from the blood into the dialysate via osmosis. Fluid removal can be increased or decreased by using different amounts of glucose in the dialysate: a 'heavy' bag contains more glucose and therefore more water will move by osmosis. Infection control is paramount to avoid peritonitis.

Haemodialysis (HD)
This method of RRT uses diffusion to create solute clearance. Dialysate fluid is passed through the filter counter-current to blood flow (i.e. in the opposite direction) and solutes will move from areas of high concentration to those of low concentration (Figure 3.4).

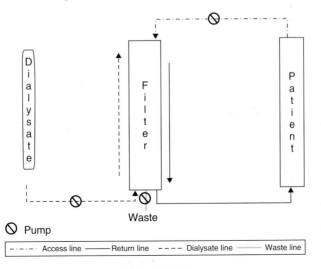

Figure 3.4   Continuous veno-venous haemodialysis (CVVHD).

Therefore, if the patient's serum $[K^+]$ is greater than the potassium concentration in the dialysate fluid, potassium will move from the blood, across the membrane, into the dialysate fluid. The 'waste' is the dialysate after it has passed through the filter and will contain the solutes that have moved across the filter. Any ultrafiltrate that is collected corresponds to the amount of fluid that the haemofilter is programmed to remove – therefore, manipulation of fluid balance can occur. HD can be performed intermittently as is seen in renal units or continuously as may be seen in critical care. In critical care, if a veno-venous line is used, this mode of RRT would be termed *continuous veno-venous haemodialysis* (CVVHD). Clearance is largely limited to small solutes.

Haemofiltration (HF)

This method of RRT uses ultrafiltration and convection (solute drag) for clearance. Blood is passed through a highly permeable filter: plasma water is pushed across the membrane by the blood hydrostatic pressure and solutes are dragged across within the ultrafiltrate. Replacement fluid is used to return volume and solutes to the patient. Replacement fluid can be added to the blood before the filter (pre-dilution) or after the filter (post-dilution) (Figure 3.5). In critical care, if this mode is used continuously via a veno-venous line, then continuous veno-venous haemofiltration (CVVH) is undertaken. Clearance of solutes is convective and equals the ultrafiltration rate.

In pre-dilution, some of the replacement fluid will be lost within the ultrafiltrate but as the blood is haemodiluted, it is less likely to clot within the filter. However, predilution is 10–15% less effective in solute removal because of dilution of the blood with the replacement fluid (Clark and Ronco, 1999). This, though, Clark and Ronco (1999) feel can be overcome by the use of a relatively high ultrafiltration rate. When post-dilution replacement fluid is used, the patient will receive all of the replacement fluid but the blood is more likely to clot. Uchino *et al.* (2003) found that the use of post-dilution replacement fluid was associated with a statistically significant reduction in filter life without any benefit to daily urea and creatinine levels.

Haemodiafiltration (HDF)

In haemodiafiltration, both convective and diffusive methods are used for clearance of solutes. Blood and dialysate are circulated counter-current to each other; however, fluid, the form of ultrafiltrate, is also removed from the patient (Figure 3.6). Solutes are therefore

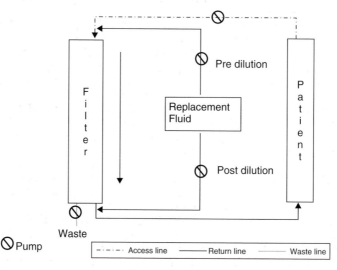

Figure 3.5 Continuous veno-venous haemofiltration (CVVH).

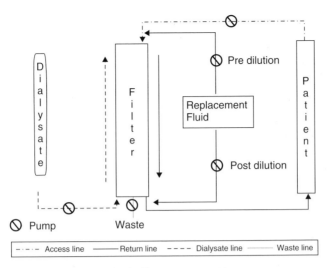

Figure 3.6   Continuous veno-venous haemodiafiltration (CVVHDF).

also dragged through the membrane as in haemofiltration. Replacement fluid is used to replace water and the required solutes. In critical care, if this mode is used continuously and blood flow is via a veno-venous line, then CVVHDF is utilised. Clearance includes small and larger molecules.

Slow continuous ultrafiltration (SCUF)
Slow continuous ultrafiltration is used to remove fluid from overloaded patients but solute removal does not occur. The ultrafiltrate is not replaced.

Dosage of CRRT

Currently, there are no standardised protocols for prescribing CRRT or quantifying adequacy of solute removal in CRRT (Tolwani *et al.*, 2008). Nor is there consensus about which clearance method (diffusion vs. convection) is best. However, several studies have been undertaken to determine this.

Ronco *et al.* (2000) found by using post-dilution CVVH that a dosage of 35 ml/kg/hr (effluent rate) had a survival benefit compared with 20 ml/kg/hr. The RRT was commenced early and the patient group largely consisted of post-surgical patients who had developed ARF. Bouman *et al.* (2002) investigated the effect of dosage and timing of treatment on survival using post-dilution CVVH. They found no difference for either dosage (25 ml/kg/hr vs. 48 ml/kg/hr) or timing (early being a BUN <46 mg/dl or late BUN being >105 mg/dl). Saudan *et al.* (2006) assigned patients to either receive CVVH or CVVHDF (predilution). Those who received CVVH had a prescribed effluent dose of 25 ml/kg/hr whereas the CVVHDF patients received an overall dosage of 42 ml/kg/hr. Survival at 28 days was better in the CVVHDF patient group. This trial, suggests Kellum (2007), indicates that patients with ARF should be treated with at least 35 ml/kg/hr of RRT. Tolwani *et al.* (2008) utilised a predilution CVVHDF approach and patients either received high-dose (35 ml/kg/hr) or low-dose (20 ml/kg/hr) CRRT. They did not find a significantly different result in relation to survival or renal recovery between the two patient groups.

These studies illustrate the difficulties in conducting research, in critical care, on RRT: the varied approaches to CRRT as well as the diversity of patients make conducting randomised controlled trials in different units difficult. However, it does seem that factors such as sepsis, presence of pre-existing renal disease, delivered dosage, technique for solute clearance and timing of initiation of treatment all contribute to the patient outcome. Pannu *et al.* (2008), following a systematic review of the literature, agree with the dose of 35 ml/kg/min as a target dose. This is also recommended by the Intensive Care Society (2009).

Anticoagulation

During RRT, anticoagulation is required to avoid the formation of clots with the CRRT circuit. Contact of blood to the tubing and filtration membrane will activate the clotting cascade leading to clot formation. The greater the flow rates, the less likely clots will form; similarly the more often the circuit stops, the more likely it will be for clots to form. Thus patency of the access line is important to ensure good flow through the circuit, and kinking of the lines needs to be avoided. Air within the venous bubble trap also increases the incidence of clot formation as air:blood contact initiates clot formation. Therefore, to avoid the clotting of filter and blood loss, anticoagulation is often required.

Heparin

Heparin is widely available and most practitioners are familiar with it. During RRT, it can be used in several ways:

Low-dose pre-filter heparin
This would be a dose of 5 IU/kg/hr and rarely has any effect on activated partial thromboplastin time (aPTT), international normalised ratio (INR) or activated clotting time (ACT).

Medium-dose pre-filter heparin
This would be a dose of 8–10 IU/kg/hr and may produce a slight effect on aPTT.

Systemic heparinisation
This may be useful for patients who require IV heparin infusion following, for example, mechanical valve repair, but generally IV heparin would not be used solely to prolong the life of the filter.

Regional heparinisation
In this situation, heparin is administered into the circuit pre-filter but at the end of the circuit before the blood returns to the patient, protamine is administered. This reverses the effect of the heparin, thereby minimising the risk of systemic heparinisation of the patient. The aPTT may become slightly prolonged and the monitoring of this enables careful manipulation of the heparin/protamine infusions. This may be useful in patients who have limited circuit duration but whose vascular access seems to be adequate (Bellomo and Ronco, 2002b).

Low molecular weight heparinoids

If a patient develops heparin-induced thrombocytopenia, heparinoids may be useful in avoiding the clotting of the filter but can also reduce the risk of the patient bleeding. Low molecular weight heparinoids may be a useful alternative for circuit anticoagulation.

Prostacyclin (PGI$_2$)

Prostacyclin is a potent inhibitor of platelet aggregation and can be used on its own, or in combination with heparin, to prolong the life of the filter. However, PGI$_2$ can induce hypotension and is expensive.

Citrate

Citrate chelates calcium, thereby preventing clot formation. If citrate is used, calcium-free and sodium citrate replacement/dialysate fluid is used and administered at such a rate as to achieve an ACT of 200–250 or an aPTT of 60–90 (Bellomo and Ronco, 2002b). Calcium chloride is administered separately to replace the chelated, dialysed calcium, thereby avoiding hypocalcaemia. This approach prolongs the life of the filter and compares favourably to heparin, whilst avoiding the risk of thrombocytopenia and systemic anticoagulation. However, there is a risk of hypocalcaemia and metabolic alkalosis.

No anticoagulation

If a patient has a low platelet count (<50,000), a high INR (>2 sec) and an aPTT > 60 seconds or is actively bleeding, anticoagulation may not be required. In certain clinical situations, such as fulminant liver failure, a 'trial of no anticoagulation' may be justified. A high blood flow speed, though, may be required.

Choice of replacement/dialysate fluid

Commercially prepared solutions will contain required electrolytes in appropriate concentrations; however, different buffers can be used in RRT. The alkaline substance used must replace bicarbonate lost during buffering of acid but also bicarbonate lost across the haemofilter. Lactate, citrate, acetate and bicarbonate can all be used as the buffer within replacement and dialysate fluid (Macias, 1996). Lactate and acetate are both metabolised into bicarbonate; however, situations of shock or severe hypoxia may inhibit their metabolism. This could lead to bicarbonate deficits as well. Large amounts of lactate can also increase urea generation. If bicarbonate is used as the buffer, it must be added to the bag just prior to administration to avoid formation of calcium and magnesium salts (Macias, 1996). Bicarbonate bags are useful for patients in liver failure as they will have difficulty clearing lactate; otherwise, lactate bags can be used for most critically unwell patients.

Conclusion

This chapter has demonstrated how a patient with a MI can go on to develop cardiogenic shock and, as a consequence of the cardiogenic shock, can develop ARD. Robert will require a high level of assessment and intervention to help improve his cardiac output and perfusion: this will require the full integration of the critical care team and coordination between different clinical areas as Robert's care requirements develop and alter.

References

Albarran J (2002) The language of chest pain. *Nursing Times* 98 (4) 38–40.

Allender S, Peto V, Scarborough B, Kaur A and Rayner M (2008) *Coronary Heart Disease Statistics.* BHF, London.

Antman E, Bassand JP, Klein W, *et al.* (2000) Myocardial infarction redefined – a consensus document of The Joint European Society of Cardiology/American College of Cardiology committee for the redefinition of myocardial infarction. *Journal of the American College of Cardiology* 36 (3) 959–969.

Aymong ED, Ramanathan K and Buller CE (2007) Pathophysiology of cardiogenic shock complicating myocardial infarction. *Medical Clinics of North America* 91 (4) 701–712.

Bell M, Lijestam E, Granath F, Fryckstedt J, Ekborn A and Martling C (2005) Optimal follow up time after continuous renal replacement therapy in actual renal failure patients stratified with the RIFLE criteria. *Nephrology Dialysis Transplantation* 20 (2) 354–360.

Bellomo R (2003) Acute renal failure. Chapter 38 in Bersten A and Soni N (Eds) *Oh's Intensive Care Manual*. 5th Edition, Butterworth Heinemann, Edinburgh.

Bellomo R, Farmer M, Wright C, Parkin G and Boyce N (1995) Treatment of sepsis associated severe acute renal failure with continuous haemodiafiltration: clinical experience and comparison with conventional dialysis. *Blood Purification* 13 (5) 246–254.

Bellomo R and Ronco C (1996) Acute renal failure in the intensive care unit: adequacy of dialysis and the case for continuous therapies. *Nephrology Dialysis Transplantation* 11 (3) 424–428.

Bellomo R and Ronco C (2002a) An introduction to continuous renal replacement therapy. Chapter 1 in Bellomo R, Baldwin I, Ronco C and Golper T (Eds) *Atlas of Hemofiltration*. Saunders, London.

Bellomo R and Ronco C (2002b) Anticoagulation during CRRT. Chapter 14 in Bellomo R, Baldwin I, Ronco C and Golper T (Eds) *Atlas of Hemofiltration*. Saunders, London.

Bellomo R, Ronco C, Kellum J, Mehta R, Palevsky P and the ADQI workgroup (2004) Acute renal failure – definition, outcome measures, animal models, fluid therapy and information technology needs: the Second International Consensus Conference of the Acute Dialysis Quality Initiative (ADQI) Group. *Critical Care* 8 (4) R204–R212.

Bench S (2004) Clinical skills: assessing and treating shock: a nursing perspective. *British Journal of Nursing* 13 (12) 715–721.

Bonegio R and Lieberthal W (2002) Role of apoptosis in the pathogenesis of acute renal failure. *Current Opinion in Nephrology and Hypertension* 11 (3) 301–308.

Bonventre J and Weinberg J (2003) Recent advances in the pathophysiology of ischemic acute renal failure. *Journal of the American Society of Nephrology* 14 (8) 2199–2210.

Bouman CS, Oudermans-Van Straaten MH, Tijsswen JG, Zandstra DF and Kesecioglu J (2002) Effects of early high-volume continuous venovenous hemofiltration on survival and recovery of renal function in intensive care patients with acute renal failure: a prospective randomised trial. *Critical Care Medicine* 30 (10) 2205–2211.

Brivet FG, Kleinknecht DJ, Lorat P and Landais PJ (1996) Acute renal failure in intensive care units – causes, outcome, and prognostic factors of hospital mortality: a prospective, multicenter study. French Study Group on Acute Renal Failure. *Critical Care Medicine* 24 (2) 192–198.

Choi K, Edelstein C, Gengaro P, Schrier R and Nemenoff R (1995) Hypoxia induces changes in phospholipase A2 in rat proximal tubules: evidence for multiples forms. *American Journal of Physiology* 269 (6) F846–F853.

Clark W and Ronco C (1999) CRRT efficiency and efficacy in relation to solute size. *Kidney International* 56 (72 Suppl.) S3–S7.

Collinson P (2006) Cardiac troponins T and I: biochemical markers in diagnosing myocardial infarction. *British Journal of Cardiac Nursing* 1 (9) 418–424.

Conger J and Falk S (1993) Abnormal vasoreactivity of isolated arterioles from rats with ischemic acute renal failure [abstract]. *Journal of the American Society of Nephrology* 4 (3) 733A.

Connors A, Speroff T, Dawson NV, *et al.* (1996) The effectiveness of right heart catheterization in the initial care of critically ill patients. *JAMA* 276 (11) 889–897.

Conover MB (2002) *Understanding Electrocardiography*. 8th Edition, Mosby, London.

Darovic GO (2002) *Hemodynamic Monitoring: Invasive and Noninvasive Clinical Application*. 3rd Edition, Saunders, London.

Del Bene S and Vaughan A (2005) Acute coronary syndromes. Chapter 26 in Woods SL, Sivarajan Forelicher ES, Underhill Motzer S and Bridges EJ (Eds) *Cardiac Nursing*. 5th Edition, Lippincott Williams & Wilkins, London.

Dellinger RP, Levy MM, Carlet JM, *et al.* The International Surviving Sepsis Campaign Guidelines Committee (2008) Surviving sepsis campaign: international guidelines for management of severe sepsis and septic shock. *Critical Care Medicine* 36 (1) 296–327.

De Vries B, Matthijsen R, Wolfs T, van Bijnen A, Heeringa P and Buurman W (2003) Inhibition of complement factor C5 protects against renal ischemia-reperfusion injury: inhibition of late apoptosis and inflammation. *Transplantation* 75 (3) 375–382.

De Vriese A, Colardyn F, Phillipe J, Vanholder R, de Sutter J and Lameire N (1999) Cytokine removal during continuous hemofiltration in septic patients. *Journal of the American Society of Nephrology* 10 (4) 846–853.

DH (2000) *National Service Framework for Coronary Heart Disease.* Department of Health, London.

DH (2008) *National Infarct Angioplasty Project (NIAP) Interim Report.* Department of Health & British Cardiovascular Society, London.

Ducas J and Grech ED (2003) ABC of interventional cardiology – percutaneous coronary intervention: cardiogenic shock. *BMJ* 326 (7404) 1450–1452.

Edwards SL (2001) Shock: types, classifications and explorations of their physiological effects. *Emergency Nurse* 9 (2) 29–38.

Edwards SL (2002) Myocardial infarction: nursing responsibilities in the first hour. *British Journal of Nursing* 11 (7) 454–468.

Filer L (2007) Cardiovascular drugs. Chapter 19 in Johnson K and Rawlings-Anderson K (Eds) *Oxford Handbook of Cardiac Nursing.* Oxford University Press, Oxford.

Foxall F (2009) *Haemodynamic Monitoring and Manipulation. An Easy Learning Guide.* M&K Publishing, London.

Gan TJ (2000) The esophageal Doppler as an alternative to the pulmonary artery catheter. *Current Opinion in Critical Care* 6 (3) 214–221.

Gardner P and Altman G (2005) Pathophysiology of acute coronary syndromes. Chapter 25 in Woods SL, Sivarajan Forelicher ES, Underhill Motzer S and Bridges EJ (Eds) *Cardiac Nursing.* 5th Edition, Lippincott Williams & Wilkins, London.

Gibson T (2007) Interventional cardiology for coronary heart disease. Chapter 8 in Johnson K and Rawlings-Anderson K (Eds) *Oxford Handbook of Cardiac Nursing.* Oxford University Press, Oxford, pp. 157–183.

Golper T (2002) Solute transport in CRRT. Chapter 3 in Bellomo R, Baldwin I, Ronco C and Golper T (Eds) *Atlas of Hemofiltration.* Saunders, London.

Grech ED and Ramsdale DR (2003) ABC of interventional cardiology – acute coronary syndrome: ST segment elevation myocardial infarction. *BMJ* 326 (7403) 1379–1381.

Green S (2007) Acute coronary syndromes. Chapter 7 in Johnson K and Rawlings-Anderson K (Eds) *Oxford Handbook of Cardiac Nursing.* Oxford University Press, Oxford, pp. 137–156.

Green S and Tagney J (2007) Assessing and managing the patient with chest pain due to an acute coronary syndrome. Chapter 6 in Albarran J and Tagney J (Eds) *Chest Pain: Advanced Assessment and Management Skills.* Blackwell Publishing, Oxford, pp. 71–94.

Gregory J (2005) Using the 12-lead ECG to assess acute coronary patients. *British Journal of Nursing* 14 (21) 1135–1140.

Harvey S, Harrison DA, Singer M, *et al.* (2005) Assessment of the clinical effectiveness of pulmonary artery catheters in management of patients in intensive care (PAC-Man): a randomized controlled trial. *Lancet* 366 (9484) 472–477.

Hochman JS, Sleeper LA, Webb JG, *et al.* (2006) Early revascularization and long-term survival in cardiogenic shock complicating acute myocardial infarction. *The Journal of the American Medical Association* 295 (21) 2511–2515.

Hofer C, Senn A, Weibel L and Zollinger A (2008) Assessment of stroke volume variation for prediction of fluid responsiveness using the modified FloTrac™ and PiCCOplus™ system. *Critical Care* 12 (3) R82.

Hoste E, Vanholder R, Lameire N, *et al.* (2002) No early respiratory benefit with CVVHDF in patient with acute renal failure and acute lung injury. *Nephrology Dialysis Transplantation* 17 (12) 2153–2158.

Iakobishvili Z and Hasdai D (2007) Cardiogenic shock: treatment. *Medical Clinics of North America* 91 (4) 713–727.

Intensive Care Society (2009) *Standards and Recommendations for the Provision of Renal Replacement Therapy on Intensive Care Units in the United Kingdom.* ICS, London.

Keeley EC, Boura JA and Grines CL (2003) Primary angioplasty versus intravenous thrombolytic therapy for acute myocardial infarction: a quantitative review of 23 randomised trials. *The Lancet* 361 (9351) 13–20.

Kellum JA (2007) Renal replacement therapy in critically ill patients with acute renal failure: does a greater dose improve survival? *Commentary Nature Clinical Practice Nephrology* 3 (3) 128–129.

Kelly J (2004) Evidence-based care of a patient with a myocardial infarction. *British Journal of Nursing* 13 (1) 12–18.

Koreny M, Delle Karth G, Geppert A, *et al.* (2002) Prognosis of patients who develop acute renal failure during the first 24 hours of cardiogenic shock after myocardial infarction. *The American Journal of Medicine* 112 (2) 115–119.

Kumar S and Roberts D (2001) Intra-aortic balloon pulsation: an overview. *The British Journal of Cardiology* 8 (11) 658–663.

Laurent D and Shinn JA (2005) Acute heart failure and shock. Chapter 30 in Woods SL, Sivarajan Forelicher ES, Underhill Motzer S and Bridges EJ (Eds) *Cardiac Nursing*. 5th Edition, Lippincott Williams & Wilkins, London.

Leahy M (2006) Primary angioplasty for acute ST-elevation myocardial infarction. *Nursing Standard* 21 (12) 48–56.

Levick JR (2003) *An Introduction to Cardiovascular Physiology*. 4th Edition, Hodder Arnold, London.

Lip GY, Chin BS and Prasad N (2002) ABC of antithrombotic therapy: antithrombotic therapy in myocardial infarction and stable angina. *British Medical Journal* 325 (7375) 1287–1289.

Macias W (1996) Choice of replacement fluid/dialysate anion in continuous renal replacement therapy. *American Journal of Kidney Diseases* 28 (5 Suppl. 3) S15–S20.

Malmberg K (1997) Prospective randomised study of intensive insulin treatment on long term survival after acute myocardial infarction in patients with diabetes mellitus DIGAMI (Diabetes Mellitus Insulin Glucose Infusion in Acute Myocardial Infarction) study group. *British Medical Journal* 314 (7093) 1512–1515.

Marino P (1998) *The ICU Book*. 2nd Edition, Lippincott Williams & Wilkins, Philadelphia.

Mayer J, Boldt J, Schöllhorn T, Röhm K, Mengistu A and Suttner S (2007) Semi-invasive monitoring of cardiac output by a new device using arterial pressure waveform analysis: a comparison with intermittent pulmonary artery thermodilution in patients undergoing cardiac surgery. *British Journal of Anaesthesia* 98 (2) 176–182.

McGee W, Horswell J, Calderon J, *et al.* (2007) Validation of a continuous, arterial pressure-based cardiac output measurement: a multicenter, prospective trial. *Critical Care* 11 (5) R105.

McKendry M, McGloin H, Saberi D, Caudwell L, Brady A and Singer M (2004) Randomised controlled trial assessing the impact of a nurse delivered, flow monitored protocol for optimisation of circulatory status after cardiac surgery. *BMJ* 329 (7460) 258.

Mehta RL, Pascual MT, Gruta CG, Zhuang S and Chertow GM (2002) Refining predictive models in critically ill patients with acute renal failure. *Journal of the American Society of Nephrologists* 13 (5) 1350–1357.

Migliozzi JG (2009) Shock. Chapter 4 in Nair M and Peate I (Eds) *Fundamentals of Applied Pathophysiology. An Essential Guide for Nursing Students*. Wiley-Blackwell, Chichester.

MINAP (2008) *How the NHS Manages Heart Attacks*. Seventh Public Report. Royal College of Physicians, London.

Morgan TJ (2003) Haemodynamic monitoring. Chapter 10 in Bersten A and Soni N (Eds) *Oh's Intensive Care Manual*. 5th edition, Butterworth Heinemann, Edinburgh.

Morris F and Brady WJ (2002) ABC of clinical electrocardiography. Acute myocardial infarction – part 1. *BMJ* 324 (7341) 831–834.

Muggenthaler M, Singh A and Wilkinson P (2008) The role of coronary artery stents in PCI. *British Journal of Cardiac Nursing* 3 (1) 24–30.

Murdoch S, Cohen A and Bellamy M (2000) Pulmonary artery catheterisation and mortality in critically ill patients. *British Journal of Anaesthetics* 8 (5) 611–615.

Myerson SG, Choudhury RP and Mitchell ARJ (2006) *Emergencies in Cardiology*. Oxford University Press, Oxford.

Naik H, Sabatine MS and Lily LS (2006) Acute coronary syndromes. Chapter 7 in Lilly LS (Ed.) *Pathophysiology of Heart Disease. A Collaborative Project of Medical Students and Faculty*. 4th Edition, Lippincott Williams & Wilkins, London.

Newby DE and Grubb NR (2005) *Cardiology: An Illustrated Colour Text*. Elsevier Churchill Livingstone, London.

NICE (2002) *Guidance on the Use of Drugs for Early Thrombolysis in Acute Myocardial Infarction*. National Institute for Clinical Excellence, London.

Noiri E, Nakao A, Uchida K, *et al.* (2001) Oxidative and nitrosative stress in acute renal ischemia. *American Journal of Physiology Renal Physiology* 281 (5) F948–F957.

Page B, Vieillard-Baron A, Chergui K, *et al.* (2005) Early veno-venous haemodiafiltration for sepsis-related multiple organ failure. *Critical Care* 9 (6) R755–R763.

Pannu N, Klarenbach S, Wiebe N, Manns B and Tonelli M, The Alberta Kidney Disease Network (2008) Renal replacement therapy in patients with acute renal failure: a systematic review. *JAMA* 299 (7) 793–805.

Perry Jones AJD and Pittman JAL (2003) Arterial pressure and stroke volume variability as measurements for cardiovascular optimisation. *International Journal of Intensive Care* 10 (2) 67–72.

Pollack C (2008) Pharmacological and mechanical revascularisation strategies in STEMI: integration of the two approaches. *Journal of Invasive Cardiology* 20 (5) 231–238.

Potts K (2006) Tenecteplase: a fibrinolytic agent. *British Journal of Cardiac Nursing* 1 (7) 318–326.

Quaal S (2001) Interpreting the arterial pressure waveform in the intra-aortic balloon-pumped patient. *Progress in Cardiovascular Nursing* 16 (3) 116–118, 125.

Quinn T (2005) The role of nurses in improving emergency cardiac care. *Nursing Standard* 19 (48) 41–48.

Ronco C, Bellomo R, Homel P, *et al.* (2000) Effects of different doses in continuous veno-venous haemofiltration on outcomes of acute renal failure: a prospective randomised trial. *Lancet* 356 (9233) 26–30.

Sanborn TA, Sleeper LA, Bates ER, *et al.* (2000) Impact of thrombolysis, intra-aortic balloon pump counterpulsation, and their combination in cardiogenic shock complicating acute myocardial infarction: a report from SHOCK trial registry. Should we emergently revascularize occluded coronaries for cardiogenic shock? *Journal of American College of Cardiology* 36 (3 Suppl A) 1123–1129.

Saudan P, Niederberger M, De Seigneux S, *et al.* (2006) Adding a dialysis dose to continuous hemofiltration increases survival in patients with acute renal failure. *Kidney International* 70 (7) 1312–1317.

Schrier R, Wang W, Poole B and Mitra A (2004) Acute renal failure: definitions, diagnosis, pathogenesis and therapy. *The Journal of Clinical Investigation* 114 (1) 5–14.

Shah M, Hasselblad V, Stevenson L, *et al.* (2005) Impact of the pulmonary artery catheter in critically ill patients: meta-analysis of randomized clinical trials. *JAMA* 294 (13) 1664–1670.

Shipgood L (2006) Investigating the suitability of the intra-aortic balloon pump for patients in cardiogenic shock. *British Journal of Cardiac Nursing* 1 (11) 520–526.

Silber S, Aviles FF, Cmici PG, *et al.* Task Force for Percutaneous Coronary Interventions of the European Society of Cardiology (2005) Guidelines for percutaneous interventions. The Task Force for percutaneous coronary interventions of the European Society of Cardiology. *European Heart Journal* 26 (8) 804–847.

Stenestrand U, Lindback J and Wallentin L, RIKS-HIA Registry (2006) Long-term outcome of primary percutaneous intervention vs. pre-hospital and in-hospital thrombolysis for patients with ST-elevation myocardial infarction. *Journal of the American Medical Association* 296 (14) 1749–1756.

Sutton AGC, Campbell PG, Grech ED, *et al.* (2000) Failure of thrombolysis: experience with a policy of early angiography and rescue angioplasty for electrocardiographic evidence of failed thrombolysis. *Heart* 84 (2) 197–204.

Tillyard A, Keays R and Soni N (2005) The diagnosis of acute renal failure in intensive care: mongrel or pedigree? *Anaesthesia* 60 (9) 903–914.

Tolwani AJ, Campbell RC, Stofan BS, Lai JR, Oster RA and Wille KM (2008) Standard versus high-dose CVVHDF for ICU-related acute renal failure. *Journal of the American Society of Nephrology* 19 (6) 1233–1238.

Tortora GJ and Derrickson BH (2009) *Principles of Anatomy and Physiology: Maintenance and Continuity of the Human Body.* 12th Edition, Vol. 2, Wiley, Asia.

Tough J (2004) Assessment and treatment of chest pain. *Nursing Standard* 18 (37) 453.

Tough J (2006) Primary percutaneous coronary intervention in patients with acute myocardial infarction. *Nursing Standard* 21 (2) 47–56.

Tsikouris JP and Tsikouris AP (2002) A review of available fibrin specific thrombolytic agents used in acute myocardial infarction. *Pharmacotherapy* 21 (2) 207–217.

Uchino S (2006). The epidemiology of acute renal failure in the world. *Current Opinion in Critical Care* 12 (6) 538–543.

Uchino S, Fealy N, Baldwin I, Morimatsu H and Bellomo R (2003) Pre-dilution vs. Post-dilution during continuous veno-venous hemofiltration: impact on filter life and azotemic control. *Nephron Clinical Practice* 94 (4) c94–c98.

Uehlinger D, Jakob S, Ferrari P, *et al.* (2005) Comparison of continuous and intermittent renal replacement therapy for acute renal failure. *Nephrology Dialysis Transplantation* 20 (8) 1630–1637.

Van de Werf F, Ardissino D, Betriu A, *et al.* Task Force on the Management of Acute Myocardial Infarction of the European Society of Cardiology (2003) Management of acute myocardial infarction in patients presenting with ST-segment elevation. The Task Force of the Management of Acute Myocardial Infarction of the European Society of Cardiology. *European Heart Journal* 24 (1) 28–66.

Venkataraman R and Kellum J (2007) Defining acute renal failure: the RIFLE criteria. *Journal of Intensive Care Medicine* 22 (4) 187–193.

Wangsiripaisan A, Gengaro P, Nemenoff R, Ling H, Edelstein C and Schrier R (1999) Effect of nitric oxide donors on renal tubular epithelial cell-matrix adhesion. *Kidney International* 55 (6) 2281–2288.

Wesseling KH, Jansen JR, Settels JJ and Schreuder JJ (1993) Computation of aortic flow from pressure in humans using a nonlinear, three-element model. *Journal of Applied Physiology* 74 (5) 2566–2573.

Young JL and Libby P (2006) Atherosclerosis. Chapter 5 in Lilly LS (Ed) *Pathophysiology of Heart Disease. A Collaborative Project of Medical Students and Faculty*. 4th Edition, Lippincott Williams & Wilkins, London.

Chapter 4

The septic patient

Sarah McGloin

Introduction

It is widely agreed that severe sepsis and septic shock affects over 18 million people per annum and is increasing in incidence (Angus *et al.*, 2001). As such, international intensive care societies joined together in an attempt to improve internationally the standard of care of patients who experience severe sepsis. In 2002, the Surviving Sepsis Campaign was launched by three groups: the International Sepsis Forum, the European Society of Intensive Care Medicine and the Society of Critical Care Medicine.

Dellinger *et al.* (2004) outline the main aims of the campaign as follows:

(1) To increase the awareness of sepsis, severe sepsis and septic shock amongst health professionals as well as the general public
(2) To develop evidence-based guidelines for the management of severe sepsis
(3) To ensure that the guidelines are used in practice to create global standards of care for patients with severe sepsis
(4) To reduce the mortality rate from sepsis worldwide by 25% in the 5 years, following the guidelines published in 2004

Patient scenario

Juliette Woods, a 47-year-old, was admitted to the medical assessment unit (MAU), as recommended by her general practitioner, complaining of acute abdominal pain. The pain had started at midday during lunchtime on Monday and had been present for 2 days now. The pain was increasing in severity. On examination, it became apparent that the pain was localised to the left upper abdominal quadrant and was also radiating down Juliette's back. Juliette was also complaining of nausea although she had not vomited. Juliette's husband was with her and he reported that following the death of both her parents in the last 18 months, Juliette's alcohol consumption had increased and she was now drinking an average of one bottle of wine a day. Over the weekend she had been on a drinking binge with family and friends.

The following parameters were recorded on Juliette's examination:

BP	127/68 mmHg (MAP 87)
HR	78 BPM SR
RR	22 BPM
Temperature	37.9°C

Full blood count results were as follows:

WBC	11
CRP	55 mg/l
RBC	11
Hb	10.8
HCT	52%
Na	140
K	3.7 mmol/l
MG	1.3
Ca	7.3
Glucose	9 mmol/l
Protein	4.9
Amylase	505
Lipase	302
Alkaline phosphate	122
AST	890
LDH	893
Blood alcohol	207

Arterial blood gas results were as follows:

pH	7.35
pCO_2	4.1 kPa
pO_2	12.1 kPa
HCO_3	25
Base excess (BE)	−1
SaO_2	94

A chest X-ray showed a small left pleural effusion.
From the clinical presentation a provisional diagnosis of acute pancreatitis was made.

Underlying physiology and pathophysiology

Key consideration

What are the endocrine and exocrine functions of the pancreas?

Pancreatic physiology

In order to effectively examine the underlying pathophysiology associated with acute pancreatitis, it is useful to review the physiology relating to the pancreas.

Quite simply the word *pancreas* stands for 'all flesh' in Greek (Parker, 2004). The pancreas is an accessory organ of the gastrointestinal tract (Totora and Derrickson, 2009). Located behind the peritoneum, the pancreas appears as an elongated gland situated posterior to the stomach in the left hydrochondriac region of the abdomen (Hughes, 2004). The location of the pancreas is of particular interest to practitioners as it is positioned behind so many other structures, rendering it implicitly difficult to palpate. As a consequence, growths and lesions are notoriously difficult to diagnose, often remaining undetected until they invade co-located regions of the gastrointestinal tract (Parker, 2004).

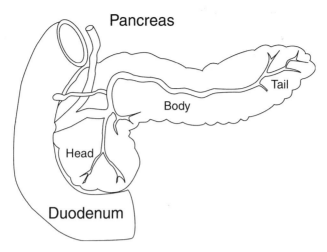

Figure 4.1   The pancreas.

Figure 4.1 illustrates the three regions of the pancreas: the head, body and tail. The gland feeds into two pancreatic ducts. The first duct, the duct of Worsung or the principle duct, extends the whole length of the pancreas (Totora and Derrickson, 2009). The second duct is the duct of Santonini or the accessory duct (Marieb, 2008). Together both ducts form the hepatopancreatic ampulla, which enters the duodenum via the common bile duct (CBD) (Parker, 2004).

The sphincter of Oddi lies at the entrance to the duodenum and facilitates the passage of pancreatic juices required for the process of digestion (Marieb, 2008). The digestion of proteins, carbohydrates and fats occurs in the presence of the hormone cholecystokinin (CKK). Importantly, the pancreas has both an endocrine and exocrine function (Totora and Derrickson, 2009).

Exocrine properties

The large majority of the gland, 98%, is associated with the exocrine activity (Parker, 2004). The exocrine portion contains small clusters called *acini*, which are collectively referred to as *acinar cells* (Totora and Derrickson, 2009). The acinar cells secrete the digestive enzymes contained within pancreatic juices; however, they are in their inactive state. These enzymes include trypsinogen which is converted into trypsin within the duodenum and is responsible for the digestion of protein. Similarly, chymotrypsinogen is converted into the active form, chymotrypsin, within the duodenum where it also digests protein. A further enzyme carboxypolypeptidase breaks down the peptide bond within proteins whilst pancreatic lipase breaks down fats into their constituent molecules of glycerol and fatty acids. Finally, pancreatic amylase digests the carbohydrate starch into the molecules of glucose, maltose and dextrin. Pancreatic amylase is also involved in the process of glycogenolysis (Totora and Derrickson, 2009).

A key function of trypsin is to act as a catalyst activating the other enzymes within the pancreas. The acinar cells actively produce and secrete trypsin inhibitor. This prevents the enzymes from becoming active before they reach the duodenum. It is when this mechanism fails that trypsin becomes activated and stimulates the activation of the other enzymes prior to reaching the duodenum. This results in the autodigestion of pancreatic tissue, and the signs and symptoms of acute pancreatitis result (Frossard *et al.*, 2008).

Endocrine properties

In contrast, the endocrine function of the gland occurs in just 1–2% of the gland. The endocrine portion is a group of small clusters of cells referred to as the *islets of Langerhan*. The islets of Langerhan are incredibly vascular, receiving approximately 15% of the total pancreatic blood volume (Marieb, 2008).

The islets of Langerhan consist of three main cell types: alpha, beta and delta cells. Another cell type is also under investigation, the pancreatic polypeptide cell; however, the function of this cell type remains unclear at present (McArdle, 2000).

The alpha, beta and delta cells secrete the hormones that contribute to the regulation of blood glucose levels. The secretion of these hormones is regulated by the parasympathetic and sympathetic branches of the autonomic nervous system (McArdle, 2000). During episodes of acute pancreatitis, this tight blood glucose level is often lost because of the autodigestion of the pancreatic tissue containing alpha, beta and delta cells.

The alpha cells secrete the hormone glucagon. Glucagon is required for the process of glycogenolysis – whereby glycogen stored in the muscle is broken down into glucose. Glucagon is also required to facilitate the process of gluconeogenesis, where glucose is synthesised from sources including amino acids during periods of limited carbohydrate supply. Both glycogenolysis and gluconeogenesis occur within the liver and kidney.

In contrast, the beta cells secrete the hormone insulin. Insulin controls protein, fat and carbohydrate metabolism. Insulin binds to specific receptors on the cell wall, which results in an increased cellular permeability to glucose, amino acids, potassium, magnesium and phosphates. This lowers blood glucose levels.

Delta cells secrete the hormone somatostatin. Somatostatin is responsible for inhibiting the release of hormones such as growth hormone, thyroid-stimulating hormone, insulin, glucagon, corticotrophin and gastrin. Somatostatin also inhibits secretion from the exocrine portion of the pancreas. Consequently, it is argued that octerotide – the synthetic form of somatostatin – may be beneficial in the treatment of the acute pancreatitis (Parker, 2004).

Pathophysiology

Having reviewed the physiology of the pancreas, the underlying pathophysiology related to Juliette's clinical presentation can now be examined.

Key considerations

What are the pathophysiological processes associated with acute pancreatitis?
What is to be understood by the term *autodigestion*?
What are the key causes of acute pancreatitis?

Pancreatitis

Classified as either acute or chronic, pancreatitis can range from a mild episode lasting a few days to a more severe episode. Mild acute pancreatitis results from localised oedema of the pancreas, whilst severe acute pancreatitis results from haemorrhage and necrosis of the gland (Holcomb, 2007).

Chronic pancreatitis

Chronic pancreatitis is the result of recurrent episodes of acute pancreatitis (Hughes, 2004). These recurring episodes result in stenosis of the ducts, thereby reducing the ability of the pancreas to release enzymes into the duodenum. Chronic pancreatitis is associated with a reduction in pain with each recurrent episode. This is the result of the progressive destruction of the acini cells responsible for the secretion of the pancreatic enzymes. In chronic pancreatitis, there is a failure to digest and absorb fats, resulting in steatorrhoea – fatty and greasy stools.

Acute pancreatitis

Acute pancreatitis is an acute yet potentially reversible inflammatory process, believed to result from the premature activation of the pancreatic enzymes (Huether, 2002). This results in cellular destruction and autodigestion of the gland. Mortality rates can be as high as 25–30% in the most severe cases (Apte and Wilson, 2003).

While it is acknowledged that mechanical factors such as cholelithiasis – gall stones passing through the common bile duct (CBD) or sepsis following cannulation during endoscopic retrograde cholangiopancreatography (ERCP) account for some of the causes of acute pancreatitis (Hughes, 2004), there remains little information as to how pancreatitis is actually stimulated although premature activation of the pancreatic enzymes remains the key as to why pancreatitis develops.

An initial event such as an acute obstruction within the pancreatic duct will obstruct the release of pancreatic juices and result in an initial injury to the acinar cells. This causes ductal hypertension, resulting in the rupture of small ducts and the release of yet more enzymes into the tissues.

As more and more enzymes are secreted, the trypsin inhibitor factor secreted by the acinar cells becomes overwhelmed, resulting in the activation of trypsinogen into trypsin (Frossard *et al.*, 2008). Trypsin in turn activates a variety of other enzymes including chymotrypsin, carboxypolypeptidase, pancreatic lipase and pancreatic amylase. These pancreatic enzymes seep into the surrounding tissues, contributing to the process of autodigestion. Autodigestion involves the activated proteins within the pancreas, digesting pancreatic tissues and cell membranes. Such a breakdown results in oedema, haemorrhage, vascular damage and fat necrosis within the pancreatic tissue (Pfrimmer, 2008).

Autodigestion

Autodigestion results in damage to the pancreatic tissue and surrounding tissue through the process of proteolysis and the release of phospholipase A, elastase and kallikrein (Huether, 2002). Such enzymes result in necrosis of the pancreatic parenchyma and the peripancreatic fat cells, thus releasing further inflammatory mediators and causing further damage to the acinar cells (Parker, 2004). Proteolysis results in the secretion of inflammatory mediators including complement, bradykinin, interleukin, tumour necrosis factor (TNF), histamine and prostaglandins (Holcomb, 2007). TNF is also secreted by the macrophages and increases the severity of pancreatitis (Frossard *et al.*, 2008). Such inflammatory mediators stimulate increased capillary permeability, which results in third space fluid loss particularly within the gastrointestinal tract. Hypovolaemia follows, resulting in volume responsive acute kidney injury (Moore and Woodrow, 2009). The hypovolaemia is also exacerbated by a change in serum osmolarity.

As autodigestion increases, the endocrine portion of the pancreas is affected. Consequently, less insulin is secreted, resulting in a raised blood sugar level. Fluid is lost from the circulating volume, resulting in a raised serum osmolarity. This results in hypovolaemia.

Causes of acute pancreatitis

Cholelithiasis

Cholelithiasis – a gall bladder disease – is recognised as a major cause in the development of acute pancreatitis (Hughes, 2004). Cholelithiasis affects four times more women than men, with pregnancy, diabetes and obesity being predisposing factors (Burkitt *et al.*, 1998). Gall stones leave the CBD, getting lodged within the main pancreatic duct outlet. This results in pancreatic duct obstruction. Bile accumulates, entering the duct of Wirsung, activating the pancreatic enzymes, resulting in autodigestion (Wang *et al.*, 2009).

Alcohol

It was apparent from Juliette's initial assessment that she has high alcohol consumption, particularly following the death of her parents. Alcohol, along with gallstone obstruction, is known to account for between 66 and 75% of cases with acute pancreatitis (Carroll *et al.*, 2007) and as such alcoholic pancreatitis cannot be disregarded as a cause for Juliette's abdominal discomfort in this instance.

Alcoholic pancreatitis is thought to occur from the inflammatory effects alcohol has on the pancreatic tissue and ducts, resulting in autodigestion (Wang *et al.*, 2009). The symptoms of pancreatitis occur 12 hours following an episode of binge drinking (Beckingham and Bornman, 2001). It is thought that alcohol has an irritating effect on the sphincter of Oddi, decreasing the muscle tone of the sphincter, resulting in spasm and reflux while also obstructing the flow of secretions (Morton and Fontaine, 2008). Holt (1993) also argues that alcohol damages the acinar cells through inflammation. This accelerates both their enzyme production and autodigestion.

As autodigestion continues, the acinar secretions become thick and glutenous. Protein is precipitated in the pancreatic enzymes (Torrance and Serginson, 2000). Calcium carbonate is also deposited, and stones form over time in the pancreatic ducts (Apte and Wilson, 2003). This results in the ducts becoming obstructed. Pancreatic juices are prevented from entering the duodenum, resulting in further destruction and fibrosis of the acinar cells. The damage results in the release of cytokines – inflammatory mediators into the surrounding tissue, resulting in peritonitis (Pfrimmer, 2008). The enzymes and cytokines are then absorbed into the circulation from the abdominal cavity, via the lymphatic system. The enzymes and mediators are then circulated to other organs, resulting in multi-organ failure (Holcomb, 2007). Severe pancreatitis will ultimately result in a major inflammatory response, vasodilation, hypotension, tachycardia and bronchoconstriction (Pfrimmer, 2008).

Other causes

There are other recognised contributory factors to acute pancreatitis. These include malignancy, inflammatory infections including mumps and hepatitis, toxins, drugs such as non-steroidal anti-inflammatory drugs, hereditary factors including pancreas divisum and abdominal injuries (McArdle, 2000).

Complications associated with pancreatitis

In particular, pulmonary complications arise when the pancreatic fluid seeps via the lymphatic system or through the diaphragm into the pleural space (Pfrimmer, 2008). This results in the development of pleural effusions (Holcomb, 2007). Pain causes the splinting of the abdominal wall, thereby resulting in the patient being at greater risk of atelectasis and pneumonia. Similarly, patients are also at greater risk of developing pulmonary emboli and acute respiratory distress syndrome (ARDS) (Pfrimmer, 2008).

Pancreatic pseudocysts are collections of pancreatic juices enclosed by a wall of fibrous tissue. Such cysts compress the surrounding tissue. This can result in the formation of fistula, which, if sited within the liver or spleen, can result in haemorrhage or infection if situated in the bowel (Murphy *et al.*, 2002).

Assessment and diagnosis

Key considerations

What strategies should be used to assess Juliette?
What diagnostic studies should be taken?

Upon admission to the MAU, Juliette underwent a thorough physical assessment using the ABCDE approach.

Airway: Juliette was able to verbally respond to the medical and nursing staff, thereby indicating that she had a patent airway.

Breathing and ventilation: Juliette's breathing requires careful assessment. The pain associated with acute pancreatitis can increase the patient's work of breathing. Consequently, the patient can experience dyspnoea, tachycardia, decreased air entry and shoulder pain. Juliette had an increased respiratory rate with decreased air entry to the bases. Oxygen saturations should be monitored (Parker, 2004). Patients may show signs of hypoxia due to hypovolaemia secondary to hypovolaemic shock. Juliette's oxygen saturations were poor on admission at 90% on air. Her chest X-ray showed a left pleural effusion.

Friedman *et al.* (2003) argue that a thorough respiratory assessment is required as ARDS can develop secondary to acute pancreatitis.

Circulation: Considering Juliette's circulation, her pulse should be monitored for rate, strength and regularity. Whilst her blood pressure remained acceptable, her heart rate was irregular and starting to climb. Her blood pressure should be continuously monitored. Hypotension associated with hypovolaemia may occur in extreme cases of acute pancreatitis. The circulatory volume may be lost due to the action of enzymes and kinins, resulting in increased capillary permeability and vasodilation (Huether, 2002). Juliette's skin must also be assessed for dryness and reduced turgor, the result of hypovolaemia secondary to the vomiting associated with this stage of the disease.

Disability: Juliette was orientated in time, place and person. However, she may become drowsy should her respiratory function deteriorate or should she go into shock. Her blood glucose levels were elevated and therefore should also be monitored. With the destruction of pancreatic tissue during an episode of acute pancreatitis coupled with the stress response to the condition, it is likely that there would be a raised blood glucose level, the result of a decrease in insulin production and secretion, affecting the uptake of glucose by the cells.

Exposure: A top to toe examination found an irregular haemorrhagic spot surrounding Juliette's umbilicus. This is referred to as *Cullen's sign* and is associated with the actions of kinins and enzymes released through the acute pancreatitis. Sometimes, Grey-Turner's sign, a bluish colour, may also be detected around the flanks and lower back during a top to toe examination; however, this does tend to be in response to prolonged hypovolaemia and so Parker (2004) argues that this is not often seen as an early diagnostic tool.

Steer *et al.* (2000) found that the pain associated with acute pancreatitis is of sudden onset and located in the upper left abdominal quadrant. This is true of the pain experienced by Juliette. The pain associated with acute pancreatitis can also be found in the mid epigastric area and it radiates to the back and flank regions. Juliette found it more comfortable to either sit up or lie in the foetal position to relieve her pain.

An abdominal assessment found that Juliette had decreased bowel sounds. Her abdomen was distended, she was guarding against pain and her abdomen was particularly tender to palpate.

Identification of risk factors

Holcomb (2000) recommends a thorough history to be taken at the time of admission to identify the risk factors associated with acute pancreatitis. Such history taking should focus on gall bladder disease, recent abdominal surgery or trauma, hyperlipidaemia, medications including thiazides, acetaminophen, tetracyclines and oestrogen-based oral contraceptives. Allergies should also be explored as should recent viral infections. The patient's alcohol intake must also be assessed. Juliette, as we have already ascertained, has a high alcohol consumption and has recently been on a binge with friends and family.

Diagnostic studies

Serum amylase and lipase measurement

Serum amylase would be expected to rise within 2 hours following the onset of symptoms and decrease within the next 36 hours. Being a small molecule, serum amylase is easily cleared by the renal system, and its high serum levels tend to be short-lived. However, amylase levels are not specific to pancreatitis, with other conditions also causing a rise in amylase levels including perforated viscera, renal insufficiency and salivary gland inflammation. Therefore, this result should not be taken in isolation.

In contrast, it is argued that serum lipase provides a more useful historical indicator to amylase as it takes longer to clear from the blood (Agarwal *et al.*, 1990). Lipase rises within 4–8 hours following the start of symptoms. It normally peaks at 24 hours and remains elevated for 14 days. Parker (2004) recommends taking the amylase and lipase results together as a means of providing 90–95% reliability for detecting acute pancreatitis.

Full blood count

A full blood count is also required to assess for the presence of the disease. The results would be expected to show a raised white cell count, haemoconcentration secondary to hypovolaemia and thrombocytopaenia due to reduced platelet levels. It is likely that there will be a reduced serum albumin level secondary to increased capillary permeability. The electrolyte profile will be dependent upon the patient's fluid status and renal function. Liver function tests are likely to be raised.

Arterial blood gases

Arterial blood gases provide an important marker for the disease. With reduced insulin levels, large quantities of fatty acids are released into the circulation, following the breakdown of stored triglycerides. These fatty acids are converted into acetoacetic acid in the liver, which cannot be metabolised, thereby resulting in a metabolic acidosis. To compensate, patients increase their respiratory rate in an attempt to excrete carbon dioxide. Pancreatitis will also reduce the levels of bicarbonate, a buffer that can affect the acid–base balance.

Radiological investigations

Further diagnostic tests include plain chest and abdominal X-rays. Such films will exclude alternative pathophysiologies such as bowel perforation and obstruction. Abdominal X-rays will also show gallstones. Chest X-rays are very useful as left-sided pleural effusions, which can be the result of toxins released by the pancreas, are often detected through such X-rays. Indeed, Juliette was seen to have a pleural effusion on her admission chest X-ray.

Electrocardiogram

Electrocardiograms (ECGs) are important as pancreatitis can result in hypocalcaemia. Such low levels of calcium result in arrhythmias.

Ultrasound

Ultrasound scans have been seen to be largely inconclusive, with it being hard to visualise the pancreas in up to 50% of cases. With obesity and bowel gas, Gandolifi (2003) argues against the use of the ultrasound scan; however, the advantage is that the scan can diagnose CBD disorders or gallstones.

CT scan

The abdominal computed tomography (CT) scan is regarded to be the gold standard diagnostic tool. However, again it may be negative in up to 30% of cases. The CT does, however, show inflammation, fluid collections, necrosis, pseudocysts or tumours (Fosmark, 2000).

Scoring systems

There are a variety of scoring systems available to aid the diagnosis of acute pancreatitis. These include Ranson's criteria, the CT Severity Score, the Imrie scoring system (or modified Glasgow score) and the Acute Physiology and Chronic Health Evaluation II (APACHE II) scale.

Ranson's criteria

Ranson's criteria (Ranson, 1982) uses 11 factors to assess the severity of the inflammatory process (Box 4.1). For each positive item there is a score of one point. The highest score achieved using this tool is 11 points.

Modified Glasgow scoring system

The modified Glasgow scoring system (Box 4.2) is the easiest and quickest tool to use to diagnose the severity of acute pancreatitis (Parker, 2004).

Box 4.1 Ranson's criteria

Severe pancreatitis is defined by the presence of three or more of the following features:

On presentation:

Age >55 (non-gallstone pancreatitis) or >70 (gallstone pancreatitis)
Leucocyte count >16,000/mm^3
Blood glucose >10 mmol/l (if not diabetic)
Lactate dehydrogenase >350 IU/l
Serum glutamic oxaloacetic transaminase levels >250 μ/l

During the first 48 hours:

Haematocrit decrease by <10%
Serum urea increase by >10 mmol/l despite adequate intravenous therapy
Hypocalcaemia: corrected serum concentrations of calcium <2 mmol/l
Low arterial oxygen partial pressure pO$_2$ <8 kPa or 60 mmHg
Metabolic acidosis: base deficit >4 mEq/l
Fluid deficit >6 l

(Adapted from Ranson, 1982)

Box 4.2 The modified Glasgow scoring system

Severe pancreatitis is defined by the presence of three or more of the following features:

Age	>55
White cell count	>15,000 mm^3
Blood glucose	>10 mmol/l
Urea	>16 mmol/l
Arterial oxygen partial pressure	<8 kPa
Albumin	<32 g/l
Calcium	<2 mmol/l
Lactate dehydrogenase	>600 IU/l

(Adapted from Blamey *et al.*, 1984)

APACHE II criteria

The APACHE II criteria (Larvin and McMahon, 1989) is highly sensitive in the diagnosis of acute pancreatitis. An APACHE II score greater than 8 in the first 24 hours indicates the presence of disease. However, the APACHE II criteria is notoriously time-consuming to apply (Parker, 2004) and requires computer software.

Computerised tomography severity index

The Computerised Tomography (CT) severity index (Balthazar *et al.*, 1994), as seen in Box 4.3, has been seen to provide a more reliable predictor of severe pancreatitis than Ranson's criteria or the APACHE II scale (Neoptolemos *et al.*, 2000). This could be due to the fact that the data is collected 72 hours post admission (Carroll *et al.*, 2007).

With so many tools available to aid the diagnosis of acute pancreatitis, the Atlanta classification of severe acute pancreatitis has become widely used as a predictor for patient outcome (Carroll *et al.*, 2007). However, the UK guidelines for the management of acute pancreatitis (2005) identify the features in Box 4.4 to predict a severe attack of acute pancreatitis.

Box 4.3 CT severity index

CT grade:

A = Normal pancreas 0 points
B = Oedematous/swollen pancreas 1 point
C = B plus extra pancreatic changes 2 points
D = Severe extra pancreatic changes plus evidence of a fluid collection 3 points
E = Multiple or excessive fluid collections 4 points

Necrosis score:

None = 0 points
>one-third = 2 points
<one-third but less than one-half = 4 points
>one-half = 6 points

Scoring:

CT grade + necrosis score

(Adapted from Balthazar *et al.*, 1994)

> **Box 4.4 Features predicting a severe attack of acute pancreatitis within 48 hours of admission to hospital**
>
> | | |
> |---|---|
> | Initial assessment | Significant systemic signs |
> | | Body mass index >30 |
> | | Pleural effusion evident on chest X-ray |
> | | APACHE II score >8 |
> | | |
> | 24 hours post admission | Significant systemic signs |
> | | APACHE II score >8 |
> | | Glasgow score of 3 or more |
> | | Persisting multiple organ failure |
> | | CRP >150 mg/l |
> | | |
> | 48 hours post admission | Significant systemic signs |
> | | APACHE II score >8 |
> | | CRP >150 mg/l |
> | | Persisting organ failure for 48 hours |
> | | Multiple or progressive organ failure |
>
> (Adapted from UK Working Party on Acute Pancreatitis, 2005)

Juliette was admitted to MAU with already severe acute pancreatitis. In line with the UK Working Party on Acute Pancreatitis (2005) guidelines Juliette's clinical presentation showed an individual with pyrexia and tachycardia in severe abdominal pain. An examination revealed decreased bowel sounds and a raised respiratory rate. Whilst her blood pressure was not too low, Juliette's biochemistry was altered and there were radiological markers on the chest X-ray. It was also apparent from the history that was taken that Juliette did have a high alcohol consumption. Despite this, instead of being admitted to a high dependency unit for close monitoring as recommended in the UK Working Party for Acute Pancreatitis (2005), Juliette was admitted to a general medical ward for management of her condition.

Evidence-based care

> **Key consideration**
>
> How should Juliette's pancreatitis be managed?

Initially it is difficult to ascertain whether an individual is experiencing mild pancreatitis, which will be likely to resolve by itself spontaneously, or a more severe episode (UK Working Party on Acute Pancreatitis, 2005). Early oxygen therapy and fluid resuscitation reduce the development of organ failure and reduce mortality and morbidity from the disease (Johnson and Abu-Hilal, 2004).

Fluids

The inflammation associated with acute pancreatitis can result in up to 6 l of fluid being lost into the retroperitoneal space. The UK Working Party on Acute Pancreatitis (2005) recommends the administration of fluids to patients with acute pancreatitis, until the severity of the episode has been established and the effect on other organs has been assessed. Fluids should be given intravenously to maintain a urine output of 0.5 ml/kg/hr, haemodynamic monitoring, such as central venous pressure (CVP) monitored regularly, to evaluate the effectiveness of the fluid resuscitation (Toouli *et al.*, 2002)

Juliette was admitted to a general medical ward where she was put on an intravenous infusion via a peripheral line. Here she also had a CVP line inserted along with urinary catheter with a urometer bag.

Oxygen

The UK Working Party on Acute Pancreatitis (2005) advocate the use of oxygen therapy to maintain an arterial oxygen saturation greater than 95%. This is of particular relevance for Juliette who has a left-sided pleural effusion on admission. Continuous oxygen saturation monitoring will help achieve this goal (Jevon and Ewens, 2007).

Antibiotics

There is great debate over the use of prophylactic antibiotics with the literature remaining broadly inconclusive over the effectiveness of the therapy. Those against the practice argue that it encourages selective growth of resistant organisms (UK Working Party on Acute Pancreatitis, 2005). Indeed, a Cochrane review (Bassi *et al.*, 2003) suggested the need for further double-blind randomised controlled trials in order to ascertain the effectiveness of antibiotic therapy in acute pancreatitis. The UK Working Party on Acute Pancreatitis (2005) therefore concluded that in cases of necrosis involving less than 30% of pancreatic tissue, antibiotics are unlikely to affect the outcome, whilst cases where more than 30% of tissue is affected may benefit from the administration of prophylactic antibiotic therapy for 7–14 days. Pitchumoni *et al.* (2005) suggest the use of broad-spectrum antibiotics, which are able to penetrate the pancreatic tissue.

What is clear is that there is no statistically significant reduction in mortality rate with the use of selective decontamination of the digestive tract (SDD) along with intravenous antibiotics. Consequently, the use of SDD cannot be supported for the treatment of acute pancreatitis (UK Working Party on Acute Pancreatitis, 2005).

Because the extent of Juliette's pancreatitis was unclear, she did not receive prophylactic antibiotic therapy at this time.

Nutrition

Enteral feeding remains another contentious issue. Food was believed to have a stimulating effect on the pancreas and so traditionally it was the practice to maintain the patient nil-by-mouth in order to rest the pancreas and for total parenteral nutrition (TPN) to be administered (Carroll *et al.*, 2007). However, Marik and Zaloga (2004) found total enteral nutrition in comparison with TPN to be more beneficial to patients with acute pancreatitis, particularly as TPN has a high correlation with infection and sepsis (Pfrimmer, 2008). The type of enteral feeding, however, is under debate. Tenner (2004) argues that nasojejunal tubes prevent pancreatic enzyme release and reduce mortality and morbidity, whilst, in contrast, Eatock *et al.* (2000) found that nasogastric feeding would be possible in up to 80% of cases. In order to prevent pancreatic secretion, the feed should be low in fat and high in carbohydrate.

Pain control

The pain associated with acute pancreatitis is the result of the extravasation of kinins and enzymes into the retroperitoneal space. A further cause is the distended pancreatic ducts, obstruction of the ampulla of Vater or duodenal obstruction caused by swelling of the head of the pancreas (Frossard *et al.*, 2008).

Parker (2004) argues that pain assessment and management is essential when treating patients with acute pancreatitis. An increase in pain has a direct effect on the secretion of pancreatic juices. Therefore, it is essential that pain is appropriately managed (Holcomb, 2007). Parker (2004) advocates the use of intravenous opioids titrated to the level of pain experienced with patient-controlled analgesia. There is a debate regarding the appropriate opiate to be used in this situation. Many support the use of pethidine (Thune *et al.*, 1990; Kredo and Onia, 2005) believing that it does not affect the sphincter of Oddi. However, Pasero (1998) argues that all opioids increase smooth muscle tone, thereby reducing pancreatic secretions and increasing the bile duct pressure. This results in biliary spasm and constriction of the sphincter of Oddi. Paulson (2002) argues that there is no evidence to support the use of morphine over pethidine. The use of morphine remains a contentious issue. While morphine is more effective at longer term management of severe pain it can cause spasm in the sphincter of Oddi, and repeated administration of pethidine can result in the accumulation of the metabolite norpethidine, which may result in central nervous system irritability and potential seizures. Parker (2004) argues for further research into the use of analgesia for the management of pain associated with pancreatitis. Pasero (1998) argues that the anti-secretory agent octeritide can reduce the pain associated with pancreatitis simply by reducing the enzymes that cause autodigestion. However, larger randomised studies have found the results of octeritide disappointing (Uhl *et al.*, 1999). Similar results are associated with antiprotease agents, gabexate and anti-inflammatory agents including lexipafant.

Ongoing patient scenario

Juliette has now been in hospital for 2 days. She is now complaining of increasing pain within her left abdominal quadrant, which continues to radiate down her back. Juliette continues to feel nauseas and has now vomited three times in the last 5 hours. It is decided to do repeat blood tests.

The following parameters were recorded on Juliette's examination:

BP	110/60 mmHg (MAP 76)
HR	132 sinus tachycardia
RR	30 breaths/min
Temperature	39.5°C
Urine output	15 ml/hr
WBC	$20 \times 1/10^9$
CRP	142 mg/l
RBC	11
Hb	9.5
HCT	56%
Na	147 mmol/l
K	3.1 mmol/l
Mg	0.72 mmol/l
Ca	1.7 mmol/l
Glucose	13 mmol/l
Protein	4.9
Amylase	1253 IU/l
Lipase	520
Alkaline phosphate	257 IU/l

Arterial blood gas results are as follows:

pH   7.31
pCO_2 4 kPa 30 mmHg
pO_2 10.9 kPa 82 mmHg
HCO_3 25
BE   −3
SaO_2 89

Progressing pathophysiology

Juliette's temperature has now risen to 39.5°C. Her respiratory rate has increased and she has become oliguric. This indicates that despite initial efforts by the team, Juliette's condition has now deteriorated. She now appears to be septic.

> **Key considerations**
>
> How does severe acute pancreatitis develop into septic shock?
> How does hypovolaemic shock occur?

Severe acute pancreatitis and sepsis

The increase in temperature is associated with inflammation of the pancreas. The inflammation is the result of autodigestion of the gland by the ongoing synthesis and secretion of pancreatic enzymes. As autodigestion of the pancreas continues, the pancreatic tissue becomes increasingly necrotic, releasing further endotoxins, thereby exacerbating the inflammation further.

The inflammatory response is the result of activation of four plasma cascade systems:

(1) The complement system results in the removal of pathogens through the process of opsonisation and phagocytosis.
(2) The kinin system is responsible for vasodilation and other inflammatory effects.
(3) The coagulation system is responsible for containing the infection or injury.
(4) The fibrinolysis system counterbalances the effects of the coagulation system.

Under normal homeostatic mechanisms, these systems work alongside each other to manage an antigen. However, as severe sepsis develops there are disturbances in the inflammatory, coagulation and fibrinolysis systems and the response of these mechanisms to the presence of infection proliferate unchecked. In particular, the pro-inflammatory and pro-coagulation responses dominate, resulting in uncontrolled systemic inflammation and advanced coagulopathy (Kleinpell, 2003).

As the pancreatic tissue continues to break down in response to the inflammatory response, Juliette's pancreas begins to haemorrhage, resulting in an increase in capillary permeability. The overall result is that Juliette develops hypovolaemic shock.

Hypovolaemic shock

Hypovolaemic shock is the result of an inadequate circulating intravascular volume (McLuckie, 2003). In Juliette's case, the hypovolaemic shock occurs as a result of toxic pancreatic exudates entering into the abdominal cavity. The toxins released by the exudate result in increased capillary permeability. Proteins leak from the blood vessels, through the increasingly permeable capillary membrane into the extracellular fluid. This is referred to as a *third space fluid loss*. As proteins occupy the extracellular space, the interstitial fluid oncotic pressure increases. Increased fluid is then pulled from the capillaries into the extracellular space, resulting in a reduced circulating blood volume and interstitial oedema. The reduced circulating volume is referred to as *hypovolaemia* and ultimately leads to hypovolaemic shock.

Hypotension occurs as a result of the hypovolaemic shock. In an attempt to compensate and maintain an adequate blood pressure, the heart rate increases, resulting in a tachycardia along with systemic vasoconstriction (Bench, 2004). Such compensatory mechanisms are aimed at maintaining an adequate mean arterial blood pressure, ensuring that vital organs such as the brain and the heart remain perfused at all times. The compensatory mechanisms are stimulated by an increase in sympathetic nervous system activity coupled with the release of endogenous catecholamines such as adrenaline and noradrenaline (McLuckie, 2003).

A further compensatory mechanism is initiated by the renal system in response to an increase in circulating adrenaline and reduced renal blood flow (Totora and Derrickson, 2009). Osmoreceptors trigger the release of antidiuretic hormone (ADH) by the posterior pituitary gland as the osmolarity of blood increases. ADH stimulates the reabsorption of water by the renal tubule. Similarly, the renin–angiotensin–aldosterone system (RAAS) stimulates the release of angiotensinogen. Angiotensinogen is an enzyme that converts angiotensin I into angiotensin II. Angiotensin II is a powerful vasoconstrictor, which increases mean arterial blood pressure through vasoconstriction.

Additionally, the adrenal cortex also secretes the hormone aldosterone (Marieb, 2008). Aldosterone increases sodium reabsorption by the renal tubule. As sodium is reabsorbed into the circulation, water passively follows. The circulating volume rises, there is an increase in preload and the cardiac output increases. However, all such compensatory mechanisms are an attempt to increase mean arterial blood pressure despite the overall decreased circulating volume. Importantly, such compensation mechanisms are transitory and unsustainable.

As the autodigestion develops and further endotoxins are secreted, Juliette's condition deteriorates. As the inflammatory process progresses, Juliette's hypovolaemic shock is accompanied by the development of severe sepsis. Here the primary inflammatory response triggers a cascade effect of sepsis, which can ultimately result in multi-organ dysfunction and death (Bone *et al.*, 1992).

Sepsis

Key considerations

What are the stages of the sepsis continuum?
What is systemic inflammatory response syndrome?
What are the diagnostic criteria for sepsis and severe sepsis?

The septic response is a component of an overall continuum that ranges from infection to multiple organ failure and death. The sepsis continuum begins with an infection. The infection leads to systemic inflammatory response syndrome (SIRS). This then develops into sepsis, and then severe sepsis resulting in overall septic shock, multiple organ dysfunction syndrome and, ultimately, death.

Systemic inflammatory response syndrome

SIRS was first defined by Bone *et al.* (1992). The manifestations of SIRS can be found in Table 4.1.

Sepsis is the next stage in this continuum. Sepsis quite simply refers to the presence of an infection that stimulates a systemic response (Levy and Geenen, 2001). The diagnostic criteria for sepsis can be found in Table 4.2.

Table 4.1   Systemic inflammatory response syndrome (SIRS)

This is the body's response to a variety of insults and results in the development of two or more of the following conditions:

Pyrexia >38°C

Temperature below 36°C

Heart rate above 90 beats/min

Respiratory rate above 20 breaths/min or pCO_2 below 32 mmHg.

Raised or reduced white cell count above 12,000/μl or below 4000/μl

(Adapted from Bone *et al.*, 1992.)

Table 4.2   Diagnostic criteria for sepsis

Infection, either documented or suspected, and some of the following:

General variables:

Fever >38.3°C

Hypothermia (core temperature) <36°C

Heart rate >90 beats/min or >2 SD above the normal value for age

Tachypnoea

Altered mental status

Significant oedema or positive fluid balance (>20 ml/kg over 24 hr)

Hyperglycaemia (blood glucose >7.7 mmol/l) in the absence of diabetes

Inflammatory variables:

Leucocytes (WBC count >12,000/μl)

Leukopenia (WBC count >4000/μl)

Normal WBC count with 10% immature forms

Plasma C-reactive protein >2 SD above the normal value

Plasma procalcitonin >2 SD above the normal value

Haemodynamic variables:

Arterial hypotension (SBP < 90 mmHg; MAP < 70 mmHg or an SBP decrease >40 mmHg in adults or <2 SD below normal for age)

Organ dysfunction variables:

Arterial hypoxaemia (pO_2:F_IO_2 <300 mmHg)

Acute oliguria for no longer than 2 consecutive hours

Creatinine increase >0.5 mg/dl

Coagulation abnormalities (INR >1.5 or a PTT >60 sec)

Ileus (absent bowel sounds)

Thrombocytopenia (platelet count <100,000/μl)

Hyperbilirubinemia (plasma total bilirubin >4 mg/dl)

Tissue perfusion variables:

Hyperlactataemia (greater than upper limit of lab normal)

Capillary refill time greater than 2 sec

SBP, systolic blood pressure; INR, international normalised ratio; PTT, partial thromboplastin time. (Adapted from Levy and Geenen, 2001.)

Table 4.3   Diagnostic criteria for severe sepsis

Severe sepsis is sepsis-induced tissue hypoperfusion or organ dysfunction

Sepsis-induced hypotension

Lactate greater than the upper limits of normal laboratory results

Urine output <0.5 ml/kg/hr for >2 hr despite adequate fluid resuscitation

ALI with a pO_2: FiO_2 <33.3 kPa (250 mmHg) in the absence of pneumonia as an infection source

ALI with a pO_2: FiO_2 < 26.6 kPa (200 mmHg) in the presence of pneumonia as an infection source

Creatinine >2.0 mg/dl (176.8 μmol/l)

Bilirubin >2 mg/dl (34.2 μmol/l)

Platelet count <100,000

Coagulopathy (INR >1.5)

(Reproduced from Dellinger RP, Levy MM, Carlet JM, *et al*. (2008) Surviving sepsis campaign: international guidelines for management of severe sepsis and septic shock. *Critical Care Medicine* 36 296–327, copyright 2008, with permission of the Society of Critical Care Medicine.)

Further along the sepsis continuum, Levy and Geenen (2001) define severe sepsis as sepsis coupled with sepsis-induced organ dysfunction or tissue hypoperfusion. The overwhelming response to severe sepsis by the body includes profound hypotension, reduced urine output and hypoxaemia (Peel, 2008).

Dellinger *et al.* (2008) argue that the thresholds to define severe sepsis from sepsis vary greatly from paper to paper; however, they have summarised the typical indications for severe sepsis in Table 4.3.

Septic shock is the next stage of the continuum. Septic shock involves the presence of severe sepsis coupled with hypotension or a raised lactate that fails to improve with fluid resuscitation.

However, despite these agreed definitions of SIRS, sepsis, severe sepsis and septic shock, a study by Poeze *et al.* (2004) found that no more than 17% of doctors agreed on one specific definition. Thus, Robson and Newell (2005) argue that for sepsis to be treated effectively, it is essential that a common definition is found and supported. To such an end, the Surviving Sepsis Campaign (Dellinger *et al.*, 2008) aims to address this and reduce mortality associated with sepsis and septic shock.

Pathophysiology of sepsis

Key considerations

What are the pathological processes associated with severe sepsis?
What is the inflammatory response?
How does the complement system work?
What is the coagulation cascade?

To understand the pathophysiological response to sepsis, it is essential to have an understanding of the normal immune response.

The normal immune response

Any cell that has been damaged by infection from viruses, bacteria, chemical agents or trauma will respond in the same way. This response is an innate defensive response by the body and is non-specific. This response is known as *inflammation*.

Inflammation has the following three basic phases:

(1) Vasodilation
(2) Emigration of phagocytes
(3) Tissue repair

Vasodilation increases the blood supply to the damaged area. The increased permeability allows phagocytes and antibodies to pass out from the circulation and work on the invading organism.

Next, the clotting cascade is activated. A clot forms, which is again part of the normal immune response. The clot is believed to prevent the spread of invading organisms from one area of the body to another (Ahrens and Vollman, 2003). Quite simply, in a normal immune response to an invading organism, the inflammation and activation of the clotting system repair the tissue and prevent further damage.

However, as the endotoxins start to leak out, an immunological cascade is triggered. Inflammatory mediators called *cytokines* are released, activating the white cells, leucocytes and phagocytes. This results in a breakdown in homeostasis and the development of severe sepsis.

Severe sepsis

Severe sepsis is the result of the breakdown in homeostasis and stimulates an exaggerated and excessive inflammatory response within the body. Severe sepsis is the result of disturbances in the inflammation, coagulation and fibrinolytic systems. The pro-inflammatory and pro-coagulation responses takeover, resulting in an uncontrolled inflammatory state and advanced coagulopathy. This results in excess coagulation, an exaggerated inflammation and impaired fibrinolysis.

A variety of mechanisms occur to destroy an invading antigen. Acute inflammation is associated with specific vascular changes, including vasodilation, increased capillary permeability and a slowing of the blood flow. Vasodilation occurs first at arteriole level, then progressing to capillary level, which results in a net increase in the volume of blood present.

The inflammatory response

When an antigen enters the circulation, it is detected by circulating white cells, either monocytes or neutrophils. The antigens in the case of acute pancreatitis have been found to be *Escherichia coli*, *Enterobacter*, *Pseudomonas aeruginosa*, *Proteus* spp., *Klebsiella* and fungi (Polaków *et al.*, 2002). The leucocytes, which include the monocytes or neutrophils, then initiate an immune response.

The monocytes release inflammatory mediators and tissue factors, which stimulate a series of events that progress rapidly. The cell-derived inflammatory mediators include interleukin-1, interleukin-6 and TNF. These inflammatory mediators are referred to as *cytokines* and are secreted primarily by the macrophages. The cytokines affect a wide variety of cells to stimulate a variety of inflammatory responses. These include the development of pyrexia, chemotaxis, leucocyte adherence and activation of fibroblasts. The cytokines are responsible for symptoms such as the loss of appetite and an increased heart rate associated with the septic response.

Leucocytes are involved with the initiation of the inflammatory response. They then act to maintain the inflammatory response. The leucocytes have to move from their usual location within the circulation to the site of the infection. The process of leucocytes moving from the blood into the tissues is referred to as *extravasation*. Extravasation is divided into three main steps:

Step 1

The leucocytes are recruited to the area of the infection. This process is driven by the presence of receptors on the endothelial cell walls. These receptors are called *P-selectin* and *E-selectin*. The secretion of the receptor P-selectin onto the endothelial cell membrane is stimulated by the presence of inflammatory mediators such as histamine. The P-selectin receptor on the endothelial cell wall binds to carbohydrates on the cell wall of the leucocyte. The leucocyte then rolls along the surface of the endothelium. As it rolls along, bonds are made and broken.

The cytokines from the inflammatory response stimulate the secretion of E-selectin. E-selectin works in a similar way as the P-selectin. Once activated, the E-selectin and P-selectin receptors have the responsibility of trapping the neutrophils in the location of the infection (Ahrens and Vollman, 2003). The neutrophil can then work on destroying the antigen.

Step 2

The second stage of extravasation is referred to as *transmigration* via diapedesis. The leucocytes change their shape (diapedesis) to move between the endothelial cells to pass through the basement membrane into the tissues.

Step 3

Finally, once in the tissues, the leucocytes adhere to an extracellular matrix of proteins. Chemicals released at the site of the infection then attract the leucocyte and it moves towards the site of the infection where it can work on destroying the antigen.

The complement system

The complement system consists of about 30 circulating plasma proteins and forms a part of the specific immune system (Totora and Derrickson, 2009). These proteins act in a cascade with each protein activating the next sequentially. Complement is activated via two pathways: the classical pathway and the alternative pathway. The classical pathway is stimulated by an antibody–antigen complex, whilst the alternative pathway occurs as a result of an already activated protein binding to the surface of an antigen.

The complement system has three main purposes:

(1) The recruitment of inflammatory cells to the area of infection
(2) The oponisation of pathogens
(3) The destruction of pathogens

C3 is the central component of the complement system. When activated, C3 cleaves off into C3a and C3b. C3a is a small soluble component that leads to increased capillary permeability. C3a is also responsible for the recruitment and activation of phagocytes at the site of infection.

In contrast, C3b is a larger molecule that covers the surface of the bacteria. The C3b stimulates the phagocytes to recognise the foreign body and attach to it, thereby facilitating phagocytosis. This is referred to as *oponisation*. Here the C3b coats the foreign organism and attracts phagocytes to the area.

C5a, C4a and C3a also work by increasing capillary permeability and attracting phagocytes to the area. In contrast, C5b recruits and binds C6 and C7 to the surface of the invading pathogen. C7, C8 and C9 work together to destruct the cell membrane.

The final role of the complement system is the removal of immune complexes from the circulation.

Consequently, if the complement system is not kept under control, it can stimulate an exaggerated response, which can lead to the development of sepsis. The final pathway in response to an infection is the coagulation cascade.

The coagulation cascade

Tissue factor initiates the coagulation cascade. This causes thrombin to convert fibrinogen into fibrin. The fibrin results in the formation of a fibrin clot. It is believed that this fibrin clot formation within the microvasculature is an attempt by the immune system to seal off the antigen to a small part of the body and to prevent it from escaping and spreading its effects throughout the circulation. If there is no infection present, the endogenous tissue plasminogen activator will break down the clot. However, in the presence of an infection, plasminogen activator inhibitor-1 and thrombin-activatable fibrinolysis inhibitor are released. This allows the clot to remain in situ. With the clot trapping the antigen, the immune system can work on breaking the antigen down and destroying it.

Throughout severe sepsis, the coagulation cascade proliferates unchecked and the development of small fibrin clots spreads. The fibrin deposits interfere with blood flow to the tissues. Tissue perfusion is thus reduced despite the cardiac output being maintained.

The action of neutrophils

The neutrophil is the body's primary line of defence. Their release is stimulated by the complement system. Quite simply the neutrophil acts as a phagocyte. The phagocyte engulfs the foreign organism, while releasing chemotaxic substances such as hydrogen peroxide. Once they have performed their task, neutrophils die and form pus.

One mechanism the neutrophil uses to destroy the antigen is referred to as the *respiratory burst* (Ahrens and Vollman, 2003). This is the release of oxygen radicals into the environment surrounding the antigen. Oxygen radicals have six as opposed to eight electrons. With just six electrons, oxygen molecules become very unstable and will take two electrons from any other molecule that it comes into contact with, even an antigen! This then results in the other molecule becoming unstable. If there are just a few oxygen radicals present, this does not cause a problem. However, if there are increasing amounts of oxygen radicals present, overwhelming molecular instability results and the cell wall disintegrates.

However, with the development of severe sepsis, this response by the neutrophil does not remain localised. The excessive inflammation and coagulation spreads throughout the body. The explanation for this is that the antigen somehow enters the systemic circulation or that it could be the result of collateral damage associated with the immune response. Any organ can then be affected by excessive coagulation, impaired fibrinolysis and excessive inflammation.

As tissue perfusion reduces, tissue nutrition (including oxygenation) becomes disrupted. Blood pressure can be taken as a simple measure of tissue perfusion with a higher blood pressure being associated with increased tissue perfusion. However, this theory fails to take into account the impact of regional vasoconstriction and vasodilation. To enhance tissue perfusion at major organs such as the brain, heart and lungs, there may be localised vasodilation. This is achieved through vasoconstriction and a reduced tissue perfusion at other organs such as the gastrointestinal tract or the kidneys.

Tissue oxygenation

Analysing the oxygen saturation of mixed venous blood (SvO_2) can enlighten the practitioner as to the ultimate status of tissue perfusion in the critically sick individual.

The SvO_2 determines the amount of oxygen left in the blood once the blood has passed through the tissues. A normal SvO_2 will be about 60–75%. This means that normally only 25–40% of oxygen available in the blood is taken up by the tissues. If the tissues need more oxygen, the body will provide this by increasing the cardiac output or by simply extracting more oxygen from the haemoglobin.

As we have previously seen, if the rate of blood flow through the tissues slows down, the tissue has greater time to extract more oxygen. Consequently, the SvO_2 will be reduced. However, if the blood flow rate through the tissues is too high, the SvO_2 will remain high.

In the severely septic patient, the SvO_2 can be either high or low. An increased SvO_2 will relate to the fact that the tissues have been unable to extract the oxygen. The overwhelming cause of this is the formation of microclots within the capillaries secondary to excessive coagulation and impaired fibrinolysis. These clots consequently impede blood flow through the tissues. For some reason, when a patient like Juliette becomes severely septic, the tissues become unable to extract the oxygen from the capillaries or are unable to use the oxygen they have managed to extract. As a result tissue perfusion is compromised, leading to organ failure and ultimately death.

Ongoing assessment

The surviving sepsis campaign

The surviving sepsis campaign advocates the use of a 6-hour resuscitation bundle. This is a group of evidence-based elements, which when delivered together are seen to be more effective. To enable this, early assessment and identification of the septic patient is essential.

Early identification of the septic patient

As soon as Juliette was admitted to the ward, she should have been screened to establish whether she was developing sepsis as a result of her necrotising pancreatitis. Visible deterioration in her condition and an early warning score (EWS) resulted in her referral to the critical care outreach team. Upon assessment it was decided to transfer Juliette into the critical care unit.

Peel (2008) argues that through the early identification of patients with severe sepsis in primary care, wards, emergency assessment units and emergency department, mortality rates can be decreased. Likewise, Vincent *et al.* (2002) found that some patients with sepsis are not identified early enough or receive the appropriate care prior to transfer to critical care. Ahrens and Tuggle (2004) argue that like the 'golden hour' in trauma cases, the detection of sepsis early on will facilitate the use of aggressive treatment, which can influence the survival and severity of the illness.

Both Peel (2008) and Robson and Newell (2005) advocate the use of an EWS. These systems often follow the ALERT™ course approach (University of Portsmouth, 2003) of airway, breathing, circulation and disability (A, B, C, D), which is based upon the rationale that airway obstruction will kill first over anything else and as such should always be assessed first. In line with the National Institute for Health and Clinical Excellence (NICE, 2007) guidelines, such systems track and trigger patients who are at risk of deterioration.

Having been identified as deteriorating rapidly, Juliette was transferred to the critical care unit where the surviving sepsis campaign's severe sepsis resuscitation bundle was implemented.

Evidence-based care

The severe sepsis resuscitation bundle

The severe sepsis resuscitation bundle outlines seven interventions that should be implemented as soon as a patient presents with either severe sepsis or septic shock. This should be implemented within 6 hours of identification of severe sepsis or septic shock. This is summarised in Table 4.4.

Element 1: Serum lactate measured
Obtaining a serum lactate level is important as it identifies tissue hypoperfusion in patients who are at risk of developing severe sepsis. A raised serum lactate greater than 4 is thought to be the result of anaerobic respiration. As has already been discussed, when a patient develops severe sepsis, there is reduced tissue perfusion. As a result, the cells at the tissues have to undertake anaerobic respiration to survive. A by-product of this is the synthesis of lactic acid.

Table 4.4   The 6-hour bundle

Bundle element 1:
Measure serum lactate

Bundle element 2:
Obtain blood cultures prior to antibiotic administration

Bundle element 3:
Administer broad-spectrum antibiotics within 3 hr of emergency department admission
or 1 hr of non-emergency department admission

Bundle element 4:
In the event of hypotension and/serum lactate >4 mmol/l:
  (1) Deliver an initial minimum of 20 ml/kg crystalloid or an equivalent
  (2) Apply vasopressors for hypotension not responding to initial fluid resuscitation to
      maintain a MAP >65 mmHg
      • Treat hypotension and /or elevated lactate with fluids
      • Apply vasopressors for ongoing hypotension

Bundle element 5:
In the event of persistent hypotension despite fluid resuscitation (septic shock) and/or lactate
>4 mmol/l:
  (1) Achieve a CVP equal to or greater than 8 mmHg
  (2) Achieve a central venous oxygen saturation ($ScvO_2$) >70% or mixed venous oxygen
      saturation (SvO_2) equal to or greater than 65%
      • Maintain adequate CVP
      • Maintain adequate $ScvO_2$

(Reproduced from Dellinger RP, Levy MM, Carlet JM, *et al.* (2008) Surviving sepsis campaign:
international guidelines for management of severe sepsis and septic shock. *Critical Care Medicine* 36
296–327, copyright 2008, with permission of the Society of Critical Care Medicine.)

However, there are some limitations in solely relying on lactate level as an indicator
of tissue hypoperfusion. Some have suggested that raised lactate levels may be the result
of reduced liver function while others have suggested that the rise in serum lactate levels
could be the direct result of cellular metabolic failure (Bakker *et al.*, 1991).
   Juliette's lactate level is 6 mmol/l.

Element 2: Blood cultures obtained prior to antibiotic administration
About 30–50% of patients presenting with severe sepsis have positive blood culture results.
   Collection of cultures before antibiotics are administered provides the best chance of
identifying the organism responsible for the septic response.
   The care bundle suggests that blood cultures should be taken as soon as pyrexia
develops. Other indications of the presence of an organism are hypoalbuminaemia, acute
renal failure and a urinary tract infection; pyrexia, hypothermia, leucocytosis, neutropenia
and cardiovascular instability (Bates *et al.*, 1997) should also stimulate blood cultures to
be taken.
   Juliette has blood cultures taken and these are sent for microbiology.

Element 3: Improve time to broad-spectrum antibiotics
Antibiotics are used to treat the underlying infection. Kumar *et al.* (2006) found that for each
hour of delay in the administration of intravenous antibiotics there was a significant increase
in mortality. In particular, those with gram-positive and gram-negative bacteraemias have
a reduced mortality rate with the administration of antibiotic therapy. Thus, the initial
choice of antibiotic therapy is to cover both gram-positive and gram-negative infections.
   It is suggested that to facilitate the rapid administration of antibiotics, a premixed supply
is kept available within the critical care unit. It is also suggested that those administered

by bolus rather than by infusion would be useful in this particular situation. Again, to enhance the speed of administration it is always useful to have multiple lumens available for administration. In Juliette's case, she has a triple lumen central line in situ.

Dellinger *et al.* (2008) suggest that when choosing which antibiotics are appropriate, it is better to avoid antibiotics that have recently been administered. They also suggest that the initial choice of antibiotic should be a broad-spectrum antibiotic. This would then be broad enough to cover all the likely pathogens responsible for the sepsis. Again, failure to treat the pathogen responsible for the sepsis results in a high mortality rate.

Dellinger *et al.* (2008) also suggest that it is important to consider the patients' past medical history or the circumstances surrounding their admission. For instance, a patient may already be admitted with an ongoing fungal infection. If the patient is admitted to the critical care unit from the ward, he or she may have developed a hospital-acquired infection.

It is also important to consider the likelihood of the prevalence of methicillin-resistant *Staphylococcus aureus* (MRSA) when initiating antibiotic therapy. If MRSA is prevalent in the community or health-care setting, it is important to then use a broad-spectrum antibiotic capable of treating both the sepsis and any potential MRSA the patient may have.

Again, there are those who argue against the use of broad-spectrum antibiotics as they have the potential to increase the development of antimicrobial resistance (Vernaz *et al.*, 2009). However, a patient such as Juliette who is developing sepsis needs a broad-spectrum antibiotic, and any argument to withhold them in view of potential increased resistance is inappropriate (Dellinger *et al.*, 2008).

The antimicrobial regimen should always be reviewed after 48–72 hours. Once the pathogen responsible for the sepsis has been isolated, it may then become necessary to review the antibiotic therapy and change to a narrow-spectrum monotherapy involving just one antibiotic that is sensitive for the isolated organism.

In an attempt to reduce the development of super infections such as *Candida*, *Clostridium difficile* or vancomycin-resistant *Enterococcus faecium*, antibiotic therapy is often limited to a short duration (Vernaz *et al.*, 2009). However, Dellinger *et al.* (2008) argue that it is essential that patients receive the full course of the antibiotic. Indeed, in cases of suspected *Pseudomonas*, Dellinger *et al.* (2008) also suggest the use of a combination of antibiotic therapy in the first instance. Garnacho-Montero *et al.* (2007) argue that in such cases at least one of the antibiotics will be effective in the treatment of the *Pseudomonas* and positively affect the patient's outcome.

The suggested length of the course is 7–10 days. However, Dellinger *et al.* (2008) do agree that if the sepsis is found to be non-infective in origin then the antibiotics should be stopped. This is also to ensure that the patient does not develop an antibiotic-resistant pathogen while in hospital.

All patients receive the full loading dose of the antibiotic. However, following this in view of potential renal or hepatic impairment or the maldistribution of fluid levels within the septic patient, it is advised that the administration of the antibiotic be tailored to the individual patient's needs.

Juliette receives her loading dose on the critical care unit and then is commenced on a broad-spectrum antibiotic therapy until her blood culture results come back.

Element 4: Treat hypotension and/or elevated lactate with fluids

As the patient's sepsis develops, the volume of blood in their circulation may decrease. As we have seen, this could be due to increased capillary permeability resulting in fluid seeping into the interstitial space, profound vasodilation or an impaired cardiac output. This results in reduced tissue perfusion at the capillary bed. The reduction in perfusion can result in the occurrence of anaerobic respiration and the synthesis of lactate. If the lactate level is greater than 4 mmol/l, this is subsequently associated with an increase in the severity of sepsis and an increased mortality rate. This patient requires fluid resuscitation (Dellinger *et al.*, 2008).

It is now widely agreed that early goal-directed resuscitation improves the outcome for patients admitted as an emergency with severe sepsis (Rivers *et al.*, 2001). Rivers *et al.* (2001) found that those patients with severe sepsis who underwent early goal-directed therapy received more fluid and more packed red blood cells which was associated with a significant reduction in the mortality rate.

The primary rationale for the early intervention with fluid therapy is that while delaying resuscitation, the cells at the tissues have already become hypoxic and ischaemia will already have set in. Consequently, if the cells are already at a point where they are dysfunctioning, it remains unlikely that they will then be able to respond to any therapy aimed at improving oxygenation and enhancing tissue perfusion.

Consequently, fluid resuscitation should be commenced as early as possible (Rivers *et al.*, 2001) and should follow a goal-directed approach to resuscitation. The following are the goals suggested:

- A CVP of 8–12 mmHg
- MAP equal to or greater than 65 mmHg
- Urine output equal to or greater than 0.5 ml/kg/hr
- Central venous oxygen saturation equal to or greater than 70%
- Mixed venous oxygen saturation equal to or greater than 65%

Malbrain *et al.* (2005) suggest that should the patient be ventilated or if the patient had increased intra-abdominal pressure, the aim for the CVP should be 12–15 mmHg. As Juliette remained spontaneously ventilating, the plan was to resuscitate her with crystalloid fluid until her CVP reached 8–12 mmHg. Dellinger *et al.* (2008) also suggest that the heart rate is a useful indicator of adequate filling. If the patient is tachycardic, this could be the direct result of a poor cardiac output secondary to hypovolaemia. By increasing the circulating volume, it could be argued the heart rate will reduce as the preload increases. However, it is recognised that with the septic patient the increased heart rate may be the result of number of factors. Despite this, many studies now support early initiation of fluid resuscitation (Shapiro *et al.*, 2006; Shorr *et al.*, 2007).

While it is recommended to make use of the CVP as a guide for preload, it is recognised that such a measurement may not always be accurate. The position of the transducer, the position of the patient and calibration all affect the accuracy of the CVP as a determinate for preload (Madger, 2006). The transoesophageal Doppler, which measures flow, can provide a useful tool to measure ventricular filling, and it is now suggested that such devices are available within clinical areas other than the critical care units as a means of guiding fluid resuscitation. Other cardiac output monitors such as LiDDCO™ or PiCCO™ offer viable alternatives (Jevon and Ewens, 2007).

In order to achieve the goals, it is suggested that repeated fluid challenges are performed until the goals are achieved. If using crystalloid, it is suggested the initial bolus is 20 ml/kg. In contrast, if colloid is used, a bolus of 0.2–0.3 g/kg is administered (Dellinger *et al.*, 2008).

A fluid challenge involves large volumes of fluid being administered over a short period of time. A fluid challenge involves a clear explanation of four components:

(1) The fluid to be infused – this could be either crystalloid or colloid depending upon individual practitioner preferences.
(2) The rate of the infusion.
(3) The goal, for example, is for the CVP to be 8 mmHg or for the heart rate to be less than 100 BPM.
(4) Safety limits so as to observe for side effects such as overloading the patient.

Crystalloid versus colloid

There is an ongoing debate within critical care as to the most appropriate fluid to use for fluid resuscitation. Despite such debate, the evidence base regarding fluid resuscitation for the patient with severe sepsis remains scant. Finfer *et al.* (2004) conducted a randomised controlled trial into the effectiveness of saline versus 4% human albumin solution and while they found no statistical significance in the difference in mortality rate between those who received the colloid and those who received the crystalloid, the study did anecdotally find some benefits of colloid for the patients.

Despite this, the Cochrane review of 2001 (Cook and Guyatt, 2001) found no difference in the outcome between those who were resuscitated with crystalloid and those who were resuscitated with colloid. However, this review did find that as the volumes of crystalloid required to get the same effect as the colloid were greater, the patient was at greater risk of developing complications such as oedema with the crystalloid (Cook and Guyatt, 2001).

When aiming to enhance the tissue perfusion once fluid resuscitation has taken place, Dellinger *et al.* (2008) consider the use of packed red cells to increase the haematocrit to greater than 30%. This will then enhance the oxygen carrying capacity of the circulation, thereby improving the oxygen delivery to the tissues. Alternatively, dobutamine may be used to enhance the cardiac output and ultimately increase the delivery of oxygen to the tissues.

It is important to note, however, that while it is widely agreed that early fluid resuscitation does improve patient outcome (Rivers *et al.*, 2001), care must be taken to consider the local effects of the septic response. While fluid can treat parameters such as CVP and mixed venous oxygen saturation, such parameters do not really explain what is happening at localised capillary level, when the tissue perfusion may be poor despite apparent fluid resuscitation. As a consequence, it is essential to look at the patient's response to the interventions holistically including parameters such as respiratory rate, mean arterial pressure (MAP), urine output, skin temperature, capillary refill time and level of consciousness.

Juliette initially received a fluid bolus of crystalloid. However, as she was admitted to critical care, the fluid was changed to colloid and the fluid challenge continued to get her CVP up to 8 mmHg.

Element 5: Maintain adequate central venous oxygenation
There are times when the patient's septic response is so overwhelming that they experience prolonged hypovolaemia. Indications of this would be that patients have a consistently raised serum lactate level above 4 or experience hypotension, which fails to respond to fluid boluses. In such cases, Dellinger *et al.* (2008) suggest that the aim should be to maintain a CVP of equal to or greater than 8 mmHg with a central venous oxygen saturation equal to or greater than 70%.

The aim is to maintain an adequate CVP in order for other haemodynamic strategies to be implemented to enhance tissue perfusion. Consequently, Dellinger *et al.* (2008) advocate the use of a CVP line to provide a guide as to the success of the fluid resuscitation. Importantly, Dellinger *et al.* (2008) also advocate the administration of blood products when the central or mixed venous oxygen saturations are low. Dellinger *et al.* (2008) argue that the blood products not only assist to maintain the CVP but they also reduce the occurrence of ischaemia at the tissue bed by enhancing oxygen delivery to the tissues.

Importantly, Rivers *et al.*'s (2001) randomised controlled trail also found that those patients who received early goal-directed therapy – which included a CVP line early into their admission, initially received a greater volume of fluid, inotropic support and blood products – had an improved outcome over those in the control group who received greater fluid volumes later into their admission and had a higher mortality rate. Rivers *et al.* (2001) concluded that early goal-directed therapy, guided with the use of CVP and central venous oxygen saturation (ScvO$_2$) readings significantly improved patient outcome.

Because Juliette's sepsis has been developing for a number of days, she fails to respond to the fluid resuscitation she received. Her CVP remains stubbornly low at 5 mmHg and her lactate is elevated at 6 mmol/l. The decision is made to commence inotropic and vassopressor support to maintain her CVP.

Vasopressors and inotropes

Vasopressors should not be used without adequate fluid resuscitation being applied first. However, when fluid fails to provide an adequate arterial blood pressure and tissue perfusion fails, vasopressors are required (Dellinger *et al.*, 2008).

Vasopressors will generally result in increased blood pressure. However, it is essential that they are only applied when adequate fluid resuscitation has taken place. Applying a vasopressor to an under-filled patient will result in vasoconstriction, which will result in overall poor tissue perfusion and reduced oxygen delivery. Indeed, tissue ischaemia will be exacerbated, not relieved (Zhou *et al.*, 2002).

Even with adequate fluid resuscitation, Dellinger *et al.* (2008) argue that the benefits of applying such a therapy must be weighed against the risks to vital organs such as the kidneys and the gastrointestinal tract. Vasopressors will direct blood away from these organs to those regarded to be more vital to sustain life such as the heart, lungs and brain.

Dellinger *et al.* (2008) argue that vasopressors should be used cautiously in those with pre-existing cardiac disease. In particular, vasopressors can increase left ventricular workload, which can result in an effect that is opposite to the desired effect. The cardiac output may infact fall and organs will remain poorly perfused. Effective blood pressure monitoring is required. Jevon and Ewens (2007) support the use of the radial artery for continuous arterial blood pressure monitoring.

Administered via a central line, noradrenaline or dopamine are the vasopressors of choice (Dellinger *et al.*, 2008). Zhou *et al.* (2002) argued against the use of epinephrine as this is seen to reduce splenic blood flow, increase gastric mucosal pCO_2 and decrease gastric pH, while Reinelt *et al.* (1999) found that phenylephrine reduced the blood flow to the spleen.

An interesting development is the use of vasopressin. Vasopressin levels in patients with septic shock are lower than normal (Landry *et al.*, 1997). Being a powerful vasoconstrictor, this drug should only be advocated for use in patients for whom conventional vasopressor therapy and fluid challenge have failed. Low doses may increase blood pressure and may have some beneficial physiological effects (Holmes *et al.*, 2001; Lauzier *et al.*, 2006). However, vasopressin is still under clinical trails at present. Interestingly, O'Brien *et al.* (2002) found that terlipressin has effects that are similar to vasopressin but remain longer lasting.

Dopamine

Dopamine increases the cardiac index without affecting the systemic vascular resistance (SVR). Meier-Hellmann *et al.* (1997) found that dopamine increases blood pressure by increasing the stroke volume and heart rate. As a result cardiac output is increased.

It is thought that splanchnic perfusion and the integrity of the gut have a significant impact on the development of severe sepsis, through the translocation of bacteria. As a consequence, care must be taken that any inotropic support does not exacerbate the sepsis. The overall effect that dopamine has on the integrity of the gut mucosa remains unclear.

Interestingly, Bailey and Burchett (1997) found that dopamine alters the inflammatory response in sepsis, by reducing the number of hormones released, especially prolactin. Dopamine can also reduce gastric and duodenal motility. As a consequence, Dellinger *et al.* (2008) argue that dopamine may have potentially harmful effects on the critically ill septic patient.

Noradrenaline

Noradrenaline is a powerful receptor adrenergic agonist, which also has some beta receptor adrenergic agonist effects. As a powerful vasoconstrictor, noradrenaline has a significant effect on increasing arterial blood pressure, with little effect on the heart rate or the cardiac output (Martin *et al.*, 1993). The blood pressure is increased through significant SVR (Meadows *et al.*, 1988).

There has been concern in the past regarding the effects of noradrenaline on renal perfusion (Mills and Moyer, 1960). However, Martin *et al.* (1990) argue that by improving the MAP, noradrenaline intrinsically increases the glomerular filtration rate.

With drawbacks evident for both noradrenaline and dopamine, Zhou *et al.* (2002) and Levy *et al.* (1997) actually advocate the use of a combination of both dopamine and noradrenaline to maintain an adequate mean arterial blood pressure greater than 65 mmHg for patients with septic shock. Dellinger *et al.* (2008) also support the use of a combination of the two drugs particularly if the cardiac output is not being measured.

Dobutamine

Should the cardiac output be reduced along with raised cardiac filling pressures, Dellinger *et al.* (2008) advocate the use of the inotrope dobutamine. Indeed Gattinoni *et al.* (1995) found dobutamine enhanced outcome through improving oxygen delivery.

In accordance with the care bundle, Juliette receives invasive cardiac output monitoring. Following the fluid challenges which had little effect on the cardiac output, it was decided to commence a combination of noradrenaline to vasoconstrict Juliette's circulation, thereby increasing her SVR and ultimately her preload, while also administering dobutamine, which aims to increase the cardiac output by off loading the left ventricle. The combination of both aims to to enhance oxygen perfusion of all the vital organs (Zhou *et al.*, 2002).

Methylene blue

Methylene blue is gaining increasing popularity in treating severe hypotension (Maslow *et al.*, 2006; Weissgerber, 2008). While the exact mechanism for its effect on the blood pressure remains unclear, it is hypothesised that methylene blue inhibits the synthesis of nitric oxide, which is a powerful vasodilator (Maslow *et al.*, 2006; Viaro *et al.*, 2002).

Nitric oxide is released in response to mediators such as bradykinin and histamine. Nitric oxide activates the enzyme guanylyl cyclase, which increases the intracellular concentrations of guanosine monophosphate. The guanosine monophosphate is then responsible for causing the smooth muscle in the vasculature to relax and dilate. By inhibiting the nitric oxide, this mechanism fails and vasoconstriction occurs (Weissgerber, 2008). A study just published argues that late administration of methylene blue increases survival rates while earlier administration after the onset of sepsis can exacerbate mortality rates (Haematology Week, 2009).

To summarise, on admission to the critical care unit, Juliette went onto the 6-hourly resuscitation care bundle to manage the severe sepsis secondary to necrotising pancreatitis. Juliette's lactate levels were checked and found to be 6 mmol/l. Blood cultures were obtained and she was commenced on a broad-spectrum antibiotic, which covered both gram-positive and gram-negative organisms. Despite fluid challenges with crystalloid and colloid, and receiving a unit of packed red blood cells, Juliette's CVP failed to climb to 8 mmHg and her lactate remained above 6 mmol/l. Following cardiac output studies, it was found that Juliette's cardiac output was low at 3.3 l/min and that her SVR was also low at 650 dynes/sec/cm^5. It was decided to commence a combination of noradrenaline to increase the SVR and dobutamine to offload the left side of the heart, thereby increasing the cardiac output.

Having received the 6-hourly resuscitation care bundle, Juliette moves onto the next phase of her treatment, the 24-hour management bundle. This is summarised in Table 4.5.

Table 4.5 The 24-hour bundle

Bundle element 1:
Administer low-dose steroids for septic shock

Bundle element 2:
Administer recombinant human-activated protein C

Bundle element 3:
Maintain glucose control >70 but <150 mg/dl (<8.3 mmol/l).

Bundle element 4:
Maintain a median inspiratory plateau pressure <30 cm H$_2$O for mechanically ventilated patients

---

(Reproduced from Dellinger RP, Levy MM, Carlet JM, *et al.* (2008) Surviving sepsis campaign: international guidelines for management of severe sepsis and septic shock. *Critical Care Medicine* 36 296–327, copyright 2008, with permission of the Society of Critical Care Medicine.)

Sepsis management bundle

Element 1: Administer low-dose steroids by a standard policy

Intravenous hydrocortisone is appropriate to administer to those patients whose blood pressure remains low despite fluid and vasopressor support (Dellinger *et al.*, 2008). The theory underlying the use of steroids for the treatment of sepsis is that they play a vital role in the body's stress response to infection. Relative adrenal insufficiency (RAI) is the main rationale for low-dose steroid therapy in the treatment of severe sepsis (Annane *et al.*, 2000).

Steroids demonstrate a highly anti-inflammatory effect on the body. Despite this, there is much debate as to the suitability of the use of steroids within the critical care setting (Dellinger *et al.*, 2008). Many believe that steroids should be used with caution, particularly in view of the infection risks and the myopathies associated with their use.

Low-dose steroids actually reverse the effects of the shock response. The definitive reasons for this remain unclear, but suggested rationales include prostaglandin metabolism, modulation of receptors affecting vascular tone and the reduction in nitric oxide formation (Keh *et al.*, 2003). Keh *et al.* (2003) also found that the corticosteroid therapy also reduced both the pro- and anti-inflammatory mediators such as interleukin-6, interleukin-8, interleukin-10 and TNF, while promoting the levels of pro-inflammatory mediators such as interleukin-12. Keh *et al.*'s (2003) study found that the steroid therapy failed to have an effect on the phagocyte's action or on the respiratory burst response.

Keh *et al.* (2003) studied the effects of low-dose steroid therapy and found that both the MAP and SVR increased with the administration of the drug. However, Keh *et al.* (2003) also found that the heart rate, cardiac index and noradrenaline requirements reduced significantly throughout the therapy.

Despite a number of studies finding that steroid therapy significantly reversed the septic shock in individuals, Sprung *et al.*'s (2007) European multicentre trial failed to identify any change to mortality rates. However, trials studying the use of low-dose steroid therapy in the form of 200–300 mg of hydrocortisone daily administered for between 5 and 7 days or longer, found the therapy did help to resolve the sepsis (Annane *et al.*, 2002; Yildiz *et al.*, 2002). Annane *et al.*'s (2005) Cochrane review found that low-dose steroid therapy reduced hospital mortality and increased the number of patients for whom the septic response was reversed.

Hydrocortisone is the drug of choice as it is the synthetic version of cortisol and has an intrinsic mineral corticoid action that other drugs such as methylprednisolone and dexamethasone do not possess. Dexamethasone is particularly inappropriate as this suppresses the negative feedback system between the adrenal gland and the hypothalamus (Reincke *et al.*, 1993). Fludrocortisone may also be administered in addition to the hydrocortisone as there has been an increased survival rate (Annane *et al.*, 2002). The therapy should be weaned as soon as the patient's reliance upon vasopressors to support their blood pressure diminishes (Keh *et al.*, 2003; Yildiz *et al.*, 2002).

There is also a debate as to the effectiveness of corticotrophin stimulation tests. These tests are used to determine whether a condition referred to as RAI exists. The debate regarding testing revolves around the point whether those with no RAI should be excluded from receiving the low-dose steroid therapy. Dellinger *et al.* (2008) conclude that it is up to the individual clinician's choice as to whether they should carry out the stimulation tests, but that they should not delay commencing the therapy whilst waiting for the results of the tests. There is also an argument that those with adequate adrenocortical function may also respond to low-dose steroid therapy (Sprung *et al.*, 2007).

Element 2: Administer recombinant human-activated protein C

Recombinant human activated protein C (rhAPC) is a relatively new therapy in the treatment of severe sepsis. Dellinger *et al.* (2008) recommend that only those with multi-organ dysfunction, which is the result of the septic response and who have an APACHE score of 25 or more, should receive rhAPC. Those with an APACHE of less than 20 or one organ failure should not receive the drug.

These recommendations are based on two randomised controlled trials into the effectiveness of the drug (drotrecogin alpha) – the protein C worldwide evaluation of severe sepsis (PROWESS) (Bernard *et al.*, 2001) and administration of drotrecogin alpha in early sepsis (ADDRESS) (Riedemann *et al.*, 2003) studies. The conclusions of these studies remain limited as they both used small subgroups to analyse their findings. Despite this, the results consistently failed to identify any benefit to giving rhAPC to patients with a low risk of death or only one organ failure, while they both found that those with a high risk of death or multi-organ dysfunction do benefit from the drug.

Activated protein C is a blood protein, which needs to be converted into its active form by thrombin-T (Ahrens and Vollman, 2003; Ruffell, 2004). Activated protein C is thought to maintain homeostasis through three specific actions, the main one being the inhibition of thrombin secretion. This then prevents the formation of microclots during the septic response (Ahrens and Vollman, 2003). Activated protein C does this through inactivating factors Va and VIIIa of the clotting cascade (Ahrens and Vollman, 2003).

Activated protein C also prevents the release of plasminogen activator inhibitor-1 and blocks thrombin formation. By blocking the formation of thrombin, the release of thrombin-activatable fibrinolysis inhibitor is also reduced. Therefore, activated protein C enables the body's fibrinolytic system to breakdown microvascular clots. It is these microclots that result in the multi-organ dysfunction associated with sepsis (Esmon, 2003).

Activated protein C will also reduce the effects of the inflammatory mediators such as TNF. This then tempers the inflammatory response. Fewer neutrophils are recruited to the area, and the inflammatory response is reduced. Consequently, there is less damage to the endothelium and homeostasis is restored (Ahrens and Vollman, 2003).

Despite the obvious benefits activated protein C has in maintaining homeostasis during a septic response, it is widely acknowledged that patients who are septic have lower levels of activated protein C (Yan *et al.*, 2001). This is because as the blood vessel's endothelium becomes damaged, it fails to secrete enough thrombin-T. If there is an inadequate level of thrombin-T being secreted there is not enough to convert protein C into its activated state. Consequently, protein C remains inactivated and microclots form in the tissues and organs. The microclots result in reduced tissue perfusion at the organs; the organs then become ischaemic and develop dysfunction. When two or more organs are poorly perfused, the body develops multi-organ dysfunction and is unable to maintain homeostasis (Ruffell, 2004).

There are risks associated with the use of rhAPC. rhAPC has a short half-life, with the effects of the drug diminishing rapidly within 30 minutes following cessation of infusion. The primary risk is that of bleeding as rhAPC reduces thrombin formation and increases fibrinolysis (Ahrens and Vollman, 2003). Consequently, rhAPC should be avoided in those who have active internal bleeding or a recent haemorrhagic stroke. The drug should also be avoided in those who have recently experienced a severe head injury or have had intracranial or intraspinal surgery within the previous 2 months. Those who have had trauma, such as a pelvic fracture, that may increase their risk of bleeding and those with an epidural in situ should also not receive the drug. Finally, those patients who have an intracerebral mass should avoid the drug to prevent tentorial herniation (Ahrens and Vollman, 2003). However, despite these obvious risks associated with the drug and bleeding, it is suggested that the risk of impending death outweighs the risks of bleeding for other patients with severe sepsis.

The use of the drug within clinical practice can be contentious. The cost of the drug is high, at around £5000 for a 96-hour treatment. This has led to the development of tight protocols for its use within individual health-care trusts. Despite this Angus *et al.* (2001) considered the cost of rhAPC to be comparable with other health-care interventions. Ahrens and Vollman (2003) argue that it is unethical to limit the drug in relation to cost alone.

Element 3: Maintain adequate glycaemic control

Increased blood sugar levels are widely recognised within the critical care setting. This is the result of insulin resistance in the liver and the muscle. Until recently, hyperglycaemia was thought to be beneficial to the critically ill patient. The theory was that the increase in blood glucose levels was an adaptive response that provides sugar for the brain, erythrocytes and promotes wound healing.

However, a study by Van den Berghe *et al.* (2001) found that through tight control of blood glucose levels, the mortality and morbidity rates among the critically ill population dramatically decreased. Van den Berghe *et al.* (2001) found that intensive insulin therapy reduced blood stream infection rates, prolonged inflammation and reduced the prevalence of acute kidney injury, critical illness myopathy and blood transfusion requirements. The therapy was also seen to reduce the need for prolonged mechanical ventilation. It is important to note, however, that Van den Berghe *et al.* (2001) only studied surgical patients. The effects of tight blood sugar levels remain unstudied at the present time. However, Dellinger *et al.* (2008) believe that as the medical patient's length of stay within critical care is generally greater, they should receive greater benefit from the therapy than surgical patients do.

Hypoglycaemia remains a potential problem associated when initiating tight glycaemic control. Dellinger *et al.* (2008) advocate the target of maintaining a blood glucose level less than 8.3 mmol/l. This should prevent the risk of overzealous blood sugar control, which may result in hypoglycaemia. Van den Berghe *et al.* (2001) found that a blood sugar level of 8.3 mmol/l still improved patient outcome. Enteral nutrition is also advocated in an attempt to prevent hypoglycaemia (Dellinger *et al.*, 2008).

It is unclear whether it is the reduced blood sugar level or the insulin infusion that promotes the favourable outcome. While insulin inhibits TNF, Das (2001) found that an infusion of insulin and glucose inhibits macrophage inhibitory factor.

In contrast, by preventing hyperglycaemia, there is an increase in anti-inflammatory effects, positive effects on coagulation and fibrinolysis and on the function of macrophages (Carr, 2001). Consequently, Van den Berghe *et al.* (2001) tried to find the cause of the favourable outcome and found that it was the low blood sugar level that improved patient outcome in critical care as opposed to the insulin infusion itself, which was in fact associated with a poor patient outcome.

Element 4: Maintain a median inspiratory plateau pressure <30 cm H_2O for mechanically ventilated patients

Patients with severe sepsis are more at risk of developing acute lung injury (ALI) and ARDS and these patients frequently require intubation and mechanical ventilation. In an attempt to limit the damage to the lungs, the Surviving Sepsis Campaign (Dellinger *et al.*, 2008) advocates the use of low tidal volumes (6 ml/kg/lean body weight) along with maintaining end inspiratory plateau pressures of less than 30 cm H_2O. The ARDS network found that such a strategy reduced mortality.

To enable this strategy to work, there has to be an element of permissive hypercapnia. It is acceptable to allow an elevated pCO_2 level if the ventilator pressures and tidal volumes can be limited, thereby reducing further damage to the lung. Positive end expiratory pressure (PEEP) should also be limited in order to prevent further lung damage.

Conclusion

The management of the patient with severe sepsis provides a complex challenge to the practitioner. This is due to the multiple and interrelated effects that the presence of sepsis has on the body. Compounding such complexities has, until recently, been an inconsistent approach to the precise definition of sepsis. Consequently, if the condition itself is poorly defined, consistent approach to treatment will remain equally elusive. To address such issues the Surviving Sepsis Campaign (Dellinger *et al.*, 2008) has clearly defined sepsis and severe sepsis along with providing comprehensive evidence-based guidelines for practitioners to adopt to manage sepsis. The overall aim will then be to reduce often preventable mortality.

References

Agarwal N, Pitchumoni CS and Sivaprasad AV (1990) Evaluating tests for acute pancreatitis. *American Journal of Gastroenterology* 85 (4) 412–416.

Ahrens T and Tuggle D (2004) Surviving severe sepsis: early recognition and treatment. *Critical Care Nurse Supplement* October S2–S15.

Ahrens T and Vollman K (2003) Severe sepsis management. Are we doing enough? *Critical Care Nurse Supplement* 23 (5 Suppl.) 2–15.

Angus DC, Linde-Zwirble WT, Lidicker J, *et al.* (2001) Epidemiology of severe sepsis in the Unites States: analysis of incidence, outcome and associated costs of care. *Critical Care Medicine* 29 (7) 1303–1310.

Annane D, Bellisant E, Bollaert P, Briegel J, Keh D and Kupfer Y (2005) Corticosteroids for treating severe sepsis and septic shock. *Cochrane Database of Systematic Reviews 2004*, (1) Art. No.: CD002243. DOI: 10.1002/14651858.CD002243.pub2.

Annane D, Sebille V and Charpentier C (2002) Effect of treatment with low doses of hydrocortisone and fludrocortisone on mortality in patients with septic shock. *The Journal of the American Medical Association* 288 (7) 862–871.

Annane D Sebille V, Troche G, *et al.* (2000) A 3 level prognostic classification in septic shock based on cortisol levels and cortisol response to corticotrophin. *Journal of American Medical Association* 23 (8) 1038–1045.

Apte M and Wilson J (2003) Alcohol induced pancreatic injury. *Best practice and Research in Clinical Gastroenterology* 17 (4) 593–612.

Bailey AR and Burchett KR (1997) Effect of low-dose dopamine on serum concentrations of prolactin in critically ill patients. *British Journal of Anaesthesia* 78 (1) 97–99.

Bakker J, Coffernils M, Leon M, Gris P and Vincent JL (1991) Blood lactate levels are superior to oxygen derived variables in predicting outcome in human septic shock. *Chest* 99 (4) 956–962.

Balthazar EJ, Freeny PC and van Sonnenberg E (1994) Imaging and intervention in acute pancreatitis. *Radiology* 193 (2) 297–306.

Bassi C, Larvin M and Villatoro E (2003) Antibiotic therapy for prophylaxis against infection of pancreatic necrosis in acute pancreatitis. *Cochrane Database Systematic Review* (4) CD002941–CD002941.

Bates DW, Sands K, Miller E, *et al.* (1997) Predicting bacteremia in patients with sepsis syndrome. *Journal of Infectious Diseases* 176 (6) 1538–1551.

Beckingham IJ and Bornman PC (2001) ABC of diseases of liver, pancreas and biliary system. Acute pancreatitis. *British Medical Journal* 322 (7286) 595–598.

Bench S (2004) Clinical skills: assessing, treating shock: a nursing perspective. *British Journal of Nursing* 13 (12) 715.

Bernard GR, Vincent JL, Laterre PF, *et al.* (2001) Efficacy and safety of recombinant human activated protein C for severe sepsis. *New England Journal of Medicine* 344 (10) 699–709.

Blamey SL, Imrey CW, O'Neil J, Gilmour WH and Carter DC (1984) Prognostic factors in acute pancreatitis. *Gut* 25 (12) 1340–1346.

Bone RC, Balk RA, Cerra FB, *et al.* (1992) Definitions for sepsis and organ failure and guidelines for the use of innovative therapies in sepsis. *Chest* 101 (6) 1644–1655.

Burkitt HG, Quick CRG and Gatt D (1998) *Essential Surgery.* 2nd Edition, Churchill Livingstone, London.

Carr ME (2001) Diabetes mellitus: a hypercoaguable state. *Journal of Diabetes and its Complications* 15 (1) 44–54.

Carroll JK, Herrick B, Gipson T and Lee SP (2007) Acute pancreatitis: diagnosis, prognosis, and treatment. *American Family Physician* 75 (10) 1513–1520.

Cook D and Guyatt G (2001) Colloid use for fluid resuscitation: evidence and spin. *Annals of Internal Medicine* 135 (3) 205–208.

Das UN (2001) Is insulin an anti-inflammatory molecule? *Nutrition* 17 (5) 409–413.

Dellinger RP, Levy MM, Carlet JM, *et al.* International Surviving Sepsis Campaign Guidelines Committee; American Association of Critical-Care Nurses; American College of Chest Physicians; American College of Emergency Physicians; Canadian Critical Care Society; European Society of Clinical Microbiology and Infectious Diseases; European Society of Intensive Care

Medicine; European Respiratory Society; International Sepsis Forum; Japanese Association for Acute Medicine; Japanese Society of Intensive Care Medicine; Society of Critical Care Medicine; Society of Hospital Medicine; Surgical Infection Society; World Federation of Societies of Intensive and Critical Care Medicine. (2004) Surviving Sepsis Campaign: international guidelines for the management of severe sepsis and septic shock. *Critical Care Medicine* 32 (3) 858–873.

Dellinger RP, Levy MM, Carlet JM, *et al.* (2008) Surviving sepsis campaign: international guidelines for the management of severe sepsis and septic shock: 2008. *Critical Care Medicine* 36 (1) 296–327.

Eatock FC, Brombacher GD, Steven A, Imrie CW, McKay CJ and Carter R (2000) Nasogastric feeding in severe acute pancreatitis may be practical and safe. *International Journal of Pancreatology* 28 (1) 23–29.

Esmon C (2003) The protein C pathway. *Chest* 124 (3 Suppl.) 26S–32S.

Finfer S, Bellomo R, Boyce N and SAFE Study Investigators. (2004) A comparison of albumin and saline for fluid resuscitation in the intensive care unit. *New England Journal of Medicine* 350 (22) 2247–2256.

Fosmark CE (2000) The diagnosis of chronic pancreatitis. *Gastrointestinal Endoscopy* 52 (2) 593.

Friedman SL, McQuaid KR and Grendall JH (2003) *Current Diagnosis and Treatment in Gastroenterology*. McGraw Hill, New York.

Frossard JL, Steer ML and Pastor CM (2008) Acute pancreatitis. *The Lancet* 371 (9618) 1072.

Gandolfi L (2003) The role of the ultrasound in biliary and pancreatic disease. *European Journal of Ultrasound* 16 (3) 141–159.

Garnacho-Montero J, Sa-Borges M and Sole-Violan J (2007) Optimal management therapy for Pseudomonas aurignosa ventilator associated pneumonia: an observational, multicentre study comparing monotherapy with combination antibiotic therapy. *Critical Care Medicine* 35 (8) 1888–1895.

Gattinoni L, Brazzi L, Pelosi P, *et al.* (1995) A trial of goal-orientated haemodynamic therapy in critically ill patients. *New England Journal of Medicine* 333 (16) 1025–1032.

Haematology Week (2009). Sepsis: research from Federal University provides new data on sepsis. p. 37.

Holcomb S (2000) Reviewing acute pancreatitis. *Nursing* 30 (4) 32cc10–32cc12.

Holcomb SS (2007) Stopping the destruction of acute pancreatitis. *Nursing* 37 (6) 42–47.

Holmes CL, Patel BM, Russell JA and Walley KR (2001) Physiology of vasopressin relevant to the management of septic shock. *Chest* 120 (3) 989–1002.

Holt S (1993) Chronic pancreatitis. *Southern Medical Journal* 86 (2) 201–207.

Huether S (2002) Alterations in digestive functions. In McCance K and Huether S (Eds) *Pathophysiology: the Biological Basis for Disease in Adults and Children*. 4th Edition, Mosby, St Louis, pp. 1261–1298.

Hughes E (2004) Understanding the care of patients with pancreatitis. *Nursing Standard* 18 (18) 45–52.

Jevon P and Ewens B (2007) *Monitoring the Critically Ill Patient*. 2nd Edition, Wiley Blackwell, Oxford.

Johnson CD and Abu-Hilal M (2004) Persistent organ failure during the first week as a marker of fatal outcome in acute pancreatitis. *Gut* 53 (9) 1340–1344.

Keh D, Boehnke T, Weber-Cartens S, *et al.* (2003) Immunologic and haemodynamic effects of 'low-dose' hydrocortisone in septic shock: a double blind, randomized, placebo-controlled, crossover study. *American Journal of Respiratory and Critical Care Medicine* 167. 512–520.

Kleinpell R (2003) Advances in treating patients with severe sepsis. *Critical Care Nurse* 23 (3) 16–29.

Kredo T and Onia R (2005) Pethidine – does familiarity or evidence perpetuate its use? *South African Medical Journal* 95 (2) 100–101.

Kumar A, Roberts D, Wood KE, *et al.* (2006) Duration of hypotension prior to the initiation of effective antimicrobial therapy is the critical determinant of survival in human septic shock. *Critical Care Medicine* 34 (6) 1589–1596.

Landry DW, Levin HR, Gallant EM, *et al.* (1997) Vasopressin deficiency contributes to the vasodilation in septic shock. *Circulation* 95 (5) 1122–1125.

Larvin M and Mc Mahon MJ (1989) APACHE-II score for assessment and monitoring of acute pancreatitis. *Lancet* 2 (8656) 201–205.

Lauzier F, Levy B, Lamarre P and Lesur O (2006) Vasopressin or norepinephrine in early hyperdynaimc septic shock: a randomized clinical trial. *Intensive Care Medicine* 32 (11) 1782–1789.

Levy B, Bollaert PE, Charpentier C, *et al.* (1997) Comparison of norepinephrine and dobutamine to epinephrine for heamodynamics. Lactate metabolism, and gastric tonometric variables in septic shock: a prospective randomized controlled study. *Intensive Care Medicine* 23 (3) 282–287.

Levy M and Geenen J (2001) Idiopathic acute recurrent pancreatitis. *The American Journal of Gastroenterology* 96 (9) 2540–2555.

Madger S (2006) Central venous pressure: a useful but not so simple measurement. *Critical Care Medicine* 34 (8) 2224–2227.

Malbrain ML, Deeren D and De Potter TJ (2005) Intra-abdominal hypertension in the critically ill: it is time to pay attention. *Current Opinion in Critical Care* 11 (2) 156–171.

Marieb EN (2008) *Essentials of Human Anatomy and Physiology.* 7th Edition, Cummings, New York.

Marik PE and Zaloga GP (2004) Meta-analysis of parenteral nutrition versus enteral nutrition in patients with acute pancreatitis. *British Medical Journal* 328 (7453) 1407–1410.

Martin C, Eon B, Saux P, Aknin P and Gouin F (1990) Renal effects of norepinephrine used to treat septic shock patients. *Critical Care Medicine* 18 (3) 282–285.

Martin C, Papazian L, Perrin G, Saux P and Gouin F (1993) Norepinephrine or dopamine for the treatment of hyperdynamic septic shock? *Chest* 103 (6) 1826–1831.

Maslow AD, Stearns G, Batula P, Schwarts CS, Gough J and Singh AK (2006) The haemodynamic effects of methyleyne blue when administered at the onset of cardiopulmonary bypass. *Anaesthesiology and Analgesia* 103 (1) 2–8.

McArdle J (2000) The biological and nursing implications of pancreatitis. *Nursing Standard* 14 (48) 46–53.

McLuckie A (2003) Shock: An Overview. In Oh TE, Bersten AD and Sori N (Eds) *Oh's Intensive Care Manual.* 5th Edition, Butterworth Heinemann, London.

Meadows D, Edwards JD, Wilkins RG and Nightingale P (1988) Reversal of intractable septic shock with norepinephrine therapy. *Critical Care Medicine* 16 (7) 663–666.

Meier-Hellmann A, Reinhart K, Bredle DL, Specht M, Spies CD and Hannemann L (1997) Epinephrine impairs splanchnic perfusion in septic shock. *Critical Care Medicine* 25 (3) 399–404.

Mills LC and Moyer JH (1960) The effects of various catecholamines on specific vascular heamodynamics in hypotensive and normotensive subjects. *American Journal of Cardiology* 5 652–659.

Morton PG and Fontaine D (2008) *Critical Care Nursing: A Holistic Approach.* 9th Edition, Lippincott Williams and Wilkins, Philadelphia.

Moore T and Woodrow P (2009) *High Dependency Nursing Care Observations, Intervention and Support for Level 2 Patients.* Routledge, Oxford.

Murphy JO, Mehigan BJ and Keane FB (2002) Acute pancreatitis. *Hospital Medicine* 63 (8) 487–892.

National Institute for Health and Clinical Excellence (2007) *Acutely Ill Patients in Hospital. Recognition of and Response to Acute Illness in Adults in Hospital. Clinical Guideline 50.* National Institute for Health and Clinical Excellence, London.

Neoptolemos JP, Kemppainen EA, Mayer JM, *et al.* (2000) Early prediction of severity in acute pancreatitis by urinary trypsinogen activation peptide: a multicentre study. *Lancet* 355 (9219) 1955–1960.

O'Brien A, Clapp L and Singer M (2002). Terlipressin for norepinephrine-resistant septic shock. *Lancet* 359 (9313) 1209–1210.

Parker M (2004) Acute pancreatitis. *Emergency Nurse* 11 (10) 28–36.

Pasero CL (1998) Pain control. *American Journal of Nursing* 98 (11) 14–15.

Paulson C (2002) Meperidine or morphine for the treatment of pancreatic pain. *RN* 65 (5) 10.

Peel M (2008) Care bundles: resuscitation of patients with severe sepsis. *Nursing Standard* 23 (11) 41–47.

Pfrimmer M (2008) Acute pancreatitis. *The Journal of Continuing Education in Nursing* 39 (8) 341–342.

Pitchumoni CS, Patel NM and Shah P (2005) Factors influencing mortality in acute pancreatitis: can we alter them? *Journal of Clinical Gastroenterology* 39 (9) 798–814.

Poeze M, Ramsay G, Gerlach H, Rubulotta F and Levy M (2004) An international sepsis survey: a study of doctors' knowledge and perception about sepsis. *Critical Care* 8 (6) R409–R413.

Polaków J, Ladny JR, Serwatka W, Walecki J, Puchalski Z and Czech B (2002) Percutaneous fine-needle pancreatic pseudocyst. *Surgical Laparoscopy, Endoscopy & Percutaneous Technique* 12 (6) 437–440.

Ranson JH (1982) Etiological and prognostic factors in human acute pancreatitis: a review. *American Journal of Gastroenterology* 77 (9) 633–638.

Reincke M, Allolio B, Wurth G and Winklemann W (1993) The hypothalamic-pituitary-adrenal axis in critical illness: response to dexamethasone and corticotrophin-releasing hormone. *Journal of Clinical Endocrinal Metabolism* 77 (1) 151–156.

Reinelt H, Radermacher P, Keifer P, *et al.* (1999) Impact of exogenous beta-adrenergic stimulation on hepatosplanic oxygen kinetics and metabolic activity in septic shock. *Critical Care Medicine* 27 (2) 325–331.

Riedemann NC, Guo RF and Ward PA (2003) Novel strategies for the treatment of sepsis. *Natural Medicine* 9 (5) 517–524.

Rivers E, Nguyen B, Havstad S, *et al.* (2001) Early goal-directed treatment of severe sepsis and septic shock. *New England Journal of Medicine* 345 (19) 1368–1377.

Robson W and Newell J (2005) Assessing, treating and managing patients with sepsis. *Nursing Standard* 19 (50) 56–64.

Ruffell AJ (2004) Sepsis strategies: an ICU package. *Nursing in Critical Care* 9 (6) 257–263.

Shapiro NI, Howell MD, Talmor D, *et al.* (2006) Implementation and outcomes of the multiple urgent sepsis therapies (MUST) protocol. *Critical Care Medicine* 34 (4) 2707–2713.

Shorr AF, Micek ST and Jackson WL (2007) Economic implications of an evidence based sepsis protocol: can we improve outcomes and lower costs? *Critical Care Medicine* 35 (5) 1257–1262.

Sprung CL, Annane D and Keh D (2007) Hydrocortisone therapy for patients with septic shock. *The New England Journal of Medicine* 358 (2) 111–124.

Steer ML, Waxman I and Freedman S (2000) Chronic pancreatitis. *New England Journal of Medicine* 84 (3) 621–623.

Tenner S (2004) Initial management of acute pancreatitis: Critical issues during the first 72 hours. *The American Journal of Gastroenterology* 99 (12) 2489–2494.

Thune A, Baker RA, Saccone GT, Owen H and Toouli J (1990) Differing effects of pethidine and morphone on human sphincter of Oddi motility. *British Journal of Surgery* 77 (9) 992–995.

Toouli J, Brooke-Smith M, Bassi C, *et al.* (2002) Guidelines for the management of acute pancreatitis. *Journal of Gastroenterology and Hepatology* 17(Suppl.) S15–S39.

Torrance C and Serginson E (2000) *Surgical Nursing.* 12th Edition, Balliere-Tindall, London.

Totora GJ and Derrickson BH (2009) *Principles of Anatomy and Physiology.* 12th Edition, John Wiley and Sons, Hoboken.

Uhl W, Buchler MW, Malfertheiner P, Beger HG, Adler G and Gaus W (1999) A randomised, double blind, multicentre trial of octreotide in moderate to severe acute pancreatitis. *Gut* 45 (1) 97–104.

UK Working Party on Acute Pancreatitis (2005) UK guidelines for the management of acute pancreatitis. *Gut* 54 (Suppl. 3) iii, 1–9.

University of Portsmouth (2003) *Acute Life-threatening Events Recognition and Treatment (ALERT™).* University of Portsmouth, Portsmouth.

Van den Berghe G, Wouters P, Weekers F, *et al.* (2001) Intensive insulin therapy in critically ill patients. *New England Journal of Medicine* 345 (19) 1359–1367.

Vernaz N, Hill K, Leggeat S, *et al.* (2009) Temporal effects of antibiotic use and *Clostridium difficile* infections. *The Journal of Antimicrobial Chemotherapy* 63 (6) 1272–1276.

Viaro F, Dalio MB and Evora PR (2002) Catastrophic cardiovascular adverse reactions to protamine are nitric oxide/ cyclic guanosine monophosphate dependent and endothelium mediated: should methylene blue be treatment of choice? *Chest* 122 (3) 1061–1066.

Vincent JL, Abraham E, Bernard G, Rivers E and Van den Breghe G (2002) Reducing mortality in sepsis: new directions. *Critical Care Medicine* 6 (Suppl. 3) S1–S18.

Wang G, Gao C, Wei D, Wang C and Ding S (2009) Acute pancreatitis: etiology and common pathogenesis. *World Journal of Gastroenterology* 15 (12) 1427–1430.

Weissgerber AJ (2008) Methylene blue for refractory hypotensin. A case report. *AANA Journal* 76 (4) 271–274.

Yan B, Helterebrand J, Hartmann D, Wright T and Bernard GR (2001) Low levels of protein C are associated with poor outcome in severe sepsis. *Chest* 120 (3) 915–922.

Yildiz O, Doğanay M, Aygen B, Güven M, Keleştimur F and Tutuş A (2002) Physiological-dose steroid therapy in sepsis. *Critical Care Medicine* 6 (3) 251–259.

Zhou SX Qiu HB, Huang YZ, Yang Y and Zheng RQ (2002) Effects of norepinephrine, epinephrine and norepinephrine-dobutamine on systemic and gastric mucosal oxygenation in septic shock. *Acta Pharmacologica Sinica* 23 (7) 654–658.

Chapter 5

The patient with acute respiratory failure

Anne McLeod

Introduction

Acute respiratory distress syndrome (ARDS) is a severe form of hypoxic respiratory failure and has high morbidity and mortality (10–90%) (Bernard *et al.*, 1994). It also entails high emotional and financial cost. The patient with ARDS can pose a challenge to the critical care team whose aim is to maintain oxygenation and tissue perfusion, but this may prove to be difficult to achieve because the underlying physiological changes evolve and develop. Brun-Buisson *et al.* (2004) found that acute lung injury (ALI) was a common occurrence in intensive care (incidence 7.1%), with one-third of patients presenting with mild ALI within 4 hours after admission. However, one-half of these cases quickly developed into ARDS. In view of the incidence and high costs, it is imperative that the team caring for the patient has a clear understanding of the underlying physiological changes as well as recommended treatment strategies.

This chapter introduces a patient scenario which will develop through the chapter, in line with typical patient presentation and disease progression. Underlying pathophysiology of ARDS, assessment and respiratory support treatment (mechanical ventilation) will be explored. This will be in line with current recommendations and strategies.

Patient scenario

Susan was a 45-year-old woman who was admitted to the ICU with type 1 respiratory failure due to pneumonia. She weighs 65 kg.

Her initial assessment yielded the following findings:

HR   130 BPM SR
BP   110/65 (MAP = 80)
RR   28 BPM
Temp   37.8°C
CVP   6 mmHg

She had reduced air entry and coarse crackles throughout her lung fields. She was using her accessory muscles and was extremely distressed. Diaphoresis was evident, although she felt cold.

Blood gas analysis was as follows:

pH   7.33
pO_2 6.5 kPa
pCO_2 5.9 kPa
HCO_3 18 mmol/l
BE   −4

A decision was made to intubate and mechanically ventilate Susan. The mode of ventilation was synchronised intermittent mandatory ventilation (pressure control) (SIMV(PC))
and pressure support (PS). She was sedated with midazolam and was receiving morphine.

Once intubated and ventilated, her assessment findings were as follows:

HR   130 BPM SR
BP   80/35 mmHg (MAP = 50)
Temperature   37.8°C
CVP   4 mmHg

She had equal, reduced air entry and coarse crackles throughout her lung fields. Her
post-intubation chest X-ray showed generalised 'white out'.

Blood gas analysis was as follows:

pH   7.30
pO_2 6.5 kPa
pCO_2 7.8 kPa
HCO_3 15 mmol/l
BE   −8

Her ventilation observations were as follows:

RR   12 BPM
PC   18
PS   18
PEEP   8
TV   350 ml
MV   4.2 l
AP   26 cm H_2O
F_1O_2 0.6

Susan was demonstrating clear signs of respiratory distress and compromise. She was
hypoxic, becoming hypercapnic and had an acidosis. The underlying alterations in lung
structure and function are the primary contributing factors to her clinical picture. Therefore,
it is essential that the health-care professionals involved in her management and care have
a clear understanding of why this clinical picture had developed.

Underlying physiology and pathophysiology

Key considerations

What are the underlying physiological changes associated with the exudative stage of ARDS?
Why do these changes create the clinical picture outlined in the scenario?

In view of Susan's clinical presentation, a provisional diagnosis of ARDS can be made.
ARDS is a form of type 1 respiratory failure (hypoxic respiratory failure) and is similar
to ALI, apart from the severity of the oxygen deficit (Table 5.1). Susan's oxygen index

Table 5.1 Definitions of acute lung injury and acute respiratory distress syndrome

Condition	Timing	Oxygen index (pO_2/F_IO_2)	Chest X-ray	PaOP
ALI	Acute	≥40 kPa (300 mmHg)	Bilateral infiltrates	≥18 mmHg; no clinical evidence of elevated right atrial pressures
ARDS	Acute	≥26.6 kPa (200 mmHg)	Bilateral infiltrates	≥18 mmHg; no clinical evidence of elevated right atrial pressures

PaOP, Pulmonary artery occlusion pressure. (Adapted from Bernard *et al.*, 1994.)

was 10.8 kPa (81.25 mmHg), thereby supporting the diagnosis of ARDS and signifying a significant degree of right to left shunt and ventilation/perfusion (V/Q) mismatching. The ensuing hypoxaemia had the consequence of reduced tissue perfusion and therefore tissue hypoxia with the development of acidosis.

Causes of ARDS

For effective gaseous exchange, there must be an intact alveolar–capillary network within the lungs. However, in situations of ARDS that fundamental physiological feature becomes disrupted, leading to a clinical picture that has been illustrated by Susan. ALI/ARDS occurs within the wider situation of multi-organ dysfunction syndrome (MODS). There is usually a definite initiating event that may cause direct injury to the lungs, for example, pneumonia, as in Susan's case (Table 5.2). However, there maybe an indirect cause, for example, systemic inflammatory response syndrome (SIRS), which can accompany, for example, acute pancreatitis. Therefore, the clinical situation analysed in Chapter 4 could have included the development of ARDS as part of the septic process.

Inflammatory response

According to Bellingan (2002), the pathophysiology of ALI/ARDS is 'driven by an aggressive inflammatory reaction'. It is uncertain why some patients develop ALI/ARDS. However, the result of the inflammatory reaction is disruption of the alveolar epithelium and endothelial damage, with the release of mediators causing capillary permeability, neutrophil and platelet aggregation and pulmonary vasoconstriction. This then leads to the disruption of pulmonary microcirculation and V/Q mismatch as seen with Susan.

Table 5.2 Examples of causes of ALI/ARDS

Direct	Indirect
Pneumonia	Sepsis
Aspiration	Pancreatitis
Smoke inhalation	Massive blood transfusion
Lung contusion	Multiple trauma
Near drowning	Post cardiopulmonary bypass
Fat embolism	

Inflammatory mediators

Many of the inflammatory mediators are thought to be involved in ALI/ARDS. Within bronchoalveolar lavage (BAL), fluid and histological specimens taken from patients with ALI/ARDS, neutrophils are the dominant leucocytes (Bellingan, 2002). Neutrophils cause cellular damage through the production of inflammatory mediators, free radicals and proteases. In addition to these, neutrophil products including, amongst other things, elastase, collagenase and cytokines such as tumour necrosis factor (TNF), have been found in patients with ALI/ARDS. Neutrophils bind to the pulmonary endothelium in the presence of adhesion molecules. This then promotes leukocyte-induced lung injury as well as activation of neutrophils by adhesion molecules and mediator release by neutrophils.

Neutrophils do not create ALI/ARDS in isolation. Alveolar macrophages are also involved in the development of lung injury as well as the release of nitric oxide (Tsukahara *et al.*, 1999). Even so, it is thought that cytokines including TNF, interleukin (IL)-1, IL-6 and IL-8 drive the inflammatory response. The release of these promotes neutrophil–endothelial adhesion, microvascular leakage and augments other proinflammatory responses. However, their role in ALI/ARDS is unclear, despite being found in BAL fluid, and when administered to rodents can elicit an ARDS type of response. Nevertheless, research into the effectiveness of anti-TNF and IL-1 therapies has been disappointing. Conversely, although substances such as endotoxin, proinflammatory cytokines, thrombin and vascular endothelial growth factor have not been found in BAL fluid, they may be involved in the increased vascular permeability seen in ALI/ARDS.

Free radicals

Free radicals are fundamental to the tissue damage seen during inflammatory responses. Normally, antioxidants such as superoxide dismutase protect against free radicals; however, in ALI/ARDS, antioxidant levels are reduced but oxidative stress is increased (Zhang *et al.*, 2000). Therefore, there is increased oxygen-derived free radical production but a lack of the scavengers that catalyse them into hydrogen peroxide and molecular oxygen. This can lead to cell membrane lipid peroxidation resulting in a failure of normal fluid and ionic balance between intracellular and extracellular fluid compartments (Woolf, 1995). This results in eventual cell death through the failure of the cell membrane. Platelet-activating factor (PAF) activates both neutrophils and platelets and is thought to contribute to the increased capillary permeability seen in ALI/ARDS.

Apoptosis

Finally, cell apoptosis regulation is altered during the inflammatory phase. Soluble Fas ligand has been found in the lung epithelial cells of patients with ARDS and can stimulate airway and alveolar epithelial cell apoptosis. Therefore, it is thought to cause excess apoptosis in the parenchymal cells leading to lung injury but in contrast reduce the rate of apoptosis in neutrophils, thereby increasing the inflammatory load (Bellingan, 2002).

Exudative phase of ARDS

ALI/ARDS itself occurs in three phases. Currently, Susan is in the exudative phase where there is evidence of diffuse alveolar damage, with the lungs being heavy and rigid. This stage is characterised by alveolar oedema resulting from endothelial damage leading to progressive pulmonary capillary permeability. The pulmonary microcirculation and alveolar membranes have focal areas of damage, with the alveolar membranes becoming oedematous. Although at this stage the basal membrane is intact, areas of necrosis within the alveolar epithelial lining are evident. In addition, increasing amounts of neutrophils are found within the capillaries, interstitial tissues and progressively within the airspaces (Bellingan, 2002).

Altered pulmonary vascular tone

Susan was experiencing refractory hypoxaemia caused by the altered lung pathology. Also, a loss of normal pulmonary vascular tone is usually seen, which contributes to hypoxaemia. Hypoxic pulmonary vasoconstriction can lead to mild pulmonary hypertension. Studies show that nitric oxide has a central role in the normal regulation of pulmonary vascular tone, but it is uncertain as to how this regulation is lost during ARDS/SIRS. It has been determined that endotoxin stimulates cyclo-oxygenase-2 (COX-2) and inducible nitric oxide synthase (iNOS) expression within the pulmonary blood vessels. This should result in vasodilation as prostaglandin and nitric oxide are released, both of which are potent vasodilators; however, pulmonary hypertension is observed. Therefore, it is thought that the production of the powerful vasoconstrictors endothelin-1 and thromboxane B_2, which are known to be released during the septic process, may underpin the hypertension seen (Bellingan, 2002). COX inhibitors have been shown to reduce the early pulmonary hypertension induced by endotoxin, although they are not used in practice.

Alterations in surfactant

In undamaged lungs, type II alveolar cells secrete surfactants, which inhibit surface tension forces created by the presence of water within the alveoli. Surfactants therefore help to prevent alveolar collapse. However, inflammation can lead to surfactant dysfunction in ALI/ARDS; this is a secondary process in ARDS rather than a causative process as in infant respiratory distress syndrome. Damage and loss of type II cells also leads to a reduction in surfactant production. In addition, hypoxia within the lungs reduces the ability of the type II alveolar cells to produce surfactant, thereby also causing alveolar collapse and atelectasis. Finally, the oedema found in ALI/ARDS, through an uncertain mechanism, contaminates the surfactant, diminishing its effectiveness. The degree to which this dysfunction contributes to ARDS is unclear, but lack of surfactant will reduce lung compliance, thereby making spontaneous and mechanical ventilation difficult.

Assessment and diagnosis

A systematic approach to patient assessment should be undertaken. This is usually undertaken using an ABCDE process. Before intubation and ventilation, Susan's ABCDE assessment was as follows:

Airway

Susan was able to verbally respond to questions; however, she could only talk in very short sentences because she was breathless.

Breathing and ventilation

In situations of respiratory distress, it is important that a thorough and accurate assessment of the respiratory system is undertaken. Susan was tachypneoic, desaturating and appeared to be distressed.

> **Key consideration**
>
> How is physical assessment of the respiratory system undertaken?

Respiratory physical assessment

Physical assessment involves four main skills.

Inspection

From the case scenario, Susan had the observable signs of respiratory distress. She was using her accessory muscles and was diaphoretic. This gave a clear indication that her work of breathing (W_B) had increased.

Work of breathing (W_B)

W_B is the sum of (1) the force required to expand the lungs against the lung and chest wall elastic forces (compliance work or elastic work), (2) the work required to overcome airway resistance and (3) the work required to overcome the resistance of the lungs/chest wall structures. Normal W_B is ~0.5 J/l of expired ventilation; however, in respiratory failure, this may be significantly increased. Intubation and ventilator tubing will also increase W_B. The consequences of increased W_B include respiratory muscle fatigue, CO_2 retention, increased O_2 consumption and acute respiratory failure (Bersten, 2003a).

   In situations of an increase in W_B, the accessory muscles assist the diaphragm and intercostal muscles to increase inspiratory effort. The sternomastoids are the most important of these and the scalenes may become visible. These muscle groups both raise the rib cage up and out, thereby increasing the horizontal diameter of the thorax. The abdominal muscles may be used to assist expiration: when they contract, the abdominal muscles push the abdominal contents against the bottom of the diaphragm, thereby increasing the force of expiration.

Respiratory rate

Susan's spontaneous respiratory rate was 28 BPM. This is considerably faster than a normal resting respiratory rate of about 10–18 BPM. This is likely to be a compensatory mechanism for the metabolic acidosis, which was evident in her arterial blood gases.

Chest expansion and depth of breathing

Symmetry of chest expansion and depth of breathing are also assessed in the inspection phase of respiratory assessment. The thorax should rise and fall gently and there should be equal expansion of the lungs. Unequal expansion could indicate lung collapse, pneumothorax or chronic fibrotic respiratory disease. Depth of breathing should also be assessed because shallow breathing could lead to basal collapse of the lungs, whereas deep breathing could be an indication of, for example, a metabolic disorder such as diabetic ketoacidosis. Susan's chest was rising equally; however, it is likely that the depth of her breathing was shallow because of underlying lung insult and the fast respiratory rate.

Palpation

When feeling or palpating the chest, the lymph nodes in the supraclavicular fossae, cervical regions and axillary areas should be palpated. If there is spread of malignant disease from the lungs/chest, the lymph nodes may be enlarged. Any obvious swelling can be localised as can painful areas. The position of the trachea should be palpated: it should be central at the suprasternal notch. If it is deviated to one side, there may be uneven pressure within the thorax such as seen with a tension pneumothorax or collapsed lung.

Rather than solely observing chest expansion, symmetry can also be assessed by feeling for differences in chest expansion. This can be achieved by placing the hands on either side of the lower rib cage, with thumbs just touching. During inspiration, the distance between the thumbs should widen: if one thumb remains closer to the midline, there is diminished expansion on that side.

Auscultation

Susan had reduced air entry and coarse crackles were heard on auscultation. Auscultation can give useful information about the condition of the lungs and involves listening to the sounds generated by breathing, listening for any added (adventitious) sounds and also listening to the sounds of the patient's spoken or whispered voice as they are transmitted through the chest.

Breath sounds are interpreted in relation to their location, intensity, pitch and duration during inspiration and expiration. There are several 'normal' breath sounds depending on where on the chest wall they are heard.

Vesicular
These are soft and low pitched. They are heard through inspiration, continue into expiration and gently fade about a third of the way through expiration. They are heard throughout the lung fields.

Bronchovesicular
These are louder with a higher pitch than vesicular breath sounds. The inspiratory and expiratory sounds are about equal. These are heard centrally around the first and second intercostal spaces.

Bronchial
These are loud and have a high pitch. Expiratory sounds may last slightly longer than the inspiratory sounds. Bronchial sounds are usually heard when the stethoscope is placed over the bronchus.

If bronchovesicular or bronchial breath sounds are heard in locations distant from where they should be heard, it is likely that the sound has been transmitted through consolidated or fluid-filled lung tissue.

Adventitious sounds
These are breath sounds that are heard in addition to normal breath sounds. The common adventitious sounds are as follows:

Crackles
These are intermittent, non-musical and brief sounds. They can either be fine (soft, high-pitched and brief) or coarse (louder, lower in pitch and are heard for longer). Crackles are heard when previously closed alveoli suddenly open when there is enough pressure inside of them. Therefore, crackles are usually caused by abnormalities in lung tissue, such as pneumonia (coarse crackles) or by fluid such as seen in pulmonary oedema (fine crackles). Susan has been admitted with pneumonia, hence the coarse crackles heard during auscultation.

Wheeze
These are musical sounds that last longer during the respiratory cycle. Wheezes are high-pitched and have a hissing or shrill quality and are associated with airway narrowing. Polyphonic wheeze is characteristic of diffuse airway obstruction such as that heard in asthma. A monophonic wheeze may also be heard if there is compression of a bronchus by, for example, a tumour.

Transmitted voice sounds

If abnormally located bronchovesicular or bronchial breath sounds are heard, it is useful to assess transmitted voice sounds, if possible. Using a stethoscope, symmetrical areas over the chest wall are auscultated as the patient

(1) says 'ninety-nine'. Normally, sounds are muffled and indistinct but if there is an area of consolidation, the sound will be louder and clearer;
(2) says 'ee'. Normally, this will sound a muffled long E sound; however, over an area of consolidation, it will be heard as 'ay'. This is known as *aegophony*;
(3) whispers 'ninety-nine'. Over an area of consolidation, this will sound louder and clearer.

This technique may be difficult to use within the critical care setting if the patient is very dyspnoeic. For this reason, Susan's transmitted breath sounds had not been used as part of her respiratory assessment. Before intensive care admission, if transmitted breath sounds had been assessed, it would have aided in determining areas of lung consolidation due to the pneumonia she had developed.

Percussion

Percussion is useful for assessing the level of fluid or areas of consolidation. The character of the sound produced on percussion varies in relation to what is underlying the area being percussed. If there is air below the percussed area, a resonant sound is heard, whereas solid tissue sounds dull on percussion. Therefore, a pleural effusion or area of consolidation will sound dull on percussion. Hyperresonance can be difficult to determine than dullness; this is heard when there is air in the pleural space as in a pneumothorax.

If percussion was done on Susan, it is likely that areas of dullness would be heard in areas of alveolar hypoinflation and atelectasis.

Chest X-ray

The chest X-ray (CXR) is an important part of respiratory assessment and also acts as a diagnostic tool. In the critical care setting, CXRs are usually taken in an anterioposterior (AP) view because the X-ray film is behind the patient and the X-ray source is in front of them. A systematic interpretation of a CXR incorporates the steps in Box 5.1.

On Susan's CXR, generalised 'white out' was found (Figure 5.2). This will be due to the fluid within the lungs, which results from the abnormal physiology as well as atelectasis that occurs during ARDS. The costophrenic angles may be ill-defined. However, her heart size should be <50% of the transthoracic diameter because the cause of the pulmonary oedema is not cardiac in origin. Therefore, her left ventricular function should be relatively normal.

Circulation

Susan was tachycardic, although her blood pressure was reasonable on admission to the ICU. She was pyrexial but also was diaphoretic and therefore her limbs may have felt clammy. On admission, it is not clear what her urine output was. Her central venous pressure (CVP) was reasonable.

Disability

Susan was responding and answering questions. It would have been useful to assess her blood sugar levels in view of her stress response.

Box 5.1 Chest X-ray interpretation

Is the patient straight or rotated? The clavicles will be asymmetrical if the patient is rotated. If the patient is rotated, the heart, mediastinum and hilar shadows will appear altered.

Is the penetration of the CXR reasonable? On an AP film, the vertebral bodies should be defined if the penetration is reasonable.

Is the shape, size and position of the heart and mediastinum normal? The heart should not be > 50% of the transthoracic diameter.

Is the trachea central or deviated to one side?

Can the diaphragm be seen on each side? Are the costophrenic angles clearly seen? The right diaphragm may be slightly higher than the left, and the costophrenic angles should be clear and well defined.

Are lung fields dark? Air on a CXR appears dark; therefore, any fluid, infection or collapse within the lungs will appear white.

Is the bony skeleton intact? Bone as well as any 'solid' structure is white on a CXR. (Figure 5.1)

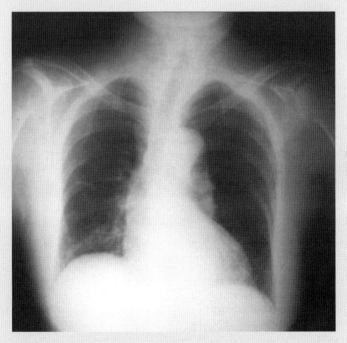

Figure 5.1   Normal chest X-ray.

Exposure

Any rashes or other signs of systemic infection would need to be assessed for.

Key considerations

What is the significance of the arterial blood gases and their interpretation?
What is the significance of the respiratory physical assessment findings?

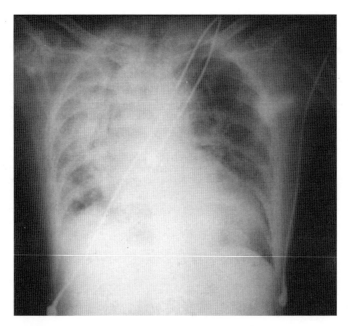

Figure 5.2   Acute respiratory distress syndrome – chest X-ray (ARDS–CXR).

Arterial blood gas analysis

Susan's first set of blood gases demonstrate the level of her hypoxaemia and that she was developing a metabolic acidosis. At that time, her CO_2 levels were within a normal range. This was largely due to her spontaneous respiratory rate of 28 BPM and this was helping to reduce the acidosis. This compensatory response is an important homeostatic mechanism to enable correction of an acid–base imbalance.

Acid–base balance

The regulation of acid–base balance, and therefore hydrogen ions, involves multiple acid–base buffering systems within blood, cells, the lungs and the kidneys. Precise hydrogen ion regulation is essential as nearly all of the activities of the different enzyme systems within the body are affected by hydrogen ion concentration. Therefore any changes in hydrogen concentration will influence nearly all cellular and body functions. Hydrogen concentration is kept at a relatively low level in comparison with other ions. For example, the sodium concentration in extracellular fluid (142 mEq/l) is almost 3.5 million times greater than the normal hydrogen concentration of 0.00004 mEq/l. Also, the concentration of hydrogen normally varies only slightly; this precise regulation of hydrogen emphasises its importance on cellular function.

Acids and bases – what are they?

Molecules, which contain hydrogen atoms that can release hydrogen ions in solutions are acids. For example, hydrochloric acid (HCl) ionises in water to form hydrogen (H^+) and chloride (Cl^-). A base is an ion or molecule that can accept, or combine with, a hydrogen ion. For example, bicarbonate (HCO_3^-) can combine with hydrogen to form H_2CO_3.

Similarly, HPO_4^+ can accept hydrogen to form $H_2PO_4^-$. Proteins are also able to accept hydrogen ions because some amino acids have a net negative charge that can accept the hydrogen ion.

The term *base* is often used interchangeably with 'alkali'. An alkali is a molecule formed by combining one or more of the alkali metals, for example, sodium, potassium and lithium, with a highly basic ion such as the hydroxyl ion (OH^-). The base portion of these molecules reacts quickly with the hydrogen ion to remove hydrogen from solution.

Strong and weak acids and bases

A strong acid is the one that rapidly disassociates and releases large amounts of hydrogen in solution. HCl is an example. Weak acids release their hydrogen ions more reluctantly and H_2CO_3 is an example of a weak acid. Likewise, a strong base is one that reacts rapidly and strongly with H^+, therefore quickly removing hydrogen from the solution. OH^-, when it combines with H^+ to form H_2O, is an example. An example of a weak base is HCO^- because it binds with H^+ more weakly. The acids and bases in extracellular fluid that are involved in the regulation of acid–base balance are weak acids/bases, with the most important being H_2CO_3 and bicarbonate.

Normal hydrogen ion concentration and pH

Normal hydrogen ion concentration is usually maintained within tight limits around a normal value of about 0.00004 mEg/l (40 nEg/l). Normal variations are only about 3–5 nEg/l but during extreme conditions, the hydrogen ion concentration can vary from as low as 10 nEg/l to as high as 160 nEg/l, without causing death.

It is usual to express hydrogen ion concentration on a logarithm scale, using pH units. Because pH is inversely related to the hydrogen ion concentration, a low pH correlates to a high hydrogen ion concentration, and a high pH indicates a lower hydrogen ion concentration. The normal pH of arterial blood is 7.4, whereas the pH of interstitial and venous blood is 7.35, because of the higher amounts of CO_2 released from the tissues to form H_2CO_3 in these fluids. Hypoxia and poor perfusion to the tissues leads to the accumulation of acid and decreased intraceullar pH.

Control of hydrogen ion concentration

There are three primary systems that regulate hydrogen ion concentration and therefore the pH.

The chemical acid–base buffer system
The acid–base buffer system prevents excessive changes in hydrogen ion concentration through the immediate combination of the buffers with acid or base. The buffer system works within a fraction of a second, should the hydrogen ion concentration alter. Buffers do not remove hydrogen but 'store' it until a balance is re-established.

The respiratory centre
The respiratory centre regulates the removal of CO_2 from extracellular fluid. This acts within a few minutes to eliminate CO_2 and therefore H_2CO_3 from the body.

The renal system
The kidneys can excrete either acid or alkaline urine, thereby influencing extracellular hydrogen ion concentration. The renal response to alterations in pH is a relatively slow response; however, the renal response is the most powerful of the three acid–base balance regulatory systems.

Buffering of hydrogen ions

A buffer is a substance that can reversibly bind with hydrogen ions. When the hydrogen ion concentration increases, the ions become bound to available buffer; if the hydrogen ion concentration decreases, hydrogen ions are then released from the buffer. Therefore, changes in hydrogen ion concentration are minimised. The bicarbonate buffer system is probably the most important extracellular buffer system.

Bicarbonate buffer system

The bicarbonate buffer system consists of a water solution that contains a weak acid (H_2CO_3) and a bicarbonate salt, such as $NaHCO_3$. H_2CO_3 is formed in the body by the reaction of CO_2 with H_2O.

$$CO_2 + H_2O \rightleftharpoons H_2CO_3$$

This reaction is slow and only small amounts of bicarbonate are made unless carbonic anydrase is present. This enzyme is present in abundant amounts in the walls of the alveoli in the lungs as well as in the epithelial cells of the renal tubules. The H_2CO_3 is then ionised to form H^+ and HCO_3^-.

$$CO_2 + H_2O \rightleftharpoons H_2CO_3 \rightleftharpoons H^+ + HCO_3^-$$

If a strong acid is added to the bicarbonate buffer solution, the increased hydrogen ions released from the acid are buffered by the HCO_3^-.

$$HCl \longrightarrow H^+ + Cl^-$$
$$\longrightarrow \uparrow H^+ + HCO_3^- \longrightarrow H_2CO_3 \longrightarrow CO_2 + H_2O$$

The excess CO_2 will then stimulate respiration in an effort to eliminate the CO_2 from extracellular fluid.

The opposite of the above reaction will occur if a strong base is added to a solution.

Henderson–Hasselbach equation

The Henderson–Hasselbach equation enables calculation of the pH of a solution if the molar concentration of bicarbonate and the pCO_2 are known.

$$pH = 6.1 + \log\frac{HCO_3^-}{0.03 \times pCO_2}$$

From this formula, it is apparent that an increase in bicarbonate ion will cause the pH to rise, whereas an increase in pCO_2 will lead to a drop in pH. This equation also provides an understanding into the physiological control of acids and bases within the extracellular fluid as a consequence of the respiratory and renal response in the maintenance of acid–base balance. The co-ordinated efforts of both these systems allow for acid–base homeostasis; however, acid–base disturbances will occur when one or both of these control mechanisms becomes impaired. If this happens, the bicarbonate concentration or the pCO_2 of the extracellular fluid will be altered. Changes in the bicarbonate concentration will lead to 'metabolic' disturbances, whereas 'respiratory' disturbances arise from changes in the pCO_2 level.

The phosphate buffer system

The phosphate buffer system is not as powerful as the extracellular fluid buffer; however, it plays an important role in the buffering of renal tubular fluid and intracellular fluids. $H_2PO_4^-$ and HPO_4^+ are the primary elements used in the phosphate buffer system. If a strong acid is added to a mixture of these two substances, the hydrogen is accepted by HPO_4^+ (base) and is converted to $H_2PO_4^-$. For example, the following occurs when HCl is added to HPO_4^+.

$$HCl + NaHPO_4 \longrightarrow NaH_2PO_4 + NaCl$$

Therefore, the strong acid (HCl) is replaced by a weak acid, minimising the decrease in pH.

If a strong base is added to the phosphate buffer system, it too will be buffered and replaced by a weaker base. This will minimise the rise in pH; for example, the following occurs if the strong base OH^- is added to the buffer solution.

$$NaOH + NaH_2PO_4 \longrightarrow Na_2HPO_4 + H_2O$$

Proteins as buffers

Because there is a high concentration, especially in cells, of proteins, these form the most plentiful buffer within the body. The intracellular pH will change in similar proportion to extracellular fluid pH changes. Hydrogen and bicarbonate can diffuse through cell membranes but this occurs in small quantities and it will take several hours before there is equilibrium between the intra- and extracellular concentrations of these ions. The exception to this is with red blood cells which have rapid equilibrium, with haemoglobin being able to buffer hydrogen ions. Even so, the diffusion of the substances involved in the bicarbonate buffer system causes the pH in intracellular fluids to change when there are changes in the extracellular pH.

Respiratory regulation of acid–base balance

The regulation of extracellular CO_2 is the second way in which acid–base balance is controlled. An increase in ventilation will increase CO_2 elimination, leading to a reduction in hydrogen ion concentration within the extracellular fluid, with the reverse happening should ventilation reduce. CO_2 is continually formed in the body as a by-product of cellular metabolic activity; therefore, changes in either pulmonary ventilation or the rate of CO_2 formation can change the extracellular fluid pCO_2. Increasing alveolar ventilation to about twice normal raises the pH of the extracellular fluid by about 0.23. Therefore if the pH of the extracellular fluids is 7.40 with normal alveolar ventilation, doubling the respiratory rate raises the pH to about 7.63. However, a decrease in ventilation to one-fourth normal reduces the pH by 0.45. Therefore, if the pH is 7.4 with normal ventilation, reducing alveolar ventilation by one-fourth (for example, if a minute volume is 8 l and it is reduced to 6 l) will reduce the pH to 6.95. Because the ventilation rate can change so markedly, it becomes evident how influential the respiratory system is in the regulation of extracellular pH. From this, it can also be seen that the respiratory system acts a negative feedback mechanism for hydrogen ion control.

The pH of extracellular fluid, in turn, affects the rate of ventilation. As pH decreases from a normal value of 7.4 to 7.0, the alveolar ventilation rate will increase to four to five times the normal value. Should the plasma pH rise above 7.4, this will lead to a decrease in respiratory rate. The change in ventilation rate will lead to a greater change in pH when there is an acidosis compared with an alkalosis. This is largely due to a hypoxaemia developing; also as the ventilation rate decreases, the drop in pO_2 will stimulate the respiratory centre to increase the respiratory rate. Therefore, the respiratory compensation for an increase in pH is not as effective as the response to a decrease in pH.

However, the respiratory system cannot return the hydrogen ion concentration completely back to normal when a disturbance outside of the respiratory system has altered the pH. Usually, the respiratory response to an altered hydrogen ion concentration is about 50–75% effective, which relates to a feedback gain of 1–3. Therefore, if the pH falls from 7.4 to 7.0, the respiratory response to this will return the pH to a value of about 7.2–7.3. However, if the response to metabolic causes of pH abnormalities become impaired or ineffective (e.g. if a patient who is very tachypneoic becomes exhausted), the normal compensatory mechanism cannot occur. In these situations, the sole remaining regulatory mechanism to control acid–base balance is the renal response.

Renal control of acid–base balance

The kidneys have a key role in acid–base balance because they can excrete acidic or alkaline urine, thereby either removing acid or base, respectively, from extracellular fluid. Bicarbonate ions are filtered continuously into the renal tubules and, if they are excreted in urine, base is removed from the extracellular fluid. However, normally, the kidneys reabsorb nearly all the bicarbonate that is filtered, thereby conserving the primary buffer of the body. The tubular epithelial cells can also secrete hydrogen ions into the filtrate, thereby removing acid from the blood. If more hydrogen ions are secreted than bicarbonate ions filtered, there will be a net loss of acid from the extracellular fluid. There will be a net loss of base if more bicarbonate ions are filtered than hydrogen ions are secreted. The lungs cannot excrete non-volatile acids because they are not formed from H_2CO_3 and therefore have to be excreted by the renal system.

When there is a reduction in the extracellular fluid hydrogen ion concentration, the kidneys do not reabsorb all the filtered bicarbonate and bicarbonate is lost in urine. This helps to increase the hydrogen ion concentration in the extracellular fluid, thereby returning the pH back towards normal. In acidosis, the kidneys do not excrete bicarbonate but rather, the bicarbonate is reabsorbed as well as manufactured by the tubular cells. This then helps to increase the pH, again back towards normal. Therefore the kidneys regulate acid–base balance through three fundamental mechanisms.

Primary active secretion of hydrogen ions

In the distal tubules (late portion) and collecting duct, the epithelium of the tubule secretes hydrogen by primary active transport (Figure 5.3). This mechanism is different from the one that occurs in the proximal tubule, loop of Henle and early portion of the distal tubule because a specific protein within the luminal membrane transports the hydrogen ions out of the cell into the filtrate. This requires ATP and only occurs in the intercalated cells of the distal tubule and collecting ducts. Secretion of hydrogen ions in these cells occurs in two steps: first, dissolved CO_2 combines with H_2O to form H_2CO_3. The H_2CO_3 then disassociates into bicarbonate, which is reabsorbed into blood and hydrogen, which is secreted into the tubule with the use of the hydrogen–ATPase mechanism. Although this only accounts for 5% of total hydrogen loss, it is an important mechanism in forming maximally acidic urine with a pH of 4.5.

Secondary secretion of hydrogen ions

The cells of the proximal tubule, the thick segment of the loop of Henle and the early distal tubule are able to secrete hydrogen ions into the filtrate by a sodium–hydrogen counter

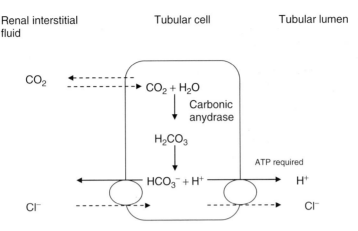

Figure 5.3   Primary active secretion of hydrogen.

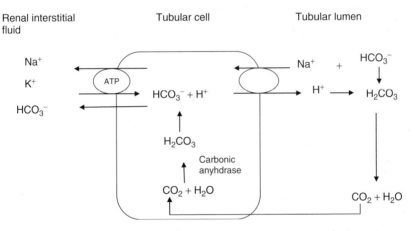

Figure 5.4   Secondary active transport of hydrogen.

transport mechanism (Figure 5.4). This secondary active transport of hydrogen is linked to the transport of sodium into the luminal membrane. This movement of hydrogen is against a concentration gradient and requires the sodium–potassium ATPase pump to enable the movement of sodium across the cell membrane, thus maintaining the gradient. CO_2 diffuses into the tubular cells or is formed during tubular cellular metabolism. Under the influence of carbonic anydrase, the CO_2 combines with H_2O to form H_2CO_3, which then disassociates into H^+ and HCO_3^-. The hydrogen ions are secreted into the tubular lumen by sodium–hydrogen counter-transport: sodium is carried across the cell membrane by a carrier protein. The hydrogen ion combines with the same carrier protein and is transported out of the cell into filtrate. The bicarbonate ion moves across the cell membrane into the renal interstitial fluid and peritubular capillaries. Therefore for every hydrogen ion that is secreted, a bicarbonate ion enters the extracellular fluid.

Reabsorption of filtered bicarbonate ions and production of new bicarbonate ions

Bicarbonate ions do not readily move across the renal cell membranes; therefore the bicarbonate ions within the ultrafiltrate cannot be directly reabsorbed. The reabsorption of bicarbonate ions is triggered by a reaction in the tubules between the filtered bicarbonate ions and the hydrogen ions, which are secreted by the tubular cells. H_2CO_3 is formed, which then disassociates into CO_2 and H_2O. The CO_2 immediately diffuses back across the cell membrane and recombines with H_2O under the influence of carbonic anydrase, thereby generating more H_2CO_3. This molecule will then disassociate to form a hydrogen ion and a bicarbonate ion: the bicarbonate diffuses across the cell membrane into the interstitial fluid and then from the peritubular capillaries into blood. Therefore, each time a hydrogen ion is formed in the tubular epithelial cells, a bicarbonate ion is also formed and released into blood. Also, the bicarbonate ion that has been filtered is actually not the one that enters the peritubular capillary blood.

The quantities of filtered hydrogen and filtered bicarbonate are almost equal, and they combine with each other in the filtrate to form CO_2 and H_2O. Therefore, to some extent they titrate each other. However, there is slightly more hydrogen ions filtered than the bicarbonates. The excess hydrogen ions help to remove the non-volatile acids produced during metabolism.

If there is an excess of bicarbonate ions over hydrogen ions in the filtrate, the excess bicarbonate is excreted because it cannot be reabsorbed. This helps to correct a metabolic alkalosis. In the situation of a metabolic acidosis, the excess amount of hydrogen allows for all the bicarbonate to be reabsorbed and any remaining hydrogen is excreted in urine. These excess hydrogen ions are buffered by phosphate and ammonia (NH_3) and are excreted as salts.

Buffering of hydrogen in the tubules

If there is an excess amount of hydrogen ions within the filtrate, in relation to bicarbonate ions, only a small amount of the hydrogen ions can be excreted as H^+ within urine. This is because of the minimal pH of urine being 4.5: this corresponds to a H^+ concentration of $10^{-4.5}$ mEq/l, or 0.03 mEq/l. Therefore for every litre of urine, the maximum amount of hydrogen that can be excreted is 0.03 mEq of free hydrogen ions. To enable the excretion of larger amounts of hydrogen, the hydrogen is buffered in the tubular fluid by, for example, phosphate and NH_3.

Phosphate buffer
Both HPO_4^+ and $H_2PO_4^-$ make up the phosphate buffer system and are found in concentrated amounts within the filtrate (Figure 5.5). Excess hydrogen can combine with HPO_4^- to form $H_2PO_4^-$; it can be excreted as a sodium salt (NaH_2PO_4), carrying with it

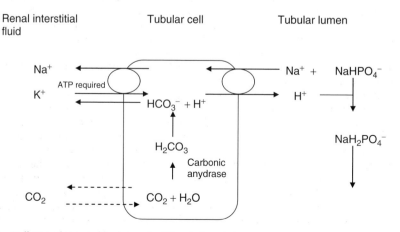

Figure 5.5   Buffering of secreted hydrogen by filtered phosphate.

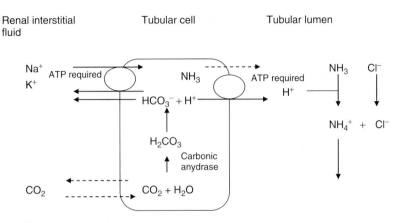

Renal interstitial fluid   Tubular cell   Tubular lumen

Figure 5.6   Buffering of secreted hydrogen by ammonia (NH_3).

the excess hydrogen. In conjunction, a new bicarbonate ion is also manufactured and added to blood.

Ammonia buffer

The NH_3 buffer system comprises of NH_3 and ammonium ion (NH_4^+) (Figure 5.6). Within the epithelial cells of the proximal tubule, thick ascending limb of the loop of Henle and distal tubules, NH_4^+ is made from glutamine. Each molecule of glutamine is metabolised to form two NH_4^+ and two HCO_3^- ions. The NH_4^+ is secreted into the tubular lumen via a sodium counter-transport mechanism, and the sodium is reabsorbed. The HCO_3^- moves into the interstitial fluid into blood. Therefore, for each glutamine molecule that is metabolised, two NH_4^+ molecules are secreted into the filtrate and two HCO_3^- ions are reabsorbed into blood.

In the collecting ducts, NH_4^+ is added to the filtrate through a different mechanism. Hydrogen is secreted by the tubular membrane into the lumen, where it combines with NH_3 to form NH_4^+, which is then excreted. Again, a bicarbonate ion is made, which moves into the interstitial fluid and into blood.

It has been shown that hydrogen ion secretion is necessary for both bicarbonate reabsorption and the manufacturing of new bicarbonate. Under normal conditions, the tubules must secrete enough hydrogen to ensure that all the bicarbonate is reabsorbed as well as the excretion of the non-volatile proteins enabled. Thus during alkalosis, the hydrogen secretion is reduced to enable excretion of bicarbonate, whereas during an acidosis, hydrogen ion secretion is increased to enhance the amount of bicarbonate within the blood. There are two important stimuli for increasing hydrogen ion secretion during acidosis: these are an increase in the pCO_2 of the extracellular fluid and an increase in the hydrogen ion concentration of extracellular fluid. In addition, aldosterone stimulates hydrogen ion secretion by the intercalated cells.

From Susan's blood gases, it would seem that she had a metabolic acidosis for which her body was attempting to compensate by increasing her respiratory rate. The metabolic acidosis has been caused by the increased formation of acids within the body due to a lack of tissue perfusion. However, the increase in her respiratory rate was not effectively compensating for the increase in the hydrogen ion concentration. Therefore, Susan actually had a mixed acidosis. Hence, in conjunction with the underlying alterations in her lung tissue, the increased work of breathing may well be contributing to the reduction in functional residual capacity (FRC) and ability of the lungs to exchange gas. Susan's ability to excrete CO_2 and to promote oxygenation of arterial blood had been significantly reduced. Her oxygen index indicates that she had right to left shunt and increased V/Q mismatching.

Evidence-based care

Mechanical ventilation

> **Key consideration**
>
> Rationalise the mode of ventilation and ventilator settings.

Mechanical ventilation is the basic life-saving supportive intervention in ARDS, and it is essential that health-care professionals have a clear understanding of the principles that underpin mechanical ventilator support.

Positive-pressure ventilation

To understand how a machine can be used to either replace or supplement spontaneous breathing, a basic understanding of the mechanics of breathing is necessary. Mechanics deals with forces, displacements and the rate of change in displacement. In relation to breathing, force is measured as pressure, displacement is volume and the rate of change is flow. Therefore, in mechanical ventilation, it is important to ascertain the pressure that is required to cause a flow of gas to pass down the airways and increase the volume of the lungs.

To develop this further by introducing variables associated with lung tissue, the equation of motion for the respiratory system can be outlined as being:

$$\text{Muscle pressure} + \text{ventilator pressure} = \text{elastance} \times \text{volume} + \text{resistance} \times \text{flow}$$

Again to simplify this further,

$$\text{Muscle pressure} + \text{ventilator pressure} = \text{elastic load} + \text{resistive load}$$

The combined respiratory muscle and ventilator pressure causes volume and flow to be delivered to the patient. If the patient is not making any spontaneous effort, then the ventilator pressure solely causes volume and flow to be delivered. Pressure, volume and flow are variable and can change in time and in different situations. Elastance and resistance are considered to be constant: elastance is viewed as the ratio of pressure change to volume change and resistance is defined as the ratio of pressure change to flow change. Therefore, the elastic load is the pressure required to overcome the elastance of the respiratory system, and the resistive load is the pressure needed to overcome the flow resistance of the airways and endotracheal tube as well as chest wall and lung tissue resistance.

In the above equation, any of the variables (pressure, volume or flow) can be predetermined, therefore making it the independent variable and the other two, the dependent variables because they will fluctuate. For example, in pressure-controlled ventilation, pressure is the independent variable, whereas volume and flow are dependent on the pressure as well as the compliance and resistance of the respiratory system. In volume-cycled ventilation, volume is the independent variable, whereas flow and pressure are dependent. It is important to remember that often 'control' is used to indicate the variable that remains constant regardless of the fluctuating variables.

Volume-cycled and pressure-cycled ventilation

This gives the basis for classifying ventilators as pressure, volume or flow controllers. By using this type of classification, interpretation of pulmonary mechanics is enabled.

For example, resistance and compliance can be calculated and taken into consideration when evaluating the effectiveness of mechanical ventilation. To allow for this, ventilators use a closed-loop control to maintain consistent inspiratory pressure or volume or flow despite changes in muscle load/function. The respiratory load can change as lung tissue undergoes pathophysiological changes as a result of lung injury; therefore, altering compliance and resistance will not influence the independent variable that has been set.

Once it is understood which variable is controlled and which are dependent (and therefore may change), the mode of ventilation can then be considered. The two general approaches to mechanical ventilation are pressure control or volume/flow control. Within these, different modes can be used to deliver mechanical breaths with some allowing for supported spontaneous breathing. The rationale for deciding which variable is controlled will ultimately depend on balancing the advantages with the disadvantages in relation to both blood gas control and impact on lung dynamics (Table 5.3).

Susan had been placed on SIMV (PC) and PS. Therefore, the pressure is the independent variable with the volumes and flow becoming dependent on the set pressure limit as well as Susan's lung tissue properties. With a pressure limit of 18 (on top of PEEP of 8), she was receiving tidal volumes of 350 ml at a respiratory rate of 12 BPM, with an airway pressure of 26. She could take spontaneous breaths if she initiated any and these would be supported by a specific pressure from the ventilator. However, is this choice of mode of ventilation supported by current recommendations?

Mechanical ventilation in ARDS

The aim of mechanical ventilation is to maintain gas exchange and promote tissue oxygenation while avoiding the adverse effects of mechanical ventilation, hyperexpansion, haemodynamic compromise and oxygen toxicity. ARDS has a mortality rate of 35–65% (Ranieri *et al.*, 1999), and, although mechanical ventilation can delay mortality by maintaining adequate oxygenation and allowing the respiratory muscles to rest, mechanical ventilation itself can worsen or cause ALI. This is especially so when large tidal volumes and high pressures are used, causing overdistension of the lungs (Esteban *et al.*, 2000). Therefore, it is recommended that overinflation and high alveolar pressures are avoided (Bersten, 2003b). These lung-protective strategies can reduce the mortality rate to 40% in comparison with the mortality rates where conventional ventilatory strategies were used (Amato *et al.*, 1998; Ranieri *et al.*, 1999).

Historically, the ventilatory management of patients with ARDS has been aimed at delivering tidal volumes of 12–15 ml/kg; however, these volumes cause lung injury because of stress factors within the lungs (Ranieri *et al.*, 1999; Ware and Matthay, 2000). Also, ventilation with large volumes causes disruption of the epithelium and endothelium and exacerbate lung inflammation, atelectasis, hypoxaemia and the release of inflammatory mediators (The Acute Respiratory Distress Syndrome Network, 2000). The release of inflammatory mediators could then cause more actual lung damage as well as cause systemic and organ dysfunction.

Lung-protection strategies are, therefore, recommended and are aimed at maintaining low inspiratory driving pressures (<20 cm H_2O above PEEP) with low tidal volumes of 6 ml/kg. This strategy, in a trial involving 861 patients, demonstrated a 22% reduction in mortality (Ware and Matthay, 2000).

The use of pressure-cycled modes of ventilation in ARDS has gained increased interest of late. Because of the decelerating flow of pressure-cycled ventilation, there is a more 'laminar' flow at the end of inspiration, allowing for a more even distribution of ventilation in lungs of varying compliance (Esteban *et al.*, 2000). This improves oxygenation and pulmonary function (Armstrong and MacIntyre, 1995; Davis *et al.*, 1996). Rappaport *et al.* (1994) compared early use of pressure-cycled ventilation and volume-cycled ventilation in patients with acute hypoxic respiratory failure and found that those who were ventilated on

Table 5.3 Modes of ventilation

	Mode of ventilation	Principles	Indications	Benefits	Drawbacks
Volume cycled	Controlled mechanical ventilation (CMV) or volume control	Pre-set respiratory rate and tidal volume; if the patient triggers the ventilator, he or she will not receive any support on the spontaneous effort	Mechanical ventilation required; critical gas exchange when it would be undesirable for the patient to take spontaneous breaths	pCO_2 controlled	Intrathoracic pressures are uncontrolled and can lead to the following: • Barotrauma • Pneumothorax • Reduced cardiac output Patient needs to be sedated and muscle relaxed
	Synchronised intermittent mandatory ventilation (SIMV) or SIMV (VC)	Pre-set respiratory rate and tidal volume. Patient can take spontaneous breaths within a trigger window and the ventilator will synchronise with spontaneous efforts	Mechanical ventilation required.	pCO_2 controlled; muscle relaxants not required	Intrathoracic pressures are uncontrolled. Can lead to: • Barotrauma • Pneumothorax • Reduced cardiac output
Pressure cycled	Pressure control (PC)	Pre-set respiratory rate. Pre-set pressure level–tidal volume delivered depends on lung compliance and pressure level. If the patient triggers the ventilator, he/she will not receive any support on the spontaneous effort	Mechanical ventilation required. Critical gas exchange when it would undesirable for the patient to take spontaneous breaths	Intrathoracic pressures are controlled. Pressure delivered more evenly within alveoli, therefore lung protective and helps to recruit alveoli	Variable tidal volumes as lung compliance alters. May lead to poorly controlled pCO_2. Patient needs to be sedated and muscle relaxed
	SIMV (PC)	Set respiratory rate and pressure level. Patient can take spontaneous breaths during a trigger window and the ventilator will synchronise with spontaneous efforts.	Mechanical ventilation required	Intrathoracic pressures are controlled. Pressure delivered more evenly within alveoli, therefore lung protective and helps to recruit alveoli. Muscle relaxants not required	Tidal volumes and minute volume can be variable leading to poor pCO_2 control

Bi-phasic positive airway pressure (BiPAP) Bilevel BiVent	Set upper and lower pressure levels. Mechanical breaths alternate between the two pressure levels according to • set respiratory rate; • set I:E ratio; • set times at the different pressure levels.	Mechanical ventilation required	Intrathoracic pressures are controlled. Pressure delivered evenly within alveoli, therefore lung protective and recruits alveoli. One mode can be used throughout ICU stay from complete ventilation to weaning. Enables unlimited spontaneous effort; maintains respiratory muscle integrity, enhances patient comfort and less sedation required	Tidal volumes and minute volume can be variable leading to poor pCO_2 control.
Dual control Pressure regulated volume control/pressure-limited SIMV	Set respiratory rate and tidal volume. Upper pressure level set: 5 cm H_2O below peak pressure OR 5 cm H_2O above plateau pressure	Situations when both minute volume and pressures need to be controlled	pCO_2 is controlled as well as intrathoracic pressures	Pressure level may still be fairly high to enable the tidal volume to be delivered
Weaning Pressure support (PS)	Spontaneous breaths supported to achieve a predetermined pressure	When spontaneous breaths are being triggered	Tidal volumes supported	Too much can lead to large spontaneous tidal volumes. Too little can lead to poor lung expansion and ultimately failure to wean
Volume control (VC)	Spontaneous breaths are supported to achieve a predetermined tidal volume	When spontaneous breaths are being triggered. Situations of potential/actual atelectasis	Tidal volumes achieved	May be uncomfortable if target tidal volume is too high

(continued)

Table 5.3 *(continued)*

Mode of ventilation	Principles	Indications	Benefits	Drawbacks
Smart modes				
Automode	Preset respiratory rate and tidal volume. Ventilator will switch to a support mode (e.g. PS) if the patient triggers spontaneous breaths. If spontaneous effort drops, will switch back into a control mode.	Mechanical ventilation required	Maintains respiratory muscle integrity, enhances patient comfort and less sedation required. Apneoa avoided	May be difficult to assess improvements in patient spontaneous effort
Adaptive support ventilation	Patients body weight, desired minute volume, F_IO_2, PEEP and maximum inspired pressure entered into ventilator. Mechanical ventilator automatically adjusts inspiratory pressure, breath cycle and frequency to achieve pre-set aims. Responds to any spontaneous effort with a PS, which can be adjusted to achieve target frequency/tidal volume combination	Mechanical ventilation required	Maintains respiratory muscle integrity, enhances patient comfort and less sedation required. Apneoa avoided	May be difficult to assess improvements in patient spontaneous effort
Autioflow©	Ventilator automatically adjusts flow of gases in relation to resistance (airway)	Mechanical ventilation required but used with a volume-cycled mode	Control of airway pressures with good control of pCO_2	Potential high airway pressures

a pressure-cycled mode had a more rapid increase in static lung compliance and were ventilated for fewer days.

Ongoing patient scenario

Susan has now been in the ICU for 12 hours and it is becoming increasingly difficult to control her blood gases, despite manipulation of her ventilation.

On assessment, the findings are as follows:

HR   105 BPM SR
BP   110/65 mmHg (MAP = 80)
Temperature   38.3°C
CVP   8 mmHg

Blood gases:

pH   7.32
pO_2 7.5 kPa
pCO_2 8.0 kPa
HCO_3 15 mmol/l
BE   −7

Her ventilation observations are as follows:

RR   16 BPM
PC   20
PS   20
PEEP   10
TV   280 ml
MV   4.4 l
AP   30 cm H_2O
F_1O_2 0.9

During the ward round, the following decisions are made.

(1) To increase the PEEP to 15
(2) To allow the pCO_2 to rise if necessary
(3) To aim for a pO_2 > 8 kPa
(4) To aim for tidal volumes of 390 ml, with a plateau pressure < 30 cm H_2O
(5) To prone her
(6) To consider the use of prostacyclin nebulisers

It is evident that Susan's condition has worsened. This is demonstrated by the continuing hypoxaemia despite the increases in F_1O_2 and strategies to enhance gas exchange. It is then important to consider how the underlying pathophysiology is evolving as well as further strategies to improve oxygen content and perfusion.

Progressing pathophysiology

Key considerations

What stage of ARDS is Susan in?
What are the physiological changes that occur within this stage?

Fibroproliferative phase

As ARDS progresses, the fibroproliferative response to the lung injury commences. Although fibroproliferation is a normal process within tissue repair, within ARDS it can have serious consequences. This phase is stimulated by mediators which encourage local fibroblasts to migrate, replicate and to produce excess connective tissues. It is unclear as to which profibrotic factor is responsible for this. The expression of TNF-α can lead to a T-lymphocyte alveolitis, which can progress into pulmonary fibrosis. Expression of transforming growth factor alpha (TGF-α) can also induce pulmonary fibrosis. Cytokines may have a role and both IL-4 and IL-3 levels are increased in fibrosis. Levels of both TGF-α and a platelet-derived growth factor (PDGF)-like factor are increased in BAL fluid in patients with ARDS; also products of the clotting cascade, which are important mediators of the pulmonary profibrotic response, such as fibrin, thrombin and factor Xa, are increased in patients with ARDS. However, there are limited studies investigating into the effect of mediators which regulate collagen metabolism in pulmonary fibrosis.

TGF-β has three closely related isoforms (TGF-β 1, 2 and 3), which all modulate inflammation, inhibit growth and proliferation and regulate production of the extracellular matrix. Studies suggest that TGF-β is important in the pathogenesis of pulmonary fibrosis (Martin, 1999). In normal tissue repair, TGF-β 1 is important for tissue repair; however, when its expression is persistent or excessive, it promotes pathological fibrosis.

The fibrosis that occurs in this stage of ARDS contributes significantly to the reduced lung compliance that is seen. Lungs are stiff and difficult to inflate without a significant increase in intrathoracic pressure. Shunt and V/Q mismatching are exacerbated, leading to further tissue hypoxia and organ dysfunction.

Ongoing assessment

Key consideration

How can the degree of shunt be assessed?

In similar situations as those being experienced by Susan, it is useful to calculate the level of hypoxaemia more thoroughly than just relying on the oxygen index. This can be accomplished through the calculation of A−a gradient.

A−a gradient

The A−a gradient gives an indication of the efficiency of alveolar:capillary oxygen transfer and takes into account the alveolar pO_2 in relation to the arterial pO_2. To be able to calculate the alveolar pO_2, it is first important to take into consideration the inspired oxygen tension (P_1O_2) of humidified gas: this is determined by the F_1O_2, the barometric pressure and saturated vapour pressure of water.

$$P_1O_2 = F_1O_2 \times (\text{barometric pressure} - 47)$$

(NB: at sea level barometric pressure = 760 mmHg)

Alveolar pO_2 in the ideal lung unit (PAO_2) is calculated from the following formula:

$$PAO_2 = P_1O_2 - (1 - F_1O_2 \times (1 - R)) \times pCO_2/R$$

where R is the respiratory exchange ratio, which can either be measured by indirect calorimetry or assumed to be 0.8. To enable easier calculation, the following approximation can be used:

$$PAO_2 = P_IO_2 - pCO_2/0.8$$

(NB: pCO_2 must be in mmHg not kPa)
In Susan's case, her PAO_2 was therefore calculated as follows:

$$PAO_2 = (0.9 \times (760 - 47)) - 60/0.8$$

Therefore,

$$PAO_2 = 641.7 - 75$$

$$PAO_2 = 566.7$$

To determine the A–a gradient, the difference between the PAO_2 and pO_2 is then calculated:

$$A-a \text{ gradient} = PAO_2 - pO_2$$

In Susan's case, this then is

$$A-a \text{ gradient} = 566.7 - 56.25$$

$$A-a \text{ gradient} = 543.45 \text{ mmHg}$$

(NB: A normal A–a gradient is < 20 mmHg)
This indicates considerable V/Q mismatching and shunt and is more exact than just using the $pO_2:F_IO_2$ ratio (oxygen index) because it can distinguish hypoxaemia from alveolar hypoventilation.

Assessing ventilation

Key consideration

How can assessment of Susan's mechanical ventilation be further enhanced?

The waveforms displayed on the mechanical ventilator can offer information about lung properties and effect of ventilator settings. The key waveforms are the pressure, volume and flow waveforms, and the gradual changes in pressure, flow and volume curves are equally dependent on the ventilator settings and lung dynamics.

Pressure curve

Volume-cycled ventilation

In volume-controlled ventilation, the airway pressure will depend on the alveolar pressure and the resistance of the airways. The pressures generated during volume delivery is largely dependent on the compliance and resistance of the lung tissue – if the flow is constant, the pressure curve gives useful information about the lung properties.

At the beginning of inspiration, there is a steep increase in pressure due to the resistance of the system; the point where the curve becomes less steep is dependent on the flow and the resistance. If the inspiratory flow is reduced and if the resistance is low, that point is reached quicker. After this point, there is a linear increase in pressure until the tidal volume

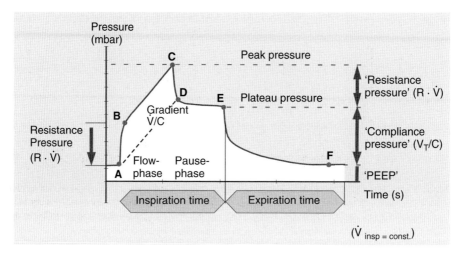

Figure 5.7   Pressure–time diagram. © Dräger Medical AG & Co. KG, Lübeck, Germany.

has been delivered and therefore, the peak pressure is reached. The gradient of this is dependent on the compliance of the system as well as the inspiratory flow. Inspiratory flow ceases at this point. As the flow stops, the pressure falls rapidly to the plateau pressure: the amount the pressure drops by is equivalent to the initial increase in pressure at the beginning of the breath. The plateau pressure is determined by the compliance and the tidal volume, with the difference between the plateau pressure and the end-expiratory pressure being obtained by dividing the tidal volume by compliance.

During the plateau time, no volume or inspiratory flow is delivered to the lungs. Expiration occurs as a passive pressure, with the elastic recoil of the thorax forcing air out of the lungs. Once expiration has occurred, the pressure in the lungs is the end-expiratory pressure. (Figure 5.7)

Pressure-cycled ventilation

In pressure-cycled ventilation, the obtained waveform is quite different to the volume-cycled one. The pressure increases rapidly from the low-pressure level until the preset upper pressure limit is reached and then remains constant for the duration of the inspiratory time that has been set. The drop in pressure during expiration is similar to the changes seen in volume-cycled ventilation. The pressure remains constant at the low-pressure level until the next inspiration occurs.

Flow time

The flow-time waveform shows inspiratory flow and expiratory flow. The volume delivered is indicated by the area under the curve. During inspiration, the mode of ventilation will dictate the flow waveform, whereas during expiration, interpretation of the waveform can give information about the compliance and resistance of the system.

Constant flow

If constant flow is applied during inspiration, the inspiratory phase of the flow-time waveform quickly rises when inspiration commences until the flow rate, as set on the

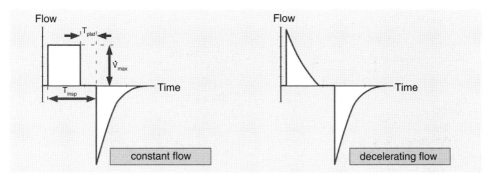

Figure 5.8 Flow–time diagram. © Dräger Medical AG & Co. KG, Lübeck, Germany. (All rights reserved. Not to be reproduced without written permission, nor stored in a data system, transmitted electronically or mechanically, by photocopying or photographing, in any way, shape, or form, in its entirety or in any part.)

ventilator, is reached. It then remains stable until the tidal volume has been delivered. At the beginning of the plateau, or pause time, the flow stops and therefore there is a sudden decrease to zero. At the end of the pause time, expiratory flow commences and the shape of the waveform will be influenced by lung and ventilator properties. Constant flow is usually used during volume-cycled ventilation.

Decelerating flow

In decelerating flow, having reached a peak during inspiration, the flow then falls at a constant rate down to zero. Even though the inspiratory phase of the breath cycle may still be occurring, the difference between the pressure in the lungs and the pressure in the breathing system is the main influence for the driving force. The pressure in the breathing system is kept fairly constant by the ventilator; therefore, as the pressure inside the lungs increases as volume is delivered, the pressures in both systems begin to equalise. As the pressures equalise the flow reduces, and ceases once the pressures are equal. Decelerating flow is used primarily in pressure-cycled ventilation (Figure 5.8).

Volume curve

The volume curve indicates the gradual changes in volume during inspiration and expiration. During the inspiratory portion of the breath cycle, the volume increases constantly. During the plateau time, the volume remains constant so that no further volume is being delivered to the lungs. During expiration, the volume drops due to passive recoil of the thorax.

The relationship of pressure, flow and volume curves needs to be taken into account and therefore the curves should not be assessed in isolation of each other (Figure 5.9).

Interpretation of changes in the waveforms

Changes in compliance

When compliance changes, the peak airway pressure and plateau airway pressure, both change (Figure 5.10). If compliance improves, the peak and plateau pressures drop, whereas they both increase if compliance worsens.

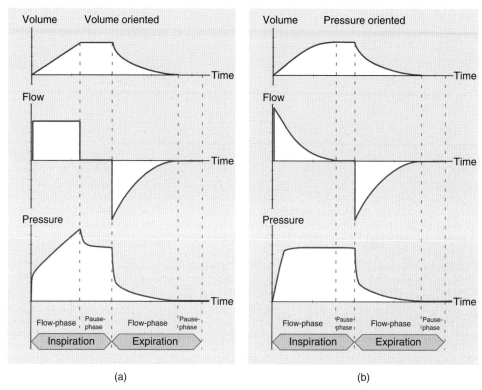

Figure 5.9 (a) Pressure, volume and flow curves for volume-cycled ventilation. (b) Pressure, volume and flow curves for pressure-cycled ventilation. © Dräger Medical AG & Co. KG, Lübeck, Germany. (All rights reserved. Not to be reproduced without written permission, nor stored in a data system, transmitted electronically or mechanically, by photocopying or photographing, in any way, shape, or form, in its entirety or in any part.)

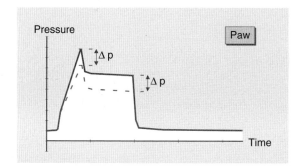

Figure 5.10 Changes in compliance. © Dräger Medical AG & Co. KG, Lübeck, Germany. (All rights reserved. Not to be reproduced without written permission, nor stored in a data system, transmitted electronically or mechanically, by photocopying or photographing, in any way, shape, or form, in its entirety or in any part.)

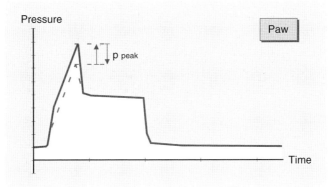

Changes in inspiratory airway resistance

Airway resistance changes are seen as alterations in the peak pressure but the plateau pressure remains the same (Figure 5.11). Therefore, if airway resistance increases, the peak pressure will increase and a reduction in airway resistance will lead to a drop in peak pressure.

Insufficient inspiratory time

If the inspiratory time is not long enough, the flow curve does not return to zero during inspiration (Figure 5.12).

Insufficient expiratory time

If the flow curve does not return to zero during expiration, there is insufficient time for full expiration to occur (Figure 5.13). This could lead to intrinsic PEEP and can be due to an increase in lung pressure during volume-cycled ventilation.

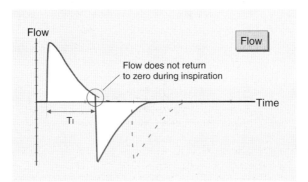

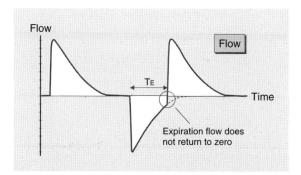

Figure 5.13 Flow curve with insufficient expiratory time. © Dräger Medical AG & Co. KG, Lübeck, Germany. (All rights reserved. Not to be reproduced without written permission, nor stored in a data system, transmitted electronically or mechanically, by photocopying or photgraphing, in any way, shape, or form, in its entirety or in any part.)

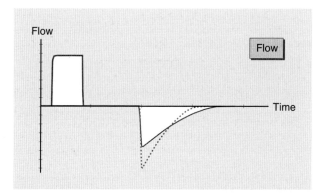

Figure 5.14 Flow curve with increased airway resistance. © Dräger Medical AG & Co. KG, Lübeck, Germany. (All rights reserved. Not to be reproduced without written permission, nor stored in a data system, transmitted electronically or mechanically, by photocopying or photgraphing, in any way, shape, or form, in its entirety or in any part.)

Changes in expiratory airway resistance

A more gentle expiratory flow curve indicates that there is an increase in expiratory airway resistance (Figure 5.14). This could lead to an increase in expiratory time and deviations from the set PEEP.

Loops

Pressure–volume loop

The pressure–volume (PV) loop, as well as the relationship between the pressure and the volume, is a good indication of lung compliance. The PV loop shows how compliance develops as volume is delivered. Initially, the pressure:volume increases rapidly and once the lower inflection point is reached, rises steeply. The lower inflection point indicates the lung opening pressure. If the lung reaches the limits of its compliance, any further pressure:volume increases will cause the loop to become bigger again. This is represented by the upper inflection point on the loop. It is generally considered that mechanical ventilation should take place within the linear compliance of the lungs – that is, between

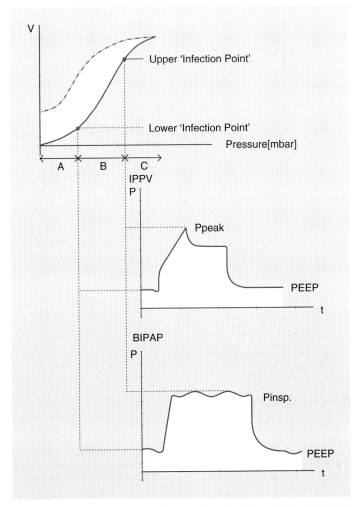

Figure 5.15 PV loop with upper and lower infection points. © Dräger Medical AG & Co. KG, Lübeck, Germany.

the lower and the upper inflection points. PEEP can overcome the lower inflection point, whereas the set volume (on volume-cycled ventilation) or pressure limit (on pressure-cycled ventilation) can be altered so that the upper inflection point is not reached. This avoids shearing forces within the lungs (Figure 5.15).

During mechanical ventilation, if the flow is constant, the PV loop can give useful information in relation to lung compliance. However, in decelerating flow, conclusions cannot be made about lung compliance because the pattern of flow delivery will contribute to the shape and 'steepness' of the PV loop.

PV loop in volume-cycled flow-constant ventilation

During inspiration, the lungs are filled with gas flow that has been pre-determined. This gradually increases the pressure in the lungs and will be equal to the pressure in the breathing system at the end of inspiration, and therefore the plateau pressure has been reached. During expiration, the exhalation valve in the ventilator is opened wide to maintain the set PEEP. Because there will be a difference between the pressure inside the lungs and the PEEP pressure, gas will flow out of the lungs and the volume will decrease. Therefore, the PV loop is anticlockwise during controlled ventilation.

PV loop in pressure-cycled decelerating flow ventilation

Again, the PV loop runs anticlockwise, but in this situation, the flow is not constant, and therefore the lungs are not filled with an even flow of gas. At the beginning of inspiration, the ventilator generates a pressure in the breathing system, which is greater than the pressure in the lungs. That pressure is maintained throughout inspiration. Because there is a difference in the pressure between the system and the lungs, gas flows into the lungs and the volume increases. This increases the pressure inside the lungs and therefore the difference between the respiratory system pressure and the lung pressure becomes smaller. Because the difference in the pressure determines the flow, as the lungs fill and the difference between the pressures becomes smaller, the flow also reduces – hence decelerating flow occurs. The PV loop is pressure cycled, and the decelerating flow is more rectangular in shape in comparison with the loop generated in volume-cycled constant flow ventilation. This is because the pressure is relatively constant throughout inspiration.

Interpretation of changes in the PV loop

Decrease in compliance

If the lungs become stiffer, the PV loop in volume-cycled ventilation becomes flatter, with the change in the steepness of the inspiratory portion of the PV loop being proportional to the change in compliance.

Changes in resistance

If there are alterations in resistance, the steepness of the inspiratory limb remains unchanged, but the position of this limb is altered.

Lung over-expansion

During volume-cycled ventilation, if the lungs are becoming over-distended, the upper part of the inspiratory limb PV loop begins to flatten.

The flow volume (FV) loop

The flow volume (FV) loop can give information about airway resistance and whether secretions are present within the endotracheal/tracheostomy tube. A sawtooth-shaped loop is seen when there is increased airway resistance – a smoother loop following suctioning would suggest that the intervention has successfully removed secretions.

Evidence-based care

Several key changes have been decided upon in Susan's care. They predominately relate to the ventilator strategies that have been introduced.

Key consideration

Rationalise the changes made to Susan's mechanical ventilation.

Alterations to mechanical ventilation

Increasing Susan's PEEP to 15 cm H_2O

PEEP improves FRC and therefore pO_2. It can also help to recruit alveoli. PEEP can reduce cardiac output; so it is important to optimise PEEP without compromising haemodynamics. Several methods to enable this have been suggested (Bersten, 2003b). For example, maximum oxygen delivery (oxygen content × flow) or the oxygen index could be used to guide PEEP. However, avoidance of repeated opening and closing of alveoli is now seen to be the primary aim, because this can help avoid the development of lung injury secondary to shear forces in the alveoli.

The lower inflection point of the pressure–volume curve of the lungs can be used to determine the level of PEEP, with PEEP set at or slightly above this point (Amato *et al.*, 1998). This can help to minimise inspiratory shear stresses, because the point of expansion on the compliance curve is already achieved through the use of PEEP and has been shown to reduce mortality (Amato *et al.*, 1998), although low tidal volumes and recruitment manoeuvres were also used.

In a multi-centred trial, the use of higher PEEP with low tidal volumes did not show any benefit or harm in comparison with lower PEEP (National Heart, Lung and Blood Institute ARDS Clinical Trials Network, 2004). However, another trial found that ARDS patients who were ventilated with high PEEP and low to moderate tidal volumes benefited in comparison with those who were ventilated with conventional tidal volumes and the least PEEP possible to obtain adequate oxygenation (Villar *et al.*, 2006).

The decision to increase Susan's PEEP to 15 cm H_2O is supported by research; however, it is recommended that there is close monitoring of blood pressure and oxygenation. If there is any deterioration in these, then this recruitment intervention should be discontinued (Dellinger *et al.*, 2008).

To aim for tidal volumes of 390 ml with a plateau pressure <30 cm H_2O

Susan weighs 65 kg and is currently receiving tidal volumes of 280 ml. It is recommended that the target tidal volume is 6 ml/kg, using the patient's predicted or ideal weight, while ensuring the plateau pressure is <30 cm H_2O (Dellinger *et al.*, 2008). Avoidance of large tidal volumes with high plateau pressures is recommended (Dellinger *et al.*, 2008) to improve mortality.

There have been a number of clinical trials that have been undertaken to establish how patients with ARDS should be ventilated (Amato *et al.*, 1998; Brochard *et al.*, 1998; The Acute Respiratory Distress Syndrome Network, 2000). Varying results have been found; however, the largest trial of a volume and pressure limited approach showed a 9% decrease in mortality when tidal volumes of 6 ml/kg (ideal weight) with a plateau pressure <30 cm H_2O were used (The Acute Respiratory Distress Syndrome Network, 2000). No specific mode of ventilation has been found to be more advantageous; therefore it is the lung-protective strategies that are of importance and which should be adhered to irrespective of the mode. There is an increased tendency, although, to use pressure-controlled ventilation because the pressures tend to be lower than those in volume-cycled ventilation, and the pressures can be well controlled, although the volumes may be variable. Also, differences in regional distribution of gas can occur in volume-cycled ventilation, leading to hyperinflation in more compliant areas of the lungs.

The above strategies have largely been introduced into clinical practice; however, consideration does need to be given to individual patients with the guidelines being adjusted as required. For example, in the situation of significantly reduced lung compliance, it may not be possible to maintain a tidal volume of 6 ml/kg within a plateau pressure of <30 cm H_2O. Then a decision will need to be made to either reduce the tidal volume or to reduce the pressure (e.g. by reducing the PEEP). It is suggested that if the plateau pressure remains >30 cm H_2O the tidal volumes could be reduced to as low as 4 ml/kg (Dellinger *et al.*, 2008), in an effort to reduce the intrathoracic pressures.

To allow the pCO_2 to rise if necessary

Permissive hypercapnia may be required if the above strategies of reduced tidal volumes and plateau pressures are introduced. Permissive hypercapnia can also occur as a consequence of inverse ratio ventilation, as the expiratory time becomes shortened, and therefore CO_2 excretion is reduced. There are consequences to elevated pCO_2 levels, such as vasodilation, tachycardia and increased cardiac output. Moderate increases in pCO_2 as a result of lower tidal volumes have been shown to be safe, although these trials were small and non-randomised (Bidani *et al.*, 1994; Hickling *et al.*, 1994). The ARDS Network (2008) suggests that respiratory rates of up to 35 BPM can be used to minimise the respiratory acidosis and that sodium bicarbonate may be required if the pH is <7.15. Permissive hypercapnia should not be introduced in situations of raised intracranial pressures.

To aim for a pO_2 > 8 kPa

The respiratory management of patients with ARDS requires a balance between the determinants of oxygenation (that is the extent of alveolar collapse and hypoxic vasocon-striction) and the target pO_2 (Bersten, 2003b). Cognitive impairment needs to be avoided; therefore, an $SaO_2 \geq 90\%$ or a $pO_2 > 8$ kPa is a reasonable target (Bersten, 2003b). However, the ARDS Network (2008) suggests that the oxygenation targets should be pO_2 of 55–80 mmHg (7.3–10.6 kPa) or SpO_2 of 88–95%.

Fraction of inspired oxygen (F_IO_2)
PEEP, as outlined, can be used to improve hypoxaemia; increases in F_IO_2 can also improve SaO_2. However, tissue damage, in the form of reduced lung compliance, oedema and fibrosis can occur with a high F_IO_2 because of oxygen toxicity. The mechanism of the toxic effects of oxygen is poorly understood, but it is thought that the oxygen directly affects the lung tissue. It is likely that oxygen free radicals are implicated in the development of the lung tissue injury (Cross *et al.*, 1994), with the protective antioxidants that are normally present within the respiratory tract becoming depleted by the prolonged oxidative challenge.

Oxygen toxicity is dependent on the concentration of oxygen as well as the duration of the exposure. However, again, it is unclear exactly how much oxygen is required to develop oxygen toxicity and for how long, as oxygen toxicity does not always develop when high concentrations of oxygen are used for a length of time. In healthy lungs, signs of oxygen toxicity usually do not occur with an F_IO_2 less than 50% (Klein, 1990) or 100% for less than 24 hours. Therefore, it is generally recommended that an initial F_IO_2 of 1.0 may be required, and then it should be titrated down, aiming for an F_IO_2 of ≤ 0.6.

Inverse ratio ventilation

Inverse ratio ventilation is often used in ARDS. This strategy increases the inspiratory time and therefore the potential for alveolar recruitment and oxygen delivery. There is a risk of the development of gas trapping and therefore intrinsic PEEP, which could compromise cardiac output as well as increase the pCO_2. The ARDS Network (2008) recommend that the inspiratory time is equal to or longer than the expiratory (i.e. an I:E ratio of 1:1 or 2:1).

Further strategies which could be considered

> **Key consideration**
>
> What other strategies could be used to enhance Susan's respiratory function and oxygenation?

To prone Susan

Prone positioning has been shown to improve alveolar recruitment of the dorsal lung as well as perfusion becoming more evenly distributed, therefore improving V/Q mismatching. The use of prone positioning is recommended in patients who require potentially injurious concentrations of oxygen or plateau pressures. Several trials have shown that pO_2 can improve when prone positioning is used (Lamm *et al.*, 1994; Stocker *et al.*, 1997; Jolliet *et al.*, 1998; Gattinoni *et al.*, 2001). Proning has not been shown to improve mortality but post hoc analysis has suggested that mortality may be reduced in patients with the most severe hypoxaemia as indicated by the oxygen index (Gattinoni *et al.*, 2001). A further multi-centred trial during which patients were proned for approximately 8 hr/day for 4 days again confirmed an improvement in oxygenation but not an improvement in survival (Guerin *et al.*, 2004). However, in a study when the patients were proned for, approximately 17 hr/day for 10 days, they had an improved mortality in relation to the control group; however, this was not statistically significant ($p = 0.12$) (Mancebo *et al.*, 2006).

The proning procedure itself has inherent risks such as accidental extubation/endotracheal tube dislodgement, cardiovascular complications and accidental removal of invasive monitoring equipment. Facial oedema can develop, and alternation of arm, leg and head positioning should be carried out.

To consider the use of prostacyclin nebulisers

Prostacyclin is a potent vasodilator and, when inhaled, is delivered to areas of well-ventilated lung. This helps to vasodilate the local pulmonary vasculature, which increases the redistribution of pulmonary blood flow away from poorly ventilated areas. This can then reduce right to left shunt and improve oxygenation.

Inhaled prostacyclin improves oxygenation as effectively as nitric oxide in ARDS patients. It needs to be continuously jet nebulised because it has a short half-life of 2–3 minutes. It may increase surfactant release (Bersten, 2003b) and avoids the noxious side effects of nitric oxide ventilation.

Mode of ventilation: dual control

Pressure-limited volume-cycled ventilation could be introduced. Modern ventilators allow closed loop control and thus control over both the tidal volume and the airway pressures, which offers the advantages of pressure-controlled and volume-controlled ventilation in combination. In dual control, there are two basic approaches.

First, the pressure waveform can be adjusted between breaths. Inspiration is pressure controlled within the breath but the pressure limit is automatically adjusted to achieve a preset target tidal volume. The initial pressure limit is set automatically on the basis of a calculated respiratory compliance. If the actual tidal volume based on the pressure limit is different from the set tidal volume, the pressure limit is adjusted up or down in an effort to achieve the set tidal volume. Although this is limited to 3 cm H_2O per breath, the process is repeated over several breaths until the desired tidal volume is achieved.

The other approach is to make adjustments within the breath to achieve the set tidal volume. The ventilator switches between pressure control and flow control within each breath, depending on whether a preset tidal volume is achieved. Therefore, for example, the ventilator may initially begin inspiration in flow control at the set flow rate. Once the airway pressure reaches the set pressure limit, the ventilator switches to pressure control at the set pressure limit, while the tidal volume is monitored. The inspiratory flow time (that is, the period from the beginning of inspiratory flow to the end of inspiratory flow) is periodically increased until the set tidal volume is achieved, provided that the set inspiratory time (the duration of time from the beginning of inspiration to the beginning of expiration) is long enough. It is important that health-care practitioners are aware of the ventilators that they use in practice and how the ventilator delivers dual controlled breaths.

Inhaled nitric oxide (iNO)

Nitric oxide (NO) is a smooth muscle relaxant and when inhaled, vasodilates the pulmonary blood vessels in well-ventilated areas of the lungs. Therefore, it acts in a similar manner to inhaled prostacyclin. Doses as low as 60 parts per billion may improve oxygenation; however, in ARDS, commonly used doses are 1 to 40 parts/billion. An improvement in $pO_2 \geq 20\%$ would be viewed as a positive response and the iNO should be administered at the lowest possible dose to obtain a positive response.

iNO can be administered continuously or using intermittent inspiratory injection. It is usually administered as NO/N_2, and both NO and NO_2 concentrations should be measured. Expired gases can be removed by a scavenging system; however, local environmental levels of NO and NO_2 are usually low. Methaemoglobin levels can be measured and monitored.

About 40–70% of ARDS patients respond favourably to iNO with an improvement in their oxygenation. When I.V. almitrine, which is a selective pulmonary vasoconstrictor in non-ventilated areas, was used in combination with iNO, oxygenation levels improved more than in the participants who received either iNO or almitrine (Gallart et al., 1998). Although the role of iNO in ARDS remains uncertain, two large clinical trials showed that iNO improved oxygenation but this response was not sustained beyond 12–24 hours (Dellinger et al., 1998; Lundin et al., 1999).

Extracorporeal membrane oxygenation (ECMO)

Extracorporeal membrane oxygenation (ECMO) has a high success rate (80%) when used in neonates with acute respiratory failure (Lewandowski, 2000); however, the same success rate has not been found when ECMO is used in adults with ARDS. The recent CESAR (Conventional Ventilation or ECMO for Severe Adult Respiratory Failure) trial in which 180 patients were recruited to either receive ECMO or conventional ventilation may give an insight into whether ECMO is beneficial to the adult patient with ARDS.

Conclusion

This chapter has illustrated that patients with ARDS need a high level of respiratory support and care to maintain oxygenation. This requires a collaborative approach to care provision and ongoing monitoring as the syndrome develops and evolves. Unconventional strategies to enable effective gas exchange may be required and this is a field of ongoing research and generation of evidence.

References

Acute Respiratory Distress Syndrome Network (2000) Ventilation with lower tidal volumes as compared with traditional tidal volumes for acute lung injury and the acute respiratory distress syndrome. *The New England Journal of Medicine* 342 (18) 1301–1308.

Amato MBP, Barbas CSV, Medeiros DM, *et al.* (1998) Effect of a protective ventilation strategy on mortality in the acute respiratory distress syndrome. *The New England Journal of Medicine* 338 (6) 347–354.

ARDS Network (2008) Mechanical Ventilation Protocol Summary NHLBI ARDS Network [online]. Available from: http://www.ardsnet.org/node/77791 [Accessed 25th September 2008].

Armstrong BW and MacIntyre NR (1995) Pressure controlled inverse ratio ventilation that avoids air trapping in the adult respiratory distress syndrome. *Critical Care Medicine* 23 (2) 279–285.

Bellingan GJ (2002) The pulmonary physician in critical care* 6: The pathogenesis of ALI/ARDS. *Thorax* 57 (6) 540–546.

Bernard GR, Artigas A, Brigham KL, *et al.* (1994) The American European Consensus Conference on ARDS: definitions, mechanisms, relevant outcomes and clinical trial coordination. *American Journal of Respiratory and Critical Care Medicine* 149 (3 pt 1) 818–824.

Bersten AD (2003a) Respiratory monitoring. Chapter 28 in Bersten AD and Soni N (Eds) *Oh's Intensive Care Manual.* 5th Edition, Butterworth Heinemann, London.

Bersten AD (2003b) Acute respiratory distress syndrome. Chapter 27 in Bersten AD and Soni N (Eds) *Oh's Intensive Care Manual.* 5th Edition, Butterworth Heinemann, London.

Bidani A, Tzouanakis RM, Cardenas VJ and Zwischenberger JB (1994) Permissive hypercapnia in acute respiratory failure. *JAMA* 272 (12) 957–962.

Brochard L, Roudot-Thoraval F, Roupie E, *et al.* (1998) Tidal volume reduction for prevention of ventilator induced lung injury in acute respiratory distress syndrome. *American Journal of Critical Care Medicine* 158 (6) 1831–1838.

Brun-Buisson C, Minelli C, Bertolini G, *et al.* (2004) Epidemiology and outcome of acute lung injury in European intensive care units results from the ALIVE study. *Intensive Care Medicine* 30 (1) 51–61.

Cross CE, van der Vliet A, O'Neill CAO and Eiserich JP (1994) Reactive oxygen species and the lung. *Lancet* 334 (8927) 930–933.

Davis K Jr , Branson RD and Campbell RS (1996) Comparison of volume control and pressure control ventilation: is flow waveform the difference? *Journal of Trauma* 41 (5) 808–814.

Dellinger RP, Levy MM, Carlet JM, *et al.* (2008) Surviving sepsis campaign: international guidelines for management of severe sepsis and septic shock. *Critical Care Medicine* 36 (1) 296–327.

Dellinger RP, Zimmerman JL, Taylor RW, *et al.* (1998) Effects of inhaled nitric oxide in patients with acute respiratory distress syndrome: results of a randomized phase II trial. *Critical Care Medicine* 26 (1) 15–23.

Esteban A, Alia I, Gordo F, *et al.* (2000) Prospective randomized trial comparing pressure-controlled ventilation and volume-controlled ventilation in ARDS. *Chest* 117 (6) 1690–1696.

Gallart L, Lu Q, Puybasset L, Umamaheswara Rao GS, Coriat P, Rouby JJ, The NO Almitrine Study Group (1998) Intravenous almitrine combined with inhaled nitric oxide for acute respiratory distress syndrome. *American Journal of Respiratory Critical Care Medicine* 158 (6) 1770–1777.

Gattinoni L, Tognoni G, Pesenti A, *et al.* Prone–Supine Study Group (2001) Effect of prone positioning on the survival of patients with Acute Respiratory Distress Syndrome. *New England Journal of Medicine* 345 (8) 568–573.

Guerin C, Gaillard S, Lemasson S, *et al.* (2004) Effects of systemic prone positioning in hypoxemic acute respiratory failure: a randomized controlled trial. *JAMA* 292 (19) 2379–2387.

Hickling KG, Henderson S and Jackson R (1994) Low mortality rate in adult respiratory distress syndrome using low volume, pressure limited ventilation with permissive hypercapnia: a prospective study. *Critical Care Medicine* 22 (10) 1568–1578.

Jolliet P, Bulpa P and Chevrolet JC (1998) Effects of the prone position on gas exchange and haemodynamics in severe acute respiratory distress syndrome. *Critical Care Medicine* 26 (12) 1977–1985.

Klein J (1990) Normobaric pulmonary oxygen toxicity. *Anesthesia and Analgesia* 70 (2) 195–207.

Lamm WJ, Graham MM and Albert RK (1994) Mechanism by which prone position improves oxygenation in acute lung injury. *Critical Care Medicine* 150 (1) 184–193.

Lewandowski K (2000) Extracorporeal membrane oxygenation for severe acute respiratory failure. *Critical Care* 4 (3) 156–168.

Lundin S, Mang H, Smithies M, Stenqvist O and Frostell C, European Study Group on Inhaled Nitric Oxide (1999) Inhalation of nitric oxide in acute lung injury: results of a European Multicentre study. *Intensive Care Medicine* 25 (9) 911–919.

Mancebo J, Fernandez R, Blanch L, *et al.* (2006) A multicenter trial of prolonged prone ventilation in severe acute respiratory distress syndrome. *American Journal of Respiratory Critical Care Medicine* 173 (11) 1233–1239.

Martin TR (1999) Lung cytokines and ARDS. *Chest* 116 2S–8S.

The National Heart, Lung and Blood Institute ARDS Clinical Trials Network (2004) Higher versus lower positive end-expiratory pressures in patients with the acute respiratory distress syndrome. *New England Journal of Medicine* 351 (4) 327–336.

Ranieri VM, Suter PM, Tortorello C, *et al.* (1999) Effect of mechanical ventilation on the inflammatory mediators in patients with acute respiratory distress syndrome: a randomized controlled trial. *JAMA* 282 (1) 54–61.

Rappaport SH, Shpiner R and Yoshihara G (1994) Randomized, prospective trial of pressure limited versus volume controlled ventilation in severe respiratory failure. *Critical Care Medicine* 22 (1) 22–32.

Stocker R, Neff T, Stein S, Ecknauer E, Trentz O and Russi E (1997) Prone positioning and low volume pressure limited ventilation improve survival in patients with severe ARDS. *Chest* 111 (4) 1008–1017.

Tsukahara Y, Morisaki T, Horita Y, Torisu M and Tanaka M (1999) Phospholipase A2 mediates nitric oxide production by alveolar macrophages and acute lung injury in pancreatitis. *Annals of Surgery* 229 (3) 385–392.

Villar J, Kacmarek RM, Perez- Mendez L and Aguirre-Jaime A, ARIES Network (2006) A high PEEP low tidal volume ventilatory strategy improves outcome in persistent ARDS: a randomized controlled trial. *Critical Care Medicine* 34 (5) 1311–1318.

Ware LB and Matthay MA (2000) Medical progress: the acute respiratory distress syndrome. *The New England Journal of Medicine* 342 (18) 1334–1349.

Woolf N (1995) *Cell, Tissue and Disease: The Basis of Pathology.* 3rd Edition, WB Saunders, London.

Zhang H, Slutsky AS and Vincent JL (2000) Oxygen free radicals in ARDS, septic shock and organ dysfunction. *Intensive Care Medicine* 26 (4) 474–476.

Chapter 6

The patient with chronic respiratory failure

Glenda Esmond and Anne McLeod

Introduction

Chronic obstructive pulmonary disease (COPD) is a major cause of morbidity and mortality and is currently the fourth leading cause of death in the world (World Health Organization, 2000). COPD is an umbrella term that includes bronchitis and emphysema, and affects the airways, lung parenchyma and pulmonary circulation. COPD is associated with bronchoconstriction of the airways, emphysema destroying gas exchange, skeletal myopathy affecting the muscle pump and pulmonary hypertension (Hurst, 2009). As the disease worsens, systemic features occur that include dyspnoea (breathlessness), muscle wasting, increased risk of cardiovascular disease, osteoporosis, anxiety and depression. The Global Initiative for Obstructive Lung Disease (GOLD) defines COPD as:

> *Chronic Obstructive Pulmonary Disease (COPD) is a preventable and treatable disease with some significant extrapulmonary effects that may contribute to the severity in individual patients. Its pulmonary component is characterized by airflow limitation that is not fully reversible. The airflow limitation is usually progressive and associated with an abnormal inflammatory response of the lung to noxious particles or gases.*
>
> (Rabe *et al.*, 2007)

Acute exacerbations of COPD trigger clinical deterioration and can result in respiratory failure due to inadequate alveolar ventilation necessitating admission to hospital and, in severe cases, may require transfer to the intensive care unit (ICU). It is a commonly held belief that patients with COPD admitted to ICU have poor outcomes. However, Breen *et al.* (2002) demonstrated that there was good survival of COPD patients who required mechanical ventilation, with 79.7% surviving to discharge. This is supported by Wildman *et al.* (2007) who identified that clinicians' prognoses were pessimistic and Davidson (2002) who identified that survival to hospital discharge of patients suffering exacerbations of COPD is better than other medical causes for ICU admission. Non-invasive ventilation (NIV) has reduced COPD admissions to ICU and even when there is a need for intubation and ventilation within ICU, it is possible to achieve extubation by using NIV as part of the weaning process. This negates the need to perform a tracheostomy and by reducing the length of time intubated, the risk of nosocomial infections also reduces.

Patient scenario

Joseph was a 68-year-old retired builder. He had a long history of COPD, which was stable but he had an acute exacerbation, necessitating hospital admission. On admission, his assessment was as follows:

HR   110 BPM
BP   150/100 mmHg (MAP 120)
RR   32 BPM
Temperature   36.8°C
SpO_2 82%

He was short of breath and only able to speak in short sentences. He was using his accessory muscles. Coarse crackles were noted in the lower bases of his lungs and he had expiratory wheeze. His arterial blood gases were as follows:

pH   7.26
pO_2 5.7 kPa (on room air)
pCO_2 9.3 kPa
HCO_3 26 mmol/l
BE   +8

Key consideration

What are the key physiological changes that occur in COPD?

Underlying physiology and pathophysiology

COPD results in airflow limitation caused by chronic inflammation with increased numbers of neutrophils, macrophages and lymphocytes, leading to mucus hypersecretion, narrowing of the small airways and destruction of the lung parenchyma, resulting in emphysemic changes. Mucus hypersecretion is a feature of chronic bronchitis and causes a chronic productive cough. In emphysemic lungs, the walls between the alveoli break down, the alveolar ducts dilate and there is loss of interstitial elastic tissue. This results in hyperinflation of the lungs and loss of normal elastic recoil, and therefore trapping and stagnation of air in the alveolar. As alveoli merge, there is loss of surface area for gaseous exchange, and this is further reduced by loss of permeability of the stretched and damaged alveolar.

As COPD progresses, gas transfer worsens, resulting in gas exchange abnormalities causing a ventilation perfusion (V/Q) imbalance or mismatch. Some gas exchanging (ventilation) parts of the lungs receive blood supply (perfusion) but no oxygen, and other parts receive oxygen but no blood supply. The severity of emphysema has been shown to correlate with arterial pO_2 and markers of V/Q imbalance. In severe disease, when peripheral airway obstruction is combined with ventilatory muscle impairment, ventilation is reduced, leading to carbon dioxide retention. The abnormalities in alveolar ventilation and a reduced pulmonary vascular bed further worsen the V/Q abnormalities.

Acute exacerbations of COPD can be triggered by both bacterial and viral infections and are clinically defined as a sustained worsening of symptoms that is beyond normal day-to-day variation and as the presence of two out of three symptoms of worsening breathlessness, cough and increased sputum purulence (National Institute for Clinical Excellence, 2004). An exacerbation of COPD causes an amplification of the inflammatory response in the airways, resulting in increased hyperinflation and air trapping with reduced expiratory flow and worsening of V/Q abnormalities. As a consequence, respiratory failure ensues and can result in hypoxaemia or type I respiratory failure ($pO_2 < 8$ kPa) or hypercapnia or type II respiratory failure ($pO_2 < 8$ kPa and $pCO_2 > 6$ kPa). This is largely the result of a shift to a rapid shallow breathing pattern and a rise in the dead space/tidal volume ratio of each breath (Calverley, 2003). The consequences of a raise in carbon dioxide is an increase in hydrogen ions (H^+), resulting in an increased acidity. As a compensatory mechanism, bicarbonate (HCO_3) is released. The acid–base status, measured by pH, depends upon the ratio of the total dissolved carbon dioxide (CO_2) and bicarbonate (HCO_3), with the body attempting to return the base:acid (HCO_3:pCO_2) ratio to 20:1. When this cannot be achieved, the pH lowers to <7.35 and, this, in combination with the raised carbon dioxide level, causes a respiratory acidosis.

Key consideration

What do the initial assessment findings indicate about Joseph's COPD?

Assessment and diagnosis

On hospital admission, Joseph was assessed using an ABCDE approach.

Airway

Joseph was talking, although not in full sentences due to his breathlessness inhibiting his ability to complete a sentence. However, despite the disruption in his speech, which can be attributed to his breathlessness, it can be assumed that his airway was patent. Talking to the patient also establishes psychological support, which for patients with COPD is important as breathlessness can cause anxiety (Bailey, 2004). Furthermore, by talking to Joseph, his level of cognition could be established, which needed to be considered in patients with an exacerbation of COPD, as severe hypoxaemia can result in cognitive impairment (Liesker *et al.*, 2004).

Breathing and ventilation

Joseph was self-ventilating; however, the quality of breathing needed to be assessed as this will indicate the presence of respiratory distress and inform the requirement of further assessment and investigations to inform treatment (Box 6.1).

From the initial physical examination, Joseph demonstrated signs of respiratory distress due to the underlying physiological changes associated with COPD. The following clinical signs and symptoms were observed.

Box 6.1 Initial respiratory assessment

Chest movement
Respiratory rate, rhythm and depth
Use of accessory muscles
Oxygen saturation (SpO_2)
Presence of central cyanosis
Auscultation
Cough ± productive
Temperature
Presence of ankle oedema
Presence of finger clubbing
Presence of CO_2 retention (facial flushing, bounding pulse, flapping tremor, headache)

Inspection

Joseph was breathless at rest with a respiratory rate of 32 BPM and 7 on the BORG dyspnoea scale (Borg, 1982). He was using his accessory muscles of breathing (sternocleidomastoid, scalenus, trapezius muscles), indicating that his work of breathing was increased. He reported having a chronic productive cough, with green sputum being expectorated, which has been gradually getting worse over 4 days. Central cyanosis was present, which is supported by oxygen saturation of 82% on air; in conjunction with this, severe finger clubbing caused by prolonged hypoxaemia was noted. Joseph had a flushed face and a bounding pulse, suggesting the possibility of carbon dioxide retention. Pitting ankle oedema was also noted, suggesting right-sided heart failure secondary to respiratory failure (*cor pulmonalae*).

Palpation and percussion

Bilateral reduction in lung expansion and increased resonance due to hyperinflated lungs were found.

Auscultation

Bilateral basal crackles were noted on auscultation as was a bilateral expiratory wheeze.

Key consideration

What further assessments/investigations will be undertaken and why?

Further assessment/investigations

Further assessment and investigations were indicated immediately, namely arterial blood gases, chest X-ray and full blood count.

Chest X-ray

The chest X-ray was undertaken to primarily exclude pneumonia although other abnormalities such as pneumothorax and focal lesions would be checked for. Figure 6.1 is Joseph's chest X-ray, which shows hyperinflated lungs but no signs of pneumonia, which was not surprising as he was apyrexial and there were no signs of consolidation on examination. The full blood count showed a raised white blood count (WBC), confirming the presence of infection and a normal haemoglobin (Hb) concentration, excluding anaemia as the cause of increased breathlessness.

Arterial blood gases

Arterial blood gas analysis was indicated by the presence of hypoxaemia, as observed by pulse oximetry and central cyanosis. However, pulse oximetry does not detect carbon dioxide levels and therefore to determine whether Joseph was in type I (hypoxaeamic) respiratory failure or type II (hypercapniac) respiratory failure arterial blood gases are required (Esmond and Mikelsons, 2009). Normal arterial blood gas values and changes that indicate type I or type II respiratory failure are shown in Table 6.1.

Joseph's arterial blood gases on air were as follows:

pH   7.26
pO_2 5.7 kPa (on room air)
pCO_2 9.3 kPa
SaO_2 82%
HCO_3 26 mmol/l

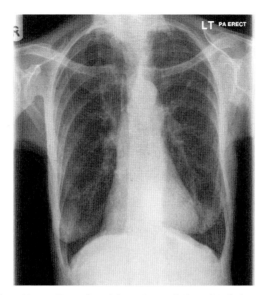

Figure 6.1   Joseph's chest X-ray. (Reproduced from Esmond G and Mikelsons C (2009) *Non-Invasive Respiratory Support Techniques: Oxygen Therapy, Non-Invasive Ventilation and CPAP.* Copyright 2009 with permission of Blackwell Publishing Ltd.)

Table 6.1   Arterial blood gas values

Value	Normal	Type I respiratory failure	Type II respiratory failure
pH	7.35–7.45	7.35–7.45	<7.35 (±)
pO_2	11–14 kPa	<8 kPa	<8 kPa
SaO_2	92–98%	<92%	<92%
pCO_2	4.5–6.0 kPa	4.5–6.0 kPa	>6.0 kPa
HCO_3	22–26	22–26	>26

The arterial blood gases show that Joseph is in type II respiratory failure as hypoxaemia and hypercapnia are present. Furthermore, there is a respiratory acidosis as the carbon dioxide (pCO_2) levels are raised and the pH is low. There is no compensation occurring as the bicarbonate (HCO_3) levels are not raised. This indicates that the changes in his blood gases are acute rather than a chronic alteration. If the respiratory acidosis is not corrected through adequate ventilatory support, the prognosis of the patient is poor (Ambrosino *et al.*, 1995).

Circulation

Joseph had a sinus tachycardia (100 BPM) and had mild hypertension (150/100 mmHg), both signs of hypoxaemia. Furthermore, the pulse was bounding, indicative of hypercapnia. There was peripheral oedema (pitting ankle oedema) and a raised jugular venous pressure (JVP), indicative of right-sided heart failure secondary to respiratory failure, also known as *cor pulmonalae*. This is caused by the pulmonary capillary vasoconstriction, requiring the right ventricle to generate higher pressures to overcome the increased right ventricular afterload. The right ventricle becomes enlarged by overworking and is unable to pump all the blood through the lung, resulting in a damming effect. Because of the high pressure in the veins, fluid is pushed out into the tissues, resulting in peripheral oedema (Wilkins *et al.*, 2000).

Disability

COPD is a major cause of disability which is linked to the impact of breathlessness and nutritional status (National Institute for Clinical Excellence, 2004). Joseph had a body mass index (BMI) of 20, which indicated that he was borderline malnourished. The impact of malnutrition is that it impairs skeletal muscle function and reduces diaphragmatic mass associated with a decrease in both strength and endurance of the respiratory muscles (Ferreira *et al.*, 2000). The level of disability caused by breathlessness can be measured using the functional Medical Research Council (MRC) dyspnoea scale. Prior to his admission to hospital, Joseph had an MRC dyspnoea score of 3 (walks slower than contemporaries on the level because of breathlessness, or has to stop for breath when walking at own pace). Joseph's level of consciousness was also assessed and his Glasgow Coma Scale (GCS) score was 15, indicating that he was not neurologically compromised.

Exposure

Joseph is a smoker and currently smokes 10 cigarettes per day; he has accumulated 42 pack years and this exposure to tobacco is the cause of his COPD. It is important to consider that nicotine withdrawal can cause agitation and therefore nicotine replacement therapy (NRT) should be considered if there are signs of withdrawal. During full examination of Joseph, it was necessary to expose his body; however, this should be undertaken to respect privacy and dignity.

Evidence-based care

> **Key considerations**
>
> Based on the clinical assessment what care is clinically indicated?
> How will Joseph's care be clinically prioritised?

The care priorities in managing Joseph are as follows:

- Oxygenation to correct hypoxaemia
- Ventilation to reduce carbon dioxide levels and to correct the respiratory acidosis
- Treatment of underlying exacerbation of COPD causing respiratory failure
- Treatment of *cor pulmonalae*

Oxygenation

Joseph was commenced on 28% oxygen via a Venturi face mask as this is a fixed performance oxygen device using the Bernoulli principle (Mitrouska *et al.*, 2006), thereby delivering precise levels of supplemental oxygen. This is necessary as Joseph's arterial blood gases show type II respiratory failure (low pO_2, high pCO_2) and therefore is sensitive to oxygen. In severe COPD, there is an increased risk of carbon dioxide retention due to a reduced hypoxic respiratory drive and increased ventilation–perfusion (V/Q) mismatch. Carbon dioxide retention is more likely to occur during exacerbations, which Rudolph *et al.* (1977) suggest, is due to a difference in hypoxic ventilatory sensitivity between stable disease state and exacerbation. If high concentrations of inspired oxygen is administered to those at risk of type II respiratory failure, this can lead to carbon dioxide retention ($pCO_2 > 6.0$ kPa) and a subsequent respiratory acidosis (pH < 7.35) through worsening V/Q mismatching and/or inducing a degree of hypoventilation (Calverley, 2003). It is relatively uncommon to have oxygen-induced carbon dioxide retention with low flow oxygen; hence patients with COPD are initiated on 24 or 28% oxygen (Georgopolous and Anthonisen, 1990). The F_IO_2 can then be titrated upwards to reach the target oxygen saturation, provided that arterial blood gases indicate that it is necessary and can be done without causing carbon dioxide retention. The British Thoracic Societies guideline for emergency oxygen use in adult patients (British Thoracic Society, 2008) recommends the following oxygen saturation target ranges:

- 94–98% for patients aged below 70
- 92–98% for those aged 70 or above
- 88–92% for those at risk of hypercapnic respiratory failure

The aim is to correct hypoxaemia, thereby preventing tissue hypoxia and secondary complication such as *cor pulmonalae*. Joseph's target saturation, therefore, was 88–92%.

Supplemental oxygen alone was not sufficient to manage Joseph's respiratory failure as his arterial blood gases showed a respiratory acidosis (high pCO_2, low pH), and therefore ventilatory support is indicated. If, however, there was carbon dioxide retention without a respiratory acidosis, then controlled supplemental oxygen therapy may be sufficient to manage the exacerbation as there is time for the medication (e.g. antibiotics, steroids and diuretics) treating the underlying exacerbation to improve respiratory function. It is therefore important in patients at risk of type II respiratory failure that arterial blood gases are used to guide the decision-making, as it is the pH that will determine what respiratory support is required. Furthermore, it will allow the most appropriate care setting (i.e. respiratory ward, high dependency unit, ICU) to be chosen so that the expected clinical outcomes are achieved. Figure 6.2 represents the decision-making process for management of type II respiratory failure using pH to guide treatment and environment.

Joseph's arterial blood gases were taken on air and on 28% oxygen therapy (Table 6.2).

The arterial blood gases showed an improvement in oxygenation, although this fell below 88–92% as recommended by the British Thoracic Societies guideline for emergency oxygen use in adult patients (British Thoracic Society, 2008). It was not possible to increase Joseph's F_IO_2 further to achieve a target saturation of 88–92%, as 28% oxygen was already causing a raise in carbon dioxide (pCO_2). This, along with the presence of a low pH, indicated the need for the addition of ventilatory support. As the pH was 7.26 and he was haemodynamically stable, therefore NIV should be considered. It should be possible to initiate the same within a respiratory ward (Plant *et al.*, 2000), although the ICU should be made aware that if there was further deterioration there may be a need for him to be intubated.

Non-invasive ventilatory support

Key consideration

Rationalise the use of NIV in the critical care setting.

NIV should be considered for patients with an acute exacerbation of COPD in whom respiratory acidosis (pH < 7.35) persists despite optimal medical management including oxygen therapy (British Thoracic Society Standards of Care Committee, 2002). There are several randomised controlled trials (RCT)s (Keenan *et al.*, 2003; Lightowler *et al.*, 2003; Ram *et al.*, 2004) that have demonstrated that NIV

- improves survival;
- reduces the need for intubation;
- reduces rate of complications;
- reduces need for ICU;
- shortens hospital and ICU lengths of stay.

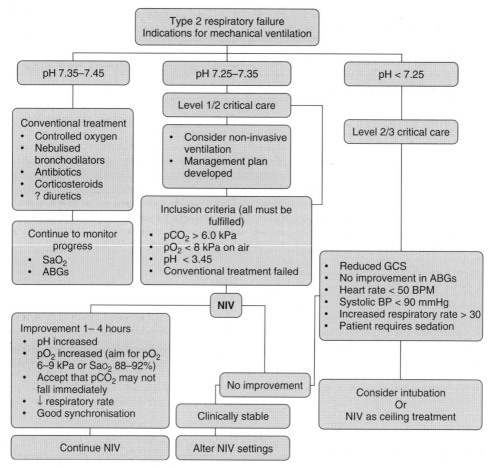

Figure 6.2 Decision-making for management of type II respiratory failure. (Reproduced from Esmond G and Mikelsons C (2009) *Non-Invasive Respiratory Support Techniques: Oxygen Therapy, Non-Invasive Ventilation and CPAP*. Copyright 2009 with permission of Blackwell Publishing Ltd.)

Table 6.2 Arterial blood gas results on air and oxygen

Value	On air	On 28% oxygen
pH	7.26	7.26
pO_2	5.7 kPa	6.9 kPa
SaO_2	82%	86%
pCO_2	9.3 kPa	9.7 kPa
HCO_3	26 mmol/l	26 mmol/l

Non-invasive ventilation and COPD

NIV is recommended for patients with acute exacerbation of COPD to avoid further deterioration necessitating admission to a level 3 (ICU) setting (Critical Care Programme Report, 2002). NIV is now widely available and should be used as a treatment strategy in COPD patients with a respiratory acidosis who meet the criteria for its use (Box 6.2).

Box 6.2 Criteria for use of non-invasive ventilation in acute respiratory failure

Acute hypercapnic respiratory failure
Respiratory acidosis (pH 7.25–7.35)
Inability to correct oxygen due to hypercapnia
Treatment of underlying condition optimised
Ability to protect airway
Conscious and cooperative
No excessive respiratory secretions
Potential for recovery to quality of life acceptable to the patient
Patient's wishes considered

Although it is not possible to predict which patients will have a successful outcome with NIV, factors that have been linked to unsuccessful episodes of treatment were associated with severely deranged baseline pH and pCO_2, a low BMI, the presence of pneumonia, a severe level of neurological deterioration and an inability to comply with ventilation (Ambrosino *et al.*, 1995).

Commencing non-invasive ventilation

The timing and place of the use of NIV will be determined by severity of the respiratory acidosis. NIV should not replace the use of intubation and ventilation where it is the most appropriate treatment. When intubation is indicated, then NIV can be used as an adjunct to weaning. However, Antonelli *et al.* (1998) found that those having invasive ventilation had more complications and more had pneumonia or sinusitis related to the endotracheal tube. Complications of intubation as identified by Ambrosino and Vagheggini (2008) are outlined in Box 6.3.

Box 6.3 Complications of intubation

Related to tube insertion
Aspiration of gastric contents
Trauma of teeth, pharynx, oesophagus, larynx and trachea
Sinusitis (nasotracheal intubation)
Need for sedation
Related to mechanical ventilation
Arrhythmias and hypotension
Barotrauma
Related to tracheostomy
Haemorrhage
Trauma of trachea and oesophagus
False lumen intubation
Stomal infections and mediastinitis
Tracheomalacia, tracheal stenoses and granulation tissue formation
Tracheo-oesophageal or tracheoarterial fistulas
Caused by loss of airway defence mechanisms
Airway colonisation with gram-negative bacteria
Pneumonia
Occurring after removal of the endotracheal tube
Hoarseness, sore throat, cough and sputum
Haemoptysis
Vocal cord dysfunction and laryngeal swelling

(Ambrosino and Vagheggini, 2008)

The use of NIV can avoid these complications and, therefore, should be used in the first instance. NIV is more likely to be effective if it is introduced earlier than when invasive ventilation would normally be clinically indicated (Critical Care Programme Report, 2002).

Therefore, Joseph was commenced on bilevel positive airway pressure (BiPAP) with the following settings:

IPAP	16 cm H_2O
EPAP	4 cm H_2O
BPM	12
F_IO_2	28%

Principles of non-invasive ventilation

As a form of pressure-cycled ventilation, BiPAP uses two alternating pressure levels to enable effective ventilation: a higher level on inspiration and a lower one on expiration. The inspiratory positive airway pressure (IPAP) provides support on inspiration so that larger inspiratory volumes are taken. The IPAP also reduces the work of breathing and increases alveolar ventilation (Tully, 2002). The expiratory positive airway pressure (EPAP) creates less resistance and discomfort on expiration as well as preventing alveolar collapse and increasing functional residual capacity. Larger tidal volumes are achieved, thereby improving carbon dioxide clearance (Calzia and Radermacher, 1997). Increasing the difference between the IPAP and the EPAP increases the pressure support (PS) for the breath and this augmentation of the tidal volume will enhance carbon dioxide clearance.

Joseph's arterial blood gases were measured after 1 hour, which is supported by studies that identified that significant changes in pH, pO_2 and pCO_2 could be achieved within 1 hour of treatment with NIV (Bott *et al.*, 1993; Brochard *et al.*, 1994; Kramer *et al.*, 1995). Although at 1 hour there was an improvement in the arterial blood gases, Joseph was becoming more fatigued and finding it difficult to tolerate the BiPAP. Four hours after commencing BiPAP, there were signs of clinical deterioration and his findings of arterial blood gases were as follows:

pH	7.22
pO_2	6.4 kPa (on 28% oxygen)
pCO_2	10.9 kPa
SaO_2	84%
HCO_3	28 mmol/l

The increase in carbon dioxide (pCO_2) has caused a worsening respiratory acidosis, hence the decision to transfer Joseph to the ICU so that he can be intubated and ventilated.

Ongoing patient scenario

On the ward round on Day 3 of being intubated and ventilated in the ICU, it is decided to wean him from mechanical ventilatory support. Joseph's acute exacerbation has been controlled; however, if weaning is unsuccessful, the medical staff feel that it is likely he will require a tracheostomy. He has been lightly sedated but is obeying commands.

His current ventilator settings are as follows:

Mode	SIMV (PC) and PS
PC level	18 cm H_2O
PEEP	8 cm H_2O
PS	18 cm H_2O
RR	10 BPM
F_IO_2	35%

His tidal volumes are 430 ml.

His blood gases are as follows:

pH   7.41
pO₂   14 kPa
pCO₂   5.5 kPa
SaO₂   98%
HCO₃   30 mmol/l
BE   +6

Weaning from ventilatory support

Key considerations

What tools can be used to assess Joseph's abilities to successfully wean from mechanical ventilatory support?
Rationalise strategies to enable Joseph's successful weaning.
What is the role of the nurse to enable successful weaning?

Weaning from mechanical ventilation is an essential component of successful ICU care but can be challenging. As prolonged ventilation is associated with significant mortality and morbidity, weaning should be considered as early as possible. This requires early and frequent assessment of readiness to wean. Boles *et al.* (2007) view weaning as a staged process made up of assessment of readiness to wean, a spontaneous breathing trial (SBT) and then onto extubation or continued mechanical support. This is a cyclic process which may need to be repeated on several occasions if the first attempt is unsuccessful.

Stage 1: Readiness to wean

Several parameters can be used to assess whether weaning should be attempted (Table 6.3). Joseph has achieved these parameters.

In addition to these parameters, there are several tools which have a greater predictive value for successful weaning.

Table 6.3   Bedside weaning parameters

Parameter	Normal range	Threshold for weaning
pO₂:F₁O₂ (oxygen index)	53.3 kPa (>400 mmHg)	20 kPa (150 mmHg)
Tidal volume	5–7 ml/kg	5 ml/kg
Respiratory rate	14–18/min	<35/min
Vital capacity	65–75 ml/kg	10 ml/kg

F₁O₂ < 0.4; PEEP ≤ 8 cm H₂O
Adequate cough
Absence of excessive tracheobronchial secretion
Resolution of acute phase of the disease for which the patient was intubated
Adequate mentation
Cardiovascular stability

(Adapted from Boles *et al.* [2007] Weaning from mechanical ventilation. *European Respiratory Journal* 29 (5) 1033–1056.)

Maximum inspiratory pressure

The strength of the respiratory muscles can be assessed by the patient exhaling and then inhaling as forcefully as possible against a closed valve. The pressure generated by doing this manoeuvre is the maximum inspiratory pressure (P_{Imax}). Normally, men can achieve a $P_{Imax} > -120$ cm H_2O whereas women achieve $P_{Imax} > -90$ cm H_2O (Marino, 1998). A P_{Imax} around -20 to -30 cm H_2O is the threshold for predicting a successful wean. However, it should be emphasised that a low P_{Imax} is useful for identifying patients who will have difficulty weaning: an acceptable P_{Imax} does not necessarily mean the patient will have a successful wean (Marino, 1998).

Frequency:volume ratio

Patients who have rapid, shallow breathing are less likely to wean successfully. Therefore, their frequency:volume ratio (or rapid shallow breathing index [RSBI]) can be assessed. An $RR:V_T$ ratio is normally less than 50 breaths/min/l, and a ratio >100 breaths/min/l normally predicts that weaning will be unsuccessful (Chao and Scheinhorn, 2007). However, Chao and Scheinhorn claim that if the RSBI is <97 breaths/min/l, the patient can progress onto a spontaneous breathing trial.

Once a patient has been assessed as ready to wean, a 30-minute SBT should be initiated (Boles *et al.*, 2007).

Stage 2: Spontaneous breathing trial (SBT)

There are two general approaches to SBTs and there appears to be no real statistic difference between them in view of patient success in the SBT or percentage of patients successfully extubated (Boles *et al.*, 2007).

T-piece SBT

In this approach, the patient is removed from ventilator support and receives humidified oxygen via a T-piece. The length of time on the T-piece will usually depend on how well the patient copes. If the patient appears to become distressed or their respiratory status deteriorates, mechanical support resumes and the patient recovers. Then the trial is repeated until mechanical support is not required.

Low levels of pressure support SBT

During this SBT, low levels of PS (for example, 8 cm H_2O) is applied. PS is often considered to help overcome the resistance of the endotracheal tube. However, Boles *et al.* (2007) identify that the assumed resistance of an endotracheal tube may be similar to the increased resistance of an inflamed upper airway: therefore, the post-extubation work of breathing is best approximated without compensation for the resistance of the endotracheal tube. Again, the duration of the SBT will depend on whether the patient copes and can maintain his or her respiratory status on the low levels of PS.

Patients who fail an SBT often do so within 20 minutes of commencing the trial (Esteban *et al.*, 1999), so success rates for SBT are similar if the trial is 30 or 120 minutes long (Boles *et al.*, 2007). Patients, like Joseph, who have COPD may benefit from an SBT with 5–7.5 cm H_2O continuous positive airway pressure (CPAP), as this has been shown to be more successful during a 30-minute SBT in this patient group (Reissmann *et al.*, 2000).

Stage 3: Proceed to extubation if SBT is successful

The aim of the SBT is then to extubate the patient if the SBT is successful. Failure of the SBT is observed through physiological signs of distress – respiratory and systemic (Table 6.4).

Table 6.4   Failure criteria of spontaneous breathing trials

Subjective signs	Objective signs
Agitation/anxiety	$pO_2 \leq 6.6-8$ kPa (50–60 mmHg) (on 0.5 F_IO_2)
Cyanosis	$SaO_2 < 90\%$
Diaphoresis	$pCO_2 > 6.6$ kPa (50 mmHg) or an increase in
Reduced level of consciousness/confusion	$pCO_2 > 1.06$ kPa (8 mmHg)
Signs of increased effort, for example,	pH < 7.32 or an decrease in pH ≥ 0.07
• Increased use of accessory muscles	RSBI > 105 breaths/min/l
• Dyspnoea	RR > 35 BPM or increase by $\geq 50\%$
• Grimacing/facial signs of distress	HR > 140 BPM or increase by $\geq 20\%$
	Systolic BP > 180 mmHg or increase by $\geq 20\%$
	Systolic BP < 90 mmHg
	Arrhythmias

(Adapted from Boles *et al.* [2007] Weaning from mechanical ventilation. *European Respiratory Journal* 29 (5) 1033–1056.)

Failure to wean

In situations of failure to wean, the patient will need to continue to receive mechanical support. Weaning failure is fairly common with an estimated occurrence of 31% (Boles *et al.*, 2007). Therefore a decision needs to be made about which mode of ventilation should be used if a patient fails his or her SBT while maintaining a balance between respiratory capacity and load, respiratory muscle function and promotion of weaning.

Pressure-support ventilation (PSV)

Pressure-support ventilation (PSV) is often used as the mode of mechanical support to aid the weaning process. Esteban *et al.* (1995) found that daily or intermittent T-piece trials resulted in a quicker weaning than using synchronised intermittent mandatory ventilation (SIMV) or PSV. However, Brochard *et al.* (1994) demonstrated that PSV, in comparison with SIMV and intermittent T-piece trials, reduced weaning times. Vitacca *et al.* (2001) similarly found that PSV reduced duration of mechanical ventilation in difficult-to-wean patients. Boles *et al.* (2007) recommended the use of PSV as a weaning mode when the initial SBT failed.

Adaptive support ventilation

Several trials evaluating adaptive support ventilation (ASV) during weaning have found that it was associated with earlier extubation and fewer ventilator adjustments (Sulzer *et al.*, 2001; Cassina *et al.*, 2003; Petter *et al.*, 2003). However, these were undertaken in patients who were post-cardiac surgery and therefore may not be transferable to other patient groups. Also, in another trial, ASV, when compared with SIMV, was shown to be the worse weaning mode (Esteban *et al.*, 1995). Therefore, further studies are required, comparing ASV to other weaning modes.

Weaning protocols

Weaning protocols have been developed to enable the identification of patients who are ready to wean and to offer a guideline as to how the weaning process should occur.

Protocols such as these should reduce the length of time the patient is mechanically ventilated. Saura *et al.* (1996) found that the use of weaning protocol reduced length of time on mechanical ventilation and ICU stay by increasing the number of safe direct extubations. They should also enable nurses to take a proactive role in the weaning process. However, Rose and Nelson (2006) feel that in the ICU environment, where there is close collaboration between nursing and medical staff, autonomous nursing practice and highly educated staff, weaning protocols may have little impact. Weaning protocols, however, do offer useful guidance to junior staff by providing a uniform method of weaning practice (Blackwood and Wilson-Barnet, 2007).

Tracheostomy formation

Key consideration

When should a tracheostomy be considered?

Tracheostomy is now a relatively common intervention in ICU, with the introduction of percutaneous techniques undertaken by the intensivist on the ICU. Timing of a tracheostomy has not been clearly defined although Rumbak *et al.* (2004) found that early tracheostomy (within 2 days of admission) halved 30-day mortality and reduced pneumonia, length of patient stay and accidental extubation. Within this trial, though, 10 of the patients ($n = 60$) in the deferred tracheostomy group weaned successfully from ventilation without the need for a tracheostomy. This emphasises the need for better predictors of dependency on ventilation. There are a number of benefits and drawbacks of tracheostomy and these would need to be carefully considered in deciding if and when a tracheostomy will be undertaken (Table 6.5).

Weaning Joseph from invasive ventilation

Joseph successfully undertook an SBT and is now extubated. Prior to his SBT, it was decided to reduce his F_1O_2 to 0.24 and his positive end-expiratory pressure (PEEP) to 5 cm H_2O, with the aim of maintaining an oxygen saturation of 92% as per the British Thoracic Society (2008) guidelines. Without this proactive reduction in his oxygen levels, Joseph is at risk of hypoventilation due to loss of his hypoxic respiratory drive.

Table 6.5 Benefits and drawbacks to a tracheostomy

Benefits	Drawbacks
Improved patient comfort	Misplacement and displacement
Improved patient communication	Haemorrhage
Less sedation required	Risk of tube obstruction
Earlier weaning from mechanical support	Impairment of swallow reflexes
Improved respiratory mechanics	Tracheal stenosis
Reduced oropharyngeal trauma	Tracheal necrosis
Prevention of ventilator-acquired pneumonia	Patients can still aspirate with a cuffed tracheostomy tube in place
Decannulation can be planned following swallow assessment	Scarring

Following his extubation, Joseph is recommenced on BiPAP with the following settings:

IPAP   16 cm H_2O
EPAP   4 cm H_2O
BPM   12
F_1O_2 28%

Joseph's arterial blood gases taken with him on BiPAP are as follows:

pH   7.41
pO_2 8.2 kPa (on 28% oxygen)
pCO_2 5.9 kPa
SaO_2 93%
HCO_3 30 mmol/l

The strategy of extubation onto NIV for patients with COPD has been shown to reduce the time spent on mechanical ventilation by patients with difficulty in weaning (Girault *et al.*, 1999). Nava *et al.* (1998) compared two weaning methods, non-invasive PS ventilation by face mask and invasive PS ventilation by an endotracheal tube, and found that non-invasive PS ventilation during weaning of patients with COPD reduces weaning time, shortens the time in the ICU, decreases the incidence of nosocomial pneumonia and improves 60-day survival rates. This is supported by Udwadia *et al.* (1992) who found that the use of NIV reduced the length of time spent on the ventilator, resulting in a reduced length of hospital stay and by Restrick *et al.* (1993) who found significant improvements in both pO_2 and pCO_2 when NIV was used in weaning from full ventilation.

Joseph can now be transferred back to the respiratory ward where he can continue to be weaned from the BiPAP. Within 24 hours of being back on the ward, he is only using the BiPAP 2 hours in the morning and afternoon and overnight. When he is off the BiPAP he uses 2 l supplemental oxygen via nasal cannulae. Forty-eight hours later, he is off BiPAP and only receiving oxygen therapy. His arterial blood gases on air are as follows:

pH   7.41
pO_2 7.1 kPa (on air)
pCO_2 5.9 kPa
SaO_2 98%
HCO_3 30 mmol/l

Joseph is clinically stable and is now in type I respiratory failure (low pO_2, normal pCO_2), indicating the need to be discharged home on oxygen therapy. He is advised to use 2 l/min oxygen via nasal cannuae for at least 15 hr/day until he is reviewed in 6 weeks time as Seemungal *et al.* (2001) demonstrated that it takes up to 6 weeks post exacerbation to regain lung function.

Ongoing care

Key consideration

What ongoing health promotion will Joseph require to avoid similar admissions in the future?

Treatment for the underlying condition needs to be optimised and will include the following:

- Smoking cessation
- Pulmonary rehabilitation

- Flu vaccine annually and a pneumococcal vaccine
- Assessment and follow-up for long-term oxygen therapy (LTOT)
- Inhaled corticosteroid plus long-acting β_2-agonist and long-acting anticholinergic, ensuring that the patient has a good inhaler technique
- Mucolytic therapy

It is always important to review what steps could be taken to prevent or reduce the risk of further episodes of type II respiratory failure, and therefore strategies to prevent acute exacerbations should be employed. The development of self-management plans including providing patients with a course of antibiotics and steroids at home will allow the patient to self-manage their exacerbation without delay.

Conclusion

This chapter has illustrated how an acute exacerbation alters the physiology of patients with COPD. It has also highlighted the treatment of acute respiratory failure and how the ICU has an important role in managing patients who have severely deranged arterial blood gases. The use of NIV both within the ward and ICU setting has also been explored as well as how its use can reduce complications associated with intubation.

References

Ambrosino N, Foglio K, Rubini F, Clini E, Nava S and Vitacca M (1995) Non-invasive mechanical ventilation in acute respiratory failure due to chronic obstructive pulmonary disease: correlates for success. *Thorax* 50 (7) 755–757.

Ambrosino N and Vagheggini G (2008) Noninvasive positive pressure ventilation in the acute care setting: where are we? *European Respiratory Journal* 31 (4) 874–886.

Antonelli M, Conti G, Rocco M, *et al.* (1998) A comparison of non-invasive positive pressure ventilation and conventional mechanical ventilation in patients with acute respiratory failure. *New England Journal of Medicine* 339 (7) 429–435.

Bailey PH (2004) The Dyspnea-Anxiety-Dyspnea Cycle – COPD patients' stories of breathlessness: "It's Scary/When you Can't Breathe" *Qualitative Health Research* 14 (6) 760–778.

Blackwood B and Wilson-Barnett J (2007) The impact of nurse-directed protocolised-weaning from mechanical ventilation on nursing practice: a quasi-experimental study. *International Journal of Nursing Studies* 44 (2) 209–226.

Boles JM, Bin J, Connors A, *et al.* (2007) Weaning from mechanical ventilation. *European Respiratory Journal* 29 (5) 1033–1056.

Borg G (1982) Psychophysical bases of perceived exertion. *Medicine and Science in Sports and Exercise* 14 (5) 377–381.

Bott J, Carroll MP, Conway JH, *et al.* (1993) Randomised controlled trial of nasal ventilation in acute ventilatory failure due to chronic obstructive airways disease. *Lancet* 341 (8860) 1555–1557.

Breen D, Churches T, Hawker F and Torzillo PJ (2002) Acute respiratory failure secondary to chronic obstructive pulmonary disease treated in the intensive care unit: a long term follow up study. *Thorax* 57 (1) 29–33.

British Thoracic Society (2008) Guideline for emergency oxygen use in adult patients. *Thorax* 63 (Suppl VI) 1–73.

British Thoracic Society Standards of Care Committee (2002) BTS guideline: non-invasive ventilation in acute respiratory failure. *Thorax* 57 192–211.

Brochard L, Rauss A, Benito S, *et al.* (1994) Comparison of three methods of gradual withdrawal from ventilatory support during weaning from mechanical ventilation. *American Journal of Respiratory Critical Care Medicine* 150 (4) 896–903.

Calverley PMA (2003) Respiratory failure in chronic obstructive pulmonary disease. *European Respiratory Journal* 22 26s–30s.

Calzia E and Radermacher P (1997) Airway pressure release ventilation and biphasic positive airway pressure. *Clinical Intensive Care* 8 (6) 296–301.

Cassina T, Chioléro R, Mauri R and Revelly JP (2003) Clinical experience with adaptive support ventilation for fast track cardiac surgery. *Journal of Cardiothoracic Vascular and Anesthesia* 17 (5) 571–575.

Chao D and Scheinhorn D (2007) Determining the best threshold of rapid shallow breathing index in a therapist-implemented patient-specific weaning protocol. *Respiratory Care* 52 (2) 159–165.

Critical Care Programme Report (2002) *Weaning and Long-Term Ventilation*. NHS Modernisation Agency, Leicester.

Davidson AC (2002) The pulmonary physician in critical care * 11: critical care management of respiratory failure resulting from COPD. *Thorax* 57 (12) 1079–1084.

Esmond G and Mikelsons C (2009) *Non-Invasive Respiratory Support Techniques: Oxygen Therapy, Non-Invasive Ventilation and CPAP*. Wiley-Blackwell, Oxford.

Esteban A, Alia I, Tobin MJ, *et al.* (1999) Effect of spontaneous breathing trial duration on outcome of attempts to discontinue mechanical ventilation. Spanish Lung Failure Collaborative Group. *American Journal of Respiratory Critical Care Medicine* 163 (2) 874–880.

Esteban A, Frutos F, Tobin MJ, *et al.* (1995) A comparison of four methods of weaning patients from mechanical ventilation. The Spanish Lung Failure Collaborative Group. *New England Journal of Medicine* 332 (6) 345–350.

Ferreira IM, Brooks D, Lacasse Y and Goldstein RS (2000) Nutritional support for individuals with COPD: a meta-analysis. *Chest* 117 (3) 672–678.

Georgopolous D and Anthonisen NR (1990) Continuous oxygen therapy for the chronically hypoxemic patient. *Annual Review of Medicine* 41 223–230.

Girault C, Daudenthun I, Chevron V, Tamion F, Leroy J and Bonmarchand G (1999) Noninvasive ventilation as a systematic extubation and weaning technique in acute-on-chronic respiratory failure: a prospective, randomized controlled study. *American Journal of Respiratory and Critical Care Medicine* 160 (1) 86–92.

Hurst J (2009) Clinical management of respiratory failure. Chapter 1 in Esmond G and Mikelsons C (Eds) *Non-Invasive Respiratory Support Techniques: Oxygen Therapy, Non-Invasive Ventilation and CPAP*. Wiley-Blackwell, Oxford.

Keenan SP, Sinuff T, Cook DJ and Hill NS (2003) Which patients with acute exacerbation of chronic obstructive pulmonary disease benefit from non invasive positive pressure ventilation? A systematic review of the literature. *Annals of Internal Medicine* 138 (11) 861–870.

Kramer N, Meyer TJ, Mehang J, Cece RD and Hill NS (1995) Randomized, prospective trial of non invasive positive pressure ventilation in acute respiratory failure. *American Journal of Respiratory and Critical Care Medicine* 151 1799–1806.

Liesker JJW, Postma DS, Beukema RJ and ten Hacken NHT (2004) Cognitive performance in patients with COPD. *Respiratory Medicine* 98 (4) 351–356.

Lightowler JV, Wedzicha JA, Elliott MW and Ram FS (2003) Non invasive positive pressure ventilation to treat respiratory failure resulting from exacerbations of chronic obstructive pulmonary disease: Cochrane systematic review and meta-analysis. *British Medical Journal* 326 (7382) 185–189.

Marino PL (1998) *The ICU Book*. 2nd Edition, Lippincott Williams and Wilkins, Philadelphia.

Mitrouska I, Tzanakis N and Siafakas NM (2006) Oxygen therapy in chronic obstructive pulmonary disease. *European Respiratory Journal* 38 302–312.

National Institute for Clinical Excellence (2004) National clinical guidelines on management of chronic obstructive pulmonary disease in adults in primary and secondary care. *Thorax* 59 (Suppl. 1) 1–232.

Nava S, Ambrosino N, Clini E, *et al.* (1998) Noninvasive mechanical ventilation in the weaning of patients with respiratory failure due to chronic obstructive pulmonary disease. A randomised controlled trial. *Annals of Internal Medicine* 128 (9) 721–728.

Petter AH, Chioléro RL, Cassina T, Chassot PG, Müller XM and Revelly JP (2003) Automatic "respirator/weaning" with adaptive support ventilation: the effect on duration of endotracheal intubation and patient management. *Anesthesia and Analgesia* 97 (6) 1743–1750.

Plant PK, Owen JL and Elliott MW (2000) Early use of non-invasive ventilation for acute exacerbations of chronic obstructive pulmonary disease on general respiratory wards: a multicentre randomised controlled trial. *Lancet* 355 (9219) 1931–1935.

Rabe KF, Hurd S, Anzueto A, *et al.* (2007) Global strategy for the diagnosis, management, and prevention of chronic obstructive pulmonary disease: GOLD executive summary. *American Journal of Respiratory and Critical Care Medicine* 176 532–555.

Ram FS, Picot J, Lightowler J and Wedzicha JA (2004) Non-invasive positive pressure ventilation for treatment of respiratory failure due to exacerbations of chronic obstructive pulmonary disease. *Cochrane Database Systematic Reviews* 3 CD004104.

Reissmann HK, Ranieri VM, Goldberg P and Gottfried SB (2000) Continuous positive airway pressure facilitates spontaneous breathing in weaning chronic obstructive pulmonary disease patients by improving breathing pattern and gas exchange. *Intensive Care Medicine* 26 (12) 1764–1772.

Restrick LJ, Scott AD, Ward AD, Feneck RO, Cornwell WE and Wedzicha JA (1993) Nasal intermittent positive-pressure ventilation in weaning intubated patients with chronic respiratory disease from assisted intermittent positive-pressure ventilation. *Respiratory Medicine* 87 (3) 199–204.

Rose L and Nelson S (2006) Issues in weaning from mechanical ventilation: a literature review. *Journal of Advanced Nursing* 54 (1) 73–85.

Rudolph M, Banks RA and Semple SJ (1977) Hypercapnia during oxygen therapy in acute exacerbations of chronic respiratory failure. Hypothesis revisited. *Lancet* 2 (8036) 483–486.

Rumbak MJ, Newton M, Truncale T, Schwartz SW, Adams JW and Hazard PB (2004) A prospective randomized study comparing early percutaneous dilational tracheostomy to prolonged intubation (delayed tracheostomy) in critically ill medical patients. *Critical Care Medicine* 32 1689–1694.

Saura P, Blanch L, Mestre J, Vallés J, Artigas A and Fernández R (1996) Clinical consequences of the implementation of a weaning protocol. *Intensive Care Medicine* 22 (10) 1052–1056.

Seemungal T, Harper-Owen R, Bhowmik A, *et al.* (2001) Respiratory viruses, symptoms, and inflammatory markers in acute exacerbations and stable chronic obstructive pulmonary disease. *American Journal of Respiratory Critical Care Medicine* 164 (9) 1618–1623.

Sulzer CF, Chioléro R, Chassot PG, Mueller XM and Revelly JP (2001) Adaptive support ventilation for fast tracheal extubation after cardiac surgery: a randomized controlled study. *Anesthesiology* 95 (6) 1339–1345.

Tully V (2002) Non-invasive ventilation: a guide for nursing staff. *Nursing in Critical Care* 7 (6) 296–299.

Udwadia ZF, Santis GF, Steven MH and Simonds AK (1992) Nasal ventilation to facilitate weaning in patients with chronic respiratory insufficiency. *Thorax* 47 (9) 715–718.

Vitacca M, Vianello A, Colombo D, *et al.* (2001) Comparison of two methods for weaning patients with chronic obstructive pulmonary disease requiring mechanical ventilation for more than 15 days. *American Journal of Respiratory and Critical Care Medicine* 164 (2) 225–230.

Wildman MJ, Sanderson C, Groves J, *et al.* (2007) Implications of prognostic pessimism in patients with chronic obstructive pulmonary disease (COPD) or asthma admitted to intensive care in the UK within the COPD and asthma outcome study (CAOS): multicentre observational cohort study. *British Medical Journal* 335 1132.

Wilkins RL, Krider SJ and Sheldon RL (2000) *Clinical Assessment in Respiratory Care.* Mosby, St Louis.

World Health Organization (2000) *World Health Report.* World Health Organization, Geneva. http://www.who.int/whr/2000/en/statistics.htm [Accessed 15th May 2009].

Chapter 7

The patient with an intracranial insult

Anne McLeod

Introduction

Traumatic brain injury is a major source of disability, death and cost (emotional and financial) to society. It is important to recognise that the neurological damage that occurs often develops after the initial impact damage and it is the control of this secondary brain injury that is imperative. With the control of secondary brain injury, the patient's prognosis improves; this has been demonstrated by progressive and significant reductions in mortality from 50 to 35 to 25% (and lower) over the last 30 years (Lu *et al.*, 2005). This has largely occurred because of a change in focus on patient management with the emphasis on promotion of adequate cerebral perfusion. To enable this, protocols that focus on maintenance of neuronal perfusion have been developed and introduced into practice. This chapter will illustrate these developments.

Patient scenario

Mark was a 30-year-old man who was involved in a road traffic accident. He was wearing a seat belt and was driving speedily when he lost control of the car and drove it into a wall. He lost consciousness after he hit his head on the windscreen. He was intubated at the scene and mechanically ventilated on volume control (VC). He was sedated at the scene. He was taken to the emergency department on a backboard with a cervical collar.

On assessment, the following were found:

HR   125 BPM SR
BP   110/70 mmHg (MAP = 83)
SpO_2 96%

His ventilation observations were as follows:

RR   12 BPM
TV   450 ml
MV   5.4 l
AP   23 cm H_2O
F_1O_2 0.3

Blood gas analysis results were as follows:

pH   7.44
pO_2 12 kPa
pCO_2 4.8 kPa
HCO_3 20 mmol/l
BE   −2

His Glasgow Coma Score (GCS) was 5/15 (E_1, V_1, M_3) and his pupils were size 3 mm and briskly reacting.

A computed tomographic (CT) scan showed frontal contusions.

Mark had a primary head injury, which had significantly reduced his level of consciousness. He was at risk of developing secondary brain injury, which may compromise his cerebral perfusion, if his cerebral blood flow (CBF) is not maintained at physiologically safe levels. Those involved in his care need to have a clear understanding of underlying physiological mechanisms and rationale for care so that his prognosis is enhanced.

Underlying physiology and pathophysiology

Key considerations

What are the mechanisms of injury in relation to intracerebral insults?
What is the difference between primary and secondary brain injury?

Primary brain injury

The severity of a primary head injury following a traumatic injury, similar to that sustained by Mark, is largely dependent on degree of neuronal injury caused by the physical forces during the event. These lead to injury of the cerebral parenchyma and vasculature. Both acceleration and deceleration injuries, and possible rotational displacement, result in shearing forces, leading to structural damage to neurones and blood vessels. These can develop into cerebral contusions and lacerations as well as diffuse axonal damage. Contusions can be contra coup, with brain tissue at the site of the injury as well as on the opposite side of the injury being involved. This occurs when the force of the injury is such that the brain moves forward and backward inside the skull, 'banging' into the skull, thereby causing injuries on both aspects of the brain. Along with contusions, haematomas (such as extradural and subdural haematomas) and haemorrhage (e.g. traumatic subarachnoid haemorrhage) can also form as part of the primary injury.

Mark's body was flung forward as he hit the wall. The velocity of the impact would have displaced his brain backward within the skull but then his brain would have moved forward again. There his primary brain injury would have been caused by acceleration and deceleration forces, with the contusions forming as a consequence.

Secondary brain injury

Secondary brain injury is largely caused by a reduction of the substances that are required to maintain cerebral perfusion. Hypotension, hypoxia, hypoglycaemia, hyperpyrexia and hypocapnia (prolonged) have been shown to significantly worsen the prognosis of those who have sustained traumatic brain injury (Myburgh, 2003). In addition to systemic causes of secondary injury, intracranial causes such as formation of haematoma, vasospasm and seizures can also lead to the development of neuronal injury. Secondary injury can occur during the initial resuscitation and transfer to hospital or later, once the patient is in the critical care setting.

Cerebral metabolic needs

The brain is a highly metabolic organ accounting for about 15% of the body's metabolic activity. The brain utilises around 3–5 ml O_2/min/100 g and 5 mg glucose/min/100 g. Normal cerebral blood is 50 ml/min/100 g and contains around 20 ml O_2/100 ml; around 35–50% of that oxygen is used during metabolism. Glucose concentration is around 5.5 mmol/l; therefore, glucose delivery to the neurones is around 50 mg/min/100 g. Glucose extraction is minimal compared to that of oxygen; however, insulin is not required for the movement of glucose into the neurones.

Most of the cerebral metabolic activity occurs within the neurones rather than the supporting glial cells, with the primary requirement being for the maintenance and restoration of ionic concentrations, during and after depolarisation. However, neurones are unable to store glucose and are therefore limited in their ability to undergo anaerobic respiration as there is no local supply of glycogen to convert into glucose. Therefore, neurones rely on a continuous supply of both oxygen and glucose; without this, unconsciousness can occur within a few seconds, as neuronal activity is reduced.

Other causes of raised intracranial pressure

> **Key consideration**
>
> What else can cause elevations in intracranial pressure?

Although Mark had sustained a head injury, cerebral injury and raised intracranial pressure (ICP) are not solely confined to intracerebral causes. There are a few extracellular causes that can increase ICP and a number of extracellular causes that can reduce the level of consciousness (Table 7.1). Many of the treatment strategies outlined in this chapter

Table 7.1   Examples of causes of raised ICP and altered level of consciousness

Raised intracranial pressure		Altered level of consciousness	
Intracranial	**Extracranial**	**Intracranial**	**Extracranial**
Tumours	Hepatic encephalopathy	Tumours	Hypoxia
Haemorrhage	Disequilibrium syndrome	Haemorrhage	Hypercapnia
Haematoma	Hyponatraemia	Haematoma	Hypocapnia
Contusions	Pre-eclampsia/eclampsia	Infarction	Carbon monoxide
Abscesses		Contusions	Hypotension
Cerebral oedema		Abscesses	Hypoglycaemia
Hydrocephalus		Cerebral oedema	Hyperglycaemia
Encephalitis		Hydrocephalus	Hypothermia
		Encephalitis	Hyperthermia
		Meningitis	Drugs
		Neurodegenerative diseases	Sepsis
		Seizures/post-ictal phase	Elevated urea levels
			Liver failure
			Embolism (fat/air/amniotic fluid)

also apply to situations where there is increased ICP, irrespective of the cause. Therefore, for example, a patient with grade IV hepatic encephalopathy would have his or her ICP monitored and controlled in a manner similar to another patient with an isolated head injury.

Cerebral insult, therefore, has many causes but the mechanisms of injury are few. The most common is the lack of the essential precursors for energy: oxygen and glucose. This can occur separately, for example, hypoxia or hypoglycaemia, or in conjunction when there is reduced/absent perfusion (e.g. during ischaemia).

Neuronal protection

The brain has a number of important mechanisms to protect the neurones from ischaemia.

Collateral blood supply

The blood supply to the brain is largely derived from two pathways: the anterior (or carotid) and the posterior (or vertebral) systems. Each provides bilateral circulation. The anterior system supplies blood to the frontal, parietal and temporal lobes and anterior diencephalon (basal ganglia and hypothalamus). The posterior circulation supplies blood to the brainstem, cerebellum, occipital lobe and thalamus. Adequacy of cerebral arterial blood supply is maintained by connections or collaterals between each system: in adults, this is the circle of Willis, which joins the large branches of the anterior and posterior circulations at the base of the brain. This arrangement allows for maintenance of CBF even in situations when one of the blood supplies becomes impaired or occluded.

Cerebral blood flow

Blood flow to the brain and through the brain is highly regulated and determined by several factors.

Cerebral perfusion pressure

Cerebral perfusion pressure (CPP) is the difference between the arterial pressure in the feeding arteries as they enter the subarachnoid space and the pressure in the draining veins before they enter the dural sinuses. As both of these pressures are difficult to measure, CPP is seen to be the difference between mean arterial pressure (MAP) and ICP (as an estimate of tissue pressure).

The cerebral blood vessels will constrict or dilate to maintain a stable CPP: this ability to autoregulate blood flow through the cerebral vasculature is a key to ensuring that perfusion is constant. The diameter of the cerebral vessels change inversely with changes in pressure: as the CPP rises, the vessels constrict and if CPP reduces, the vessels dilate. Pressure autoregulation is thought to occur through local myogenic responses to changes in pressure; this, however, can only occur in a specific range: if the arterial pressure is outside of a range of 50–150 mmHg, CPP becomes pressure passive (Figure 7.1). This means that the perfusion pressure will follow the changes in arterial pressure, increasing or decreasing proportionally. The autoregulatory range does alter with age with a shift to the left for newborns and a shift to the right for those with chronic hypertension. Although this would not be of concern with Mark as he is unlikely to have chronic hypertension, it would need to be considered in patients who are normally hypertensive as overaggressive management of their hypertension within a critical care setting could put them at risk of ischaemic stroke as their blood pressure may be reduced to beyond *their* lower limit of autoregulation. However, Mark could be at risk of acute hypertension as part of a sympathetic response to the injury, which could increase his blood pressure

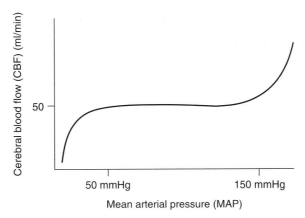

Figure 7.1 MAP–CBF diagram. (Reproduced from Mcleod A (2004) Traumatic injuries to the head and spine 2: nursing considerations, *British Journal of Nursing* 13 (17) 1041–1049, by permission of MA Healthcare Limited.)

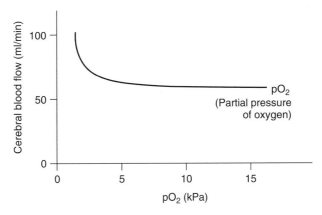

Figure 7.2 pO_2–CBF diagram. (Reproduced from Mcleod A (2004) Traumatic injuries to the head and spine 2: nursing considerations, *British Journal of Nursing* 13 (17) 1041–1049, by permission of MA Healthcare Limited.)

to above the limit of normal autoregulation: this would put him at risk of developing cerebral oedema due to increased hydrostatic pressure as well as hypertensive intracerebral haemorrhage.

pO_2 and pCO_2

Oxygen and carbon dioxide are both powerful influences of CBF. A normal pO_2 or even hyperoxic level of pO_2 leads to little change in blood flow but in situations of hypoxaemia, there is a rapid increase in CBF, which is proportional to the reduction in pO_2. This ensures that oxygen delivery remains constant despite the reduced oxygen content of arterial blood (Figure 7.2).

pCO_2 also directly influences CBF, with an increase in pCO_2 increasing blood flow. This is probably due to a requirement of the brain to maintain pH, and therefore by increasing blood flow, waste products of metabolism are removed more efficiently. pCO_2 can greatly influence blood flow as every 0.13 kPa (1.0 mmHg) change in pCO_2 alters CBF by 1–2 ml/min/100 g. This proportional correlation means that a doubling of pCO_2 will double CBF, whereas halving the pCO_2 will halve the CBF (Figure 7.3).

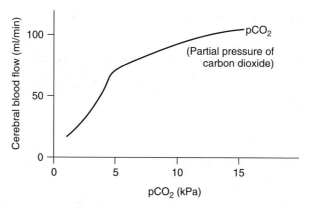

Figure 7.3 pCO_2 diagram. (Reproduced from Mcleod A (2004) Traumatic injuries to the head and spine 2: nursing considerations, *British Journal of Nursing* 13 (17) 1041–1049, by permission of MA Healthcare Limited.)

Control of intracranial pressure

> **Key consideration**
>
> How is intracranial pressure usually controlled?

Any increase in CBF and therefore cerebral blood volume can increase ICP. It is imperative that any increase in ICP is controlled to avoid cerebral ischaemia. ICP is normally a fluctuating pressure and is defined as the pressure exerted within the cerebral ventricles by the cerebrospinal fluid (CSF). A normal ICP is 0–10 cm H_2O, whereas anything more than 15 cm H_2O is considered to be raised.

Kellie–Monroe Doctrine

The brain has normal compensatory mechanisms to maintain the ICP at a normal level; this can be understood through the application of the Kellie–Monroe Doctrine, which states that as the skull has a fixed capacity, if there is an increase in one of the three intracranial contents, there must be a reciprocal reduction in one of the others if ICP is to remain stable. The three intracranial contents are brain (80%), blood (10%) and CSF (10%). The CSF is most able to reduce in volume as it can be shunted down to the lumbar theca as well as CSF production can be reduced and absorption increased. The brain is the least able to reduce in volume, and as the brain requires a constant blood flow, it may be undesirable to reduce the blood volume.

Cerebral compliance and elastance

The ability of the brain to compensate and control increases in intracranial volume is largely dependent on the compliance of the contents of the cranial vault. Cerebral compliance refers to how well the cranial contents can accommodate an increase in their volume. If compliance is high, increases in volume will not alter ICP. However, conversely, elastance refers to the stiffness of the cranial contents. If elastance is high, increases in volume are not well accommodated and will lead to deleterious changes in ICP. This can be life threatening.

Changes to cerebral blood flow following injury

As outlined, normally CBF is maintained at a constant rate despite changes in systemic pressure due to myogenic and metabolic autoregulatory mechanisms. However, these homeostatic mechanisms can become impaired following a head injury, especially the myogenic response. This has led to the recognition of distinct patterns of blood flow following a head injury.

The hypoperfusion phase

In the first 72 hours following a head injury, CBF is reduced by extrinsic and intrinsic mechanisms. This results in global and regional ischaemia. During this phase, myogenic mechanisms are significantly deranged, which means that CBF is pressure passive as autoregulation is impaired. During this phase, because of the neuronal ischaemia, cytotoxic oedema may develop, which will increase ICP. This will further reduce cerebral perfusion. It is, therefore, imperative that during this phase, cerebral perfusion is protected and any hypotension is effectively managed. Therefore, a good CPP of ≥ 70 mmHg should be aimed for (Myburgh, 2003).

The hyperaemic phase

The hypoperfusion phase is followed by the hyperaemic phase, during which normal autoregulatory responses begin to recover. This improves CBF and occurs in about one-third of patients who have sustained a head injury. It can last for up to 10 days post injury. During this time, due to the combination of inflammation, hyperaemia and altered blood–brain barrier permeability, vasogenic oedema can develop. Rather than aiming for an optimal CPP during this phase, an acceptable CPP of 60–70 mmHg should be achieved as this will reduce the risk of vasogenic oedema and raised ICP.

The vasospastic phase

In a small proportion of patients (10–15%), a vasospastic phase which is characterised by normal CBF patterns may be seen. This largely occurs in patients who have severe primary and secondary brain injury or those with significant traumatic subarachnoid haemorrhage. Cerebral perfusion is reduced as a consequence of arterial vasospasm, post-traumatic hypermetabolism and impaired autoregulation. In this situation, CPP needs to be supported by maintaining the MAP.

Assessment and diagnosis

As with any other patient, an ABCDE approach to patient assessment should be undertaken.

Airway

In Mark's case, his airway had been secured.

Breathing and ventilation

His breathing was being controlled by mechanical ventilation.

Circulation

Although Mark was tachycardic, his blood pressure was reasonable at this stage.

Disability

Mark's neurological status will need to be carefully and accurately assessed.

Glasgow Coma Score

His GCS was 5/15. This was significantly reduced and would suggest that he was in a coma, but he was being sedated in order to facilitate airway management and control of arterial blood gases. Therefore, his 'true' GCS may be higher than the level currently being demonstrated. However, he was flexing in response to central pain: if a patient is sedated, the best motor response gives a useful indication of the level of cerebral injury and prognosis (Myburgh, 2003). The GCS has limited use in the sedated, neurosurgical patient and does not necessarily accurately reflect changes in ICP or ongoing neurological injury such as development of ischaemia or infarction (Brunker, 2006): this is supported by Price *et al.*'s (2000) retrospective analysis of the use of GCS in this patient group, which suggests that the GCS is a poor predictor of changes in ICP and cerebral perfusion.

Pupillary response

Assessment of pupillary response is an essential part of neurological assessment. Brain stem compression is indicated by dilated pupils, which have a sluggish (or do not react) pupil response to bright light. This suggests dysfunction of the III cranial nerve (oculomotor) due to tentorial or tonsillar herniation as ICP increases to potentially lethal levels. Should one side of the brain stem become compressed, ipsilateral dilation of the pupils will occur. Transtentorial herniation may initially be identified as the affected pupil becomes oval in shape: this can then become a fully dilated pupil. Mark's pupils were equal and reactive to light, thereby indicating that his III cranial nerves were functioning and therefore his brain stem was not being compressed.

Exposure

Further injuries should be assessed for and care prioritised appropriately. Mark may have a chest wall injury, an abdominal injury and/or a spinal injury, in addition to the head injury. These injuries will need to be considered and managed accordingly.

The National Institute for Health and Clinical Excellence (NICE) (2007) recommends that patients with a severe head injury (GCS ≤8) should be transferred to a tertiary neurosurgical centre irrespective of the need for surgery or, if this is not possible especially if surgery is not clinically indicated, the admitting medical team should liaise closely with neurosurgical specialists. However, a transfer to a tertiary centre should not be considered should the patient have other injuries that cannot be managed in that specialist centre (NICE, 2007).

Evidence-based care

Care is directed towards maintaining CBF and therefore avoiding both ischaemia and hyperaemia. In order to achieve this, the factors that influence blood flow need to be controlled and manipulated to ensure that cerebral perfusion is maintained.

Mechanical ventilation

Mark's respiratory function was controlled. This was important for several reasons:

(1) His airway was now patent and maintained – this is necessary with patients with a reduced level of consciousness to avoid airway obstruction or aspiration of oral secretions/vomit.
(2) Respiratory gases can be controlled and manipulated to aid cerebral perfusion and reduce ICP.
(3) He can be sedated as required, which is useful for reducing cerebral metabolic requirement. Also other therapies, such as induced hypothermia, can be initiated as required, which would otherwise be impossible without sedation.

The control of respiratory gases is key in the critical care management of the person with head injury. Both carbon dioxide and oxygen influence CBF (Figures 7.2 and 7.3) and thus ICP, and both can be easily manipulated within the critical care setting.

Carbon dioxide

Traditionally, patients with raised ICP have been hyperventilated in order to reduce the pCO_2 and, as recently as 1995, a survey of US trauma centres found that 83% of the units were still aggressively hyperventilating head injured patients to reduce their ICP (Ghajar *et al.*, 1995). This should have the effect of vasoconstricting the cerebral vasculature and therefore reduce ICP. However, there is significant risk of ischaemia developing as the CBF becomes reduced due to the vasoconstriction. There is histological evidence of ischaemia in patients who die following traumatic brain injury (Graham *et al.*, 1988; Ross *et al.*, 1993), and Muizelaar *et al.* (1991) found that outcomes at 3 and 6 months were significantly worse in patients who had been hyperventilated. Therefore, the Brain Trauma Foundation (BTF) (2007) recommends limiting the use of hyperventilation in an effort to improve patient outcome and reduce the risk of developing iatrogenic cerebral ischaemia.

The impact of reducing the pCO_2 needs to be considered in the context of the alterations in CBF following a cerebral injury. Studies have shown that CBF may be as low as 18 ml/min/100 g tissue during the first 5 days following injury (Marion *et al.*, 1991; Bouma *et al.*, 1992; Sioutos *et al.*, 1995). In conjunction with this, studies have shown that different injuries have different derangements in CBF and vasoresponsiveness to CO_2. Contusions and subdural haematomas have lower CBF rates and reduced CO_2 vasoresponsiveness (Marion *et al.*, 1991; Salvant and Muizelaar, 1993; McLaughlin and Marion, 1996). Lower CBF rates are also seen in diffuse head injuries. This could lead to dangerous reductions in CBF to the areas underlying or surrounding the contusion/haematoma during and following hyperventilation.

In view of these issues, the BTF (2007) has the following recommendations:

- Prophylactic hyperventilation to <25 mmHg (3.3 kPa) should be avoided.
- Hyperventilation should be avoided for the first 24 hours post injury as CBF is often critically reduced during this time.
- Short-lived hyperventilation, as a temporary measure, is recommended to stabilise and lower elevated ICP.

Despite these concerns, control of pCO_2 remains part of the mainstay of effective management of this patient group. The 'Lund therapy' protocol recommends aiming for a 'normal' ICP of 4.6–5.2 kPa (35–39 mmHg) (Gründe, 2006) whereas NICE (2007) recommends that the pCO_2 should be maintained at 4.5–5 kPa. To this end, the mode of ventilation that is chosen for this patient group should allow for good control of the expired minute volume as it is this mode that controls the expired CO_2. This may require the use of a volume-cycled mode of ventilation rather than a pressure-cycled mode. Even so, consideration needs to be taken of the effect of raised intrathoracic pressures, which are not controlled in volume-cycled ventilation. If the intrathoracic pressures are elevated, cardiac output (and therefore cerebral perfusion) will be reduced as will venous return. Both of these could affect cerebral perfusion and cerebral haemodynamics.

Oxygen

Hypoxaemia, with or without hypotension, can cause secondary brain injury. Chesnut *et al.* (1993) found that 22.4% of patients had hypoxaemia and that this was associated with a poorer outcome. Stocchetti *et al.* (1996) found that 55% of patients with head injuries had hypoxaemia prior to intubation: this again was associated with worse outcomes and emphasises the importance of early and effective resuscitation in both pre-hospital and in-hospital settings. Additionally, hypoxaemia reduces perfusion and also increases CBF due to vasodilation, which may increase ICP. The BTF (2007) recommends that hypoxaemias <60% should be avoided and the Lund protocol (Gründe, 2006) advocates that a normal pO_2 of 12–14 kPa (90–105 mmHg) should be aimed for. This is supported by the NICE (2007) guidelines.

Positive expiratory end pressure (PEEP) may be required to ensure that a normal pO_2 is achieved. Low levels (5–10 cm H_2O) are recommended to maintain functional residual capacity and to avoid/resolve atelectasis (Myburgh, 2003). Levels higher than this may raise ICP and reduce venous cerebral drainage.

Haemodynamics

As the aim of care is to maintain neuronal perfusion, blood pressure management is an essential aspect of the head injured patient's care. Supporting and augmenting the MAP with the use of fluids and drugs is commonplace within the neurological critical care setting, and requires careful nursing observation and proactivity to avoid placing the patient at risk of cerebral ischaemia.

Avoidance of hypotension

Hypotension, both pre-hospital and in-hospital, has been shown to reduce patient outcome, with systolic blood pressure <90 mmHg being one of the main predictors of patient outcome. A single episode of pre-hospital hypotension is associated with increased morbidity and a doubling of mortality when compared with normotensive patients (Chesnut *et al.*, 1993). Hypotension and the correlation with an increase in mortality and morbidity are also reflected within in-hospital patients with traumatic head injury, especially if there are repeated episodes of hypotension.

Mean arterial pressure management

The 'aim' of a specific MAP rather than systolic blood pressure should be advocated for this patient group as it is MAP that is important when taking into consideration cerebral perfusion. Even so, a systolic BP <90 mmHg should be avoided (BTF, 2007) and any evidence of hypotension in both the pre-hospital and in-hospital setting should be promptly corrected. This will require fluids initially, with the aim to achieve normovolaemia as assessed against central venous pressure (CVP) or other haemodynamic assessment devices such as the transoesphageal Doppler or pulse contour analysis devices as available. Fluid choice will depend on local preferences – there is no evidence to recommend colloids over crystalloids (Myburgh, 2003) but both Clayton *et al.* (2004) and Grände (2006) advocate the use of colloids to resolve any hypotension. This is largely to minimise the risk of cerebral oedema developing due to large quantities of crystalloid infusions, which may be required to create a state of euvolaemia. Normal values of serum electrolytes should be aimed for, with a sodium level of 145 mmol/l maintained. Any active bleeding will need to be treated and haemoglobin level should be maintained between 8.5 and 10 g/l (Myburgh, 2003) although Clayton *et al.* (2004) suggest that the Hb should be >10 g/dl.

Cerebral perfusion pressure

Grände (2006) recommends aiming for a CPP of 60–70 mmHg for adults; however, lower CPP values (50–70 mmHg) may be required should a patient develop hyperaemia (Myburgh, 2003), whereas Clayton *et al.* (2004) suggest that a CPP >70 mmHg should be maintained. Actual aims for the CPP may depend on whether the patient is demonstrating signs of ischaemia or hyperaemia, taking into consideration the changes in CBF that can occur following certain injuries such as contusions.

Sedation, analgesia and muscle relaxants

Within the critical care setting, patients with head injuries will often require sedation and analgesics to facilitate mechanical ventilation and to reduce cerebral metabolic demand. The level of sedation and analgesia required will depend on the extent of the cerebral injury, ICP and the haemodynamic status of the patient.

Within the resuscitation phase, haemodynamic stability is paramount as it is during this time that cerebral hypoperfusion is common. Therefore, sedation should be titrated to cause the least effect on the systemic blood pressure. Short-acting drugs, such as fentanyl and propofol, are useful and may help to resolve episodes of surges of sympathetic activity, which can occur following trauma.

Within the intensive care setting, the requirements for sedation are different. In this setting, the patient should be sedated as lightly as possible so that neurological assessment can be carried out but intubation and mechanical ventilation is well tolerated. In conjunction with this, haemodynamic stability and ICP also need to be taken into consideration. Propofol is commonly used for this patient group as it provides a deep level of sedation, is effective in controlling sympathetic fluctuations and rises in ICP. It does not accumulate and neurological assessment can be undertaken promptly once administration ceases as it is quickly reversed. However, it can have a negative inotropic effect and can cause haemodynamic instability. If propofol is used for a prolonged period of time, the calories contained within the lipid solution should be taken into consideration when calculating the nutritional requirements of the patient. Tachyphylaxis can also occur with prolonged use, which will necessitate increases in dosage to achieve the same therapeutic response.

Infusions of benzodiazepines, such as midazolam, offer moderate to deep level of sedation and can be used in conjunction with propofol or instead of it. Benzodiazepines accumulate, which makes neurological assessment difficult and may lead to a prolonged period of reduced neurological function. Similarly, infusions of narcotics can supplement the effectiveness of sedation as well as have an analgesic effect. However, they too can accumulate.

On admission, Mark's arterial blood gases, cardiovascular status and sedation were satisfactory. He was tachycardic and so may be slightly hypovolaemic or may be having a stress response from the injury. He will require close observation of his haemodynamic

Table 7.2   Classification of CT scan appearance following a traumatic head injury

Category	Definition
Diffuse injury I	No visible pathology on CT scan
Diffuse injury II	Basal cisterns are open
	Midline shift 0–5 mm
	Lesion densities present
	No high/mixed density lesions >25 mm
	Bony fragments/foreign bodies may be present
Diffuse injury III (swelling)	Compressed or absent basal cisterns
	Midline shift 0–5 mm
	No high/mixed density lesions >25 mm
Diffuse injury IV (shift)	Midline shift >5 mm
	No high/mixed density lesions >25 mm
Mass lesion evacuated	Any lesion surgically removed
Non-evacuated mass lesion	High/mixed density lesion >25 mm which has not been surgically removed

(Adapted from Myburgh JA (2003) Severe head injury. Chapter 65 in Bersten AD and Soni N (Eds) *Oh's Intensive Care Manual*. 5th Edition, Butterworth Heinemann, Edinburgh).

and neurological status with the aims of management focused on maintaining his CBF and controlling influencing factors.

When is ICP monitoring required?

In view of the findings on his scan and GCS, transfer to a specialist neuroscience critical care setting should be explored (NICE, 2007). In consideration of ICP monitoring, the BTF (2007) recommends ICP monitoring in patients with traumatic coma (GCS $\leq$ 8 following non-surgical resuscitation) with either of the following:

- Abnormal CT scan:
  - Diffuse injury II–IV (see Table 7.2)
  - High or mixed density lesions >25 mm
- Normal CT scan or two or more of the following features:
  - Age > 40 years
  - Unilateral or bilateral motor posturing
  - Significant extracranial trauma with hypotension <90 mmHg

As Mark had a contusion on scan, his grade of injury was at least II and with his GCS of 5, ICP monitoring was clinically indicated.

Ongoing patient scenario

Mark has been in the ICU for 48 hours and his ICP is becoming increasingly difficult to control. His CPP is 55 mmHg despite efforts to increase it. He has also developed a very large diuresis.

On assessment, the following are found:

HR   115 BPM SR
BP   110/65 mmHg (MAP = 80)
Temperature   37.3°C
CVP   4 mmHg
ICP   30 mmHg
UOP   >300 ml/hr dilute urine for the last 3 hours

His ventilation observations on synchronised intermittent mandatory ventilation (SIMV) (VC) and pressure support (PS) are as follows:

RR   12 BPM
TV   450 ml
MV   5.4 l
AP   28 cm H_2O
PEEP   +5
PS   15 (he is not triggering the ventilator)
F_IO_2 0.3

Blood gases:

pH   7.34
pO_2 8 kPa
pCO_2 5.2 kPa
HCO_3 18 mmol/l
BE   −4
Na^+ 147 mmol/l
K^+ 3.8 mmol/l
HCT   44%
Hb   14 g/dl

His GCS is 4/15 and his pupils are size 5 mm and reacting sluggishly. He is receiving continuous infusions of propofol and fentanyl. A midazolam infusion was commenced overnight as his ICP was difficult to control and he was coughing slightly on suctioning.

Following the ward round, the following decisions are made:

 (1) To change the mode of ventilation to pressure-regulated volume control (PRVC)
 (2) To aim for a pO_2 >10 kPa and a pCO_2 4.5–5 kPa
 (3) To cool Mark to normothermia
 (4) To commence muscle relaxants
 (5) To commence noradrenaline to aim for a CPP of >60 mmHg
 (6) If his CPP does not increase to consistently >60 mmHg, a barbiturate coma would be introduced
 (7) To replace fluids to meet 80% of his fluid requirement
 (8) To aim for a CVP of 8 mmHg
 (9) To assess his serum and urine osmolality
(10) To maintain normal electrolyte balance

Mark is now demonstrating signs of raised ICP and a reduction in his cerebral perfusion. It is imperative that his CPP improves, otherwise he is at risk of cerebral ischaemia and infarction. For those looking after him, it is important that they have a clear understanding as to what is causing the increase in his ICP and subsequent reduction in perfusion. It is also important that they have to apply theory to practice by being aware of rationales for care and changes in treatment strategies.

Progressing pathophysiology

> **Key considerations**
>
> What precipitates secondary brain injury?
> What is the effect of ischaemia on cerebral cellular integrity?

Secondary brain injury

Secondary brain injury develops after the primary injury and is largely due to cerebral hypoxia or ischaemia. Therefore, it is possible to have good flow (perfusion) but no oxygen or good oxygen and no flow. Either way, ischaemia at the cellular level will occur and secondary brain injury will develop. Normally the cerebral vasculature is able to respond to these changes by increasing blood flow but this mechanism becomes limited when, for example, cerebrovascular disease exists, which restricts perfusion, or there is an intracranial mass, lesion, oedema or raised ICP, which constricts the blood vessels and therefore alters flow. It is important, though, to distinguish between global and focal hypoxic/ischaemic insults.

Global hypoxic/ischaemic insults

Hypoxaemia and cardiovascular events such as ventricular failure or cardiac arrest lead to cerebral hypoxic and reduced (or no) CBF, respectively. Usually, these events are sudden, severe and short-lived, and if there is to be recovery, oxygen delivery and blood flow need to be restored. Recovery and lasting effects will depend on the severity and duration of the insult in relation to the vulnerability of different cells. Four to six minutes of complete global ischaemia will lead to permanent histological damage and survivors will have neurological deficits. There are significant prognostic implications if the global ischaemia lasts for 15 minutes or longer.

Focal hypoxic/ischaemic insults

Focal hypoxic/ischaemic insults usually occur suddenly but usually are of longer duration than global events. Neuronal cell bodies in the area of focal ischaemia supplied by end arteries will die if perfusion is not restored rapidly. The area surrounding the infarcted area is the ischaemic penumbra; in this area, the CBF is greater than in the core of the infarcted area, but is less than in normal tissue. Infarction and irreversible damage to the brain from a focal hypoxic/ischaemic insult takes around 30–60 minutes; therefore, the focus of therapeutic interventions is to restore blood flow to the penumbral area so that there is potential for recovery. However, if blood flow is not promoted to this area, coalescing of the penumbra into the infarcted area will occur.

Brain ischaemic and infarction processes

As CBF decreases, changes in normal physiology can be found (Table 7.3). Once CBF has reduced to 10 ml/min/100 g, cell membrane failure occurs, as there is a lack of adenosine triphosphate (ATP) to maintain energy-dependent processes. If, at this stage, CBF is not restored as soon as possible, neuronal cell death will occur, which will lead to permanent neurological deficits.

Ischaemia occurs when there is insufficient oxygen and glucose for aerobic production of ATP. As identified previously, there is little storage of either oxygen or glucose within

Table 7.3   Effect of reduced cerebral blood flow

Cerebral blood flow (ml/min/100 g)	Physiological changes
50	Normal
25–50	Slowing of EEG
15–25	Reduced electrical activity
10–15	Cell membrane ion pump activity continues
<10	Cell membrane failure
<10 (prolonged)	Cell death

(Hayes M (2003) Cerebral protection. Chapter 43 in Bersten AD and Soni N (Eds) *Oh's Intensive Care Manual*. 5th Edition, Butterworth Heinemann, Edinburgh).

the brain, so ATP production during ischaemia relies on anaerobic glycolysis for as long as those stores last for. Levels of ATP become depleted within 2–3 minutes of complete ischaemia. During anaerobic glycolysis, lactic acidosis develops. When ATP production is reduced and insufficient for requirements, the energy-dependent cell membrane ion channels fail. This leads to an efflux of potassium and an influx of sodium, chloride and calcium. With the reverse in ionic concentrations, depolarisation will occur; during this, excitatory neurotransmitters (e.g. glutamate) will be released, which will cause further depolarisation of the neurones. Influx of sodium through both depolarisation and cell membrane channel failure will be followed by water, leading to intracellular oedema. Calcium influx also causes the release of excitatory neurotransmitters, which will further lead to depolarisation (Figure 7.4). In addition, the increased intracellular calcium levels will lead to the conversion of phosphorylases, with oxidative phosphorylation occurring within the mitochondria. Proteases will also be activated, which will cause intracellular proteins to be broken down and lipases to be stimulated. The lipases will release arachidonic acid and other free fatty acids which cause tissue damage through oxygen-free radical and prostaglandin production.

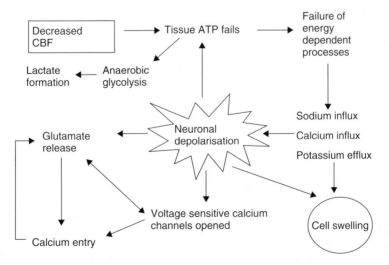

Figure 7.4   Cellular changes following cerebral ischaemia.

Extracellular events are thought to be largely due to leucocytes and it is thought that they contribute to reperfusion injury by

(1) plugging up small capillaries during the period of time when the blood flow is sluggish (these plugs will then block blood flow once blood flow is re-established) and
(2) enhancing the production of oxygen free radicals and activating inflammatory mediators.

Both of these events will lead to the development of oedema: this will worsen the ischaemia as blood vessels will be compressed and will involve tissues around the injury by mechanical compression of tissue and its blood supply.

The pathophysiological events of secondary brain injury are not predictable, so it is likely that the impact on cellular function is well established prior to intervention by the critical care team. These events can develop soon after the primary injury or a few days later. In Mark's situation, it would seem that oedema is collecting around the contusions, causing the increase in ICP and subsequent reduction in CPP. Unless remedied promptly, he is at risk of having a cerebral infarction which will considerably reduce the likelihood of a positive outcome.

Cerebral injury and neuroendocrine effects – diabetes insipidus

Neuroendocrine disorders

> **Key consideration**
>
> What is the effect of altered cerebral perfusion on the neuroendocrine system?

Mark currently has a very large diuresis. In view of the quantities of dilute urine that are being passed, he may have diabetes insipidus (DI). DI is characterised by polyuria, excessive thirst and polydipsia; however, Mark is unable to tell the nursing staff if he is thirsty. There are two main types of DI.

(1) *Central or neurogenic DI:* This is caused by a lack of antidiuretic hormone (ADH) being released in response to osmotic stimuli.
(2) *Nephrogenic DI:* This is caused by a lack of response to ADH.

Severe head injury can cause central DI, so this is the likely cause of Mark's DI.

Antidiuretic hormone

ADH is a major contributor to the maintenance of water balance, and is part of a negative feedback system involving thirst and osmotic stimuli. Normally plasma osmolality is maintained within a tight range of 275–295 mosmol/kg. A steady increase in the release of ADH occurs as osmolality increases from 280 mosmol/kg. ADH is made in the hypothalamic neurones and is transported to the pituitary gland, where it is stored in granules bound to neurophysin (carrier protein).

ADH has three main actions:

Antidiuresis
ADH acts on V_2 receptors in the distal portion of the renal tubule, mainly in the collecting duct. V_2 agonist action stimulates 3,5 cyclic adenosine monophosphate (cAMP) in the tubule cell cytoplasm. This stimulates a protein kinase to open microtubular passages for

the movement of water from the tubule filtrate. The creation of aquaporin, which is a highly selective water channel protein, allows for the reabsorption of up to 12% of filtrate, which allows for regulation of free water excretion and the maintenance of water and osmolality homeostasis.

Vasoconstriction

When high concentrations of ADH exist, stimulation of the V_{1a} receptors can lead to vasoconstriction. This is useful in hypotensive situations as ADH secretion will be stimulated and will contribute to improving the blood pressure.

Coagulation

V_2 receptors are also found extrarenally and the coagulation effects of ADH are due to extrarenal V_2 stimulation. Prostacyclin is stimulated and there is an increase in the activity of plasminogen activator, factor VIII and factor VII. Von Willebrand's factor multimers increase also. Therefore, there is an increase in coagulation activity when ADH (and its analogues) is present.

Central DI

The causes of both permanent and transient central DI include damage to the hypothalamus or pituitary gland (neurohypophysis). The nature of the injury to the neurohypophyseal tract will influence the duration and severity of the DI: for example, lesions of the pituitary stalk will lead to permanent DI, whereas vasospasm of the anterior cerebral circulation or cerebral oedema is more likely to lead to transient DI.

Central DI usually presents as sudden polyuria, excessive thirst and intake of fluids. In critical care, it is the large urine output that usually alerts the team to the development of DI: a urine output of 4–6 l/day or 3 ml/kg for 4–6 consecutive hours would suggest that DI has developed. Urine is very hypotonic, with an osmolality inappropriately low in comparison with plasma osmolality. A diagnosis is usually made when there is an elevated plasma osmolality due to hypernatraemia and an inappropriately low urine osmolality. Mark currently has an elevated sodium level and therefore, both urine and blood osmolality need to be measured to confirm the diagnosis.

Ongoing assessment

Neuromonitoring

Accurate neurological assessment of a head injured patient whilst they are in the intensive care setting requires sedation to be stopped. This may not be possible for the majority of patients with head injury as waking them could cause life-threatening changes to their neurological status (through increases in ICP), respiratory function (alterations in pCO_2 and pO_2) and cardiovascular status (tachycardia and hypertension). Ideally, neuromonitoring should provide accurate information about perfusion (CBF), ICP and cerebral function; however, no such monitor exists, but different tools can allow for assessment of these different parameters with varying degrees of accuracy and reliability. Although management of the patient with head injury is focused on maintaining an adequate CBF to avoid ischaemia or hyperaemia, currently, there is no method of directly measuring CBF at the bedside. Methods such as Xenon CT scanning, laser Doppler flowmetry and thermal diffusion flow measurement are available. However, these are largely available only in critical care units which are undertaking research studies, are labour intensive and are used intermittently rather than offering continuous minute-by-minute information. Indirect measurement of CBF, however, can be utilised in the intensive care setting and can be of use especially in conjunction with other strategies such as ICP monitoring.

Key consideration

What further monitoring devices would be of use?

Cerebral blood flow

Jugular bulb oximetry

The placement of a retrograde catheter in the jugular vein allows for the measurement of oxygen saturation of the blood leaving the brain and therefore neuronal oxygen uptake. Jugular venous saturation (SjO_2) is inversely proportional to CBF for a given metabolic rate, with changes occurring independently of changes in ICP. $SjO_2 < 55\%$ indicates low CBF and therefore cerebral hypoperfusion, whereas a saturation >85% occurs when there is hyperaemia. High saturation can also occur when there is inadequate neuronal metabolism or infarction as there is reduced oxygen extraction in both these situations. Both high and low saturations are associated with a poorer outcome. Routine use of jugular bulb catheters is currently not supported by evidence, despite both low and high saturations being associated with an adverse outcome (BTF, 2007). However, jugular bulb catheters also offer the opportunity to assess the extraction of oxygen by tissue rather than just the saturation of the blood. The measurement of arteriojugular difference in oxygen ($AJDO_2$) compares arterial pO_2 with jugular pO_2 and a higher $AJDO_2$ is associated with a better outcome (Stocchetti *et al.*, 2004). It is thought that a higher $AJDO_2$ indicates better extraction of oxygen by the brain.

There may be some clinical situations where the measurement of SjO_2 is supported (Box 7.1) (Myburgh, 2003).

Near-infrared spectrometry

This is a non-invasive technique in which a scalp oximeter is used to assess regional cerebral oxygen saturation. However, readings can be unreliable because of extracranial signals, and currently this tool is not used in routine clinical practice.

Transcranial Doppler

Transcranial Doppler allows for assessment of the velocity of blood flow through large vessels, such as the middle cerebral artery. Through this, systolic, mean and diastolic flow rates can be measured, and distinct patterns of blood flow have been recognised when hyperaemia, normal, vasospastic and absent flow exists. Even so, the routine use of a transcranial Doppler is not supported by evidence: at best it can be used intermittently, and gives useful information about blood flow through that specific blood vessel. Continuous

---

Box 7.1 Indications for SjO_2 monitoring

- To support CPP by maintaining $SjO_2 > 55\%$

    o Situations of systemic haemodynamic instability
    o Stable haemodynamics but large doses of catecholamines are required to achieve an adequate CPP

- Identification and assessment of hyperaemia in patients with a raised ICP >72 hours post injury
- Assessment and titration of supportive interventions (e.g. barbiturate coma, hypothermia) in patients with raised ICP to maintain their $SjO_2 > 55\%$

use would give a better indication of flow/velocity but that would be dependent on operator expertise in the use and interpretation of equipment.

Intracranial pressure monitoring

Raised ICP is associated with an adverse outcome and therefore the measurement of ICP allows for the injury to be quantified and facilitates assessment of the response to interventions. Indications for ICP monitoring have been previously outlined but any coagulopathy needs to be corrected prior to insertion of an ICP monitor.

An intraventricular catheter gives the most accurate measurement of ICP. This might be through an extraventricular drain and allows for CSF drainage as well as measurement of pressure. However, it may be difficult to insert especially if the ventricles are being compressed by oedema and there is an increased risk of infection as there is a direct route of entry for organisms.

Solid state system such as fibreoptic or strain-gauge tipped catheters can be placed intraparenchymally or intraventricularly. These devices transduce the pressure, providing both a real-time measurement and a waveform. Subdural and extradural catheters can be used; however, the measurement may not accurately reflect ICP, especially if the patient has undergone a craniectomy.

Once ICP is being measured, then CPP can be calculated. It is largely advocated to use the external auditory meatus as the reference point for zeroing the arterial blood pressure transducer as this is seen to be equivalent to the circle of Willis (Myburgh, 2003).

In conjunction with monitoring ICP values, the ICP waveform can be obtained. This is a pulsatile pressure with 3–4 peaks. P1 is the percussion wave and is associated with arterial pressure. P2, 3 and 4 have smaller amplitudes and are attributed to choroid plexus or venous pressure artefact. Usually these waves occur in a 'stairstep' fashion but P2 can become prominent as cerebral compliance decreases and/or ICP rises. There are three ICP waveforms.

- C waves – occur every 3–4 minutes and are related to changes in blood pressure.
- B waves – these appear as sharp rhythmic oscillation waves every 30–120 seconds. These are seen in relation to respiratory patterns. They are indicative of an unstable ICP.
- A waves – these are plateau waves and occur with rises in ICP of 60 mmHg over prolonged periods of time (5–10 minutes). These are always pathological.

The BTF (2007) recommends that treatment of raised ICP should commence if the ICP is >20 mmHg; however, they also recommend that specific ICP lowering treatment should be initiated following assessment of ICP in conjunction with CT findings and clinical signs. Small studies have demonstrated a decrease in mortality if the threshold for ICP is changed from 25 to 15 mmHg (Narayan *et al.*, 1982; Saul and Ducker, 1982). Patients can herniate at pressures less than 20–25 mmHg depending on where the intracranial mass is and pupillary changes can occur with an ICP of 18 mmHg (Marshall *et al.*, 1983). Thus, it is recommended that ICP measurements should not be considered in isolation but in conjunction with clinical signs and imaging.

Cerebral function monitoring

An assessment of cerebral function is also useful for ongoing indications of the impact of injury. They can also be helpful in assessing the effect of therapeutic interventions.

Electroencephalography

Electroencephalography (EEG) monitoring allows for the assessment of any seizure activity which is being masked by sedation or muscle relaxants as well as the degree of neuronal depression which is created by a barbiturate coma, if being used. Sub-clinical seizure activity can be a source of secondary brain injury and will only be identified through EEG monitoring; however, within the critical care setting, the reliability and validity of EEG monitoring is questionable as there may be interference from equipment (Procaccio *et al.*, 2001). EEG monitoring as well as other forms of EEG such as cerebral function activity monitors (CFAM) require skilled personnel who can both acquire and interpret the data obtained.

Microdialysis

Cerebral microdialysis measures extracellular fluid metabolites such as lactate. A microdialysis catheter is inserted into the same burr hole as the ICP monitor and the dialysate fluid obtained is analysed for the concentrations of metabolites. This technique is currently limited to research centres.

Bispectral index monitoring

Bispectral index (BIS) monitoring assesses depth of anaesthesia and can be used to assess effectiveness of sedation or barbiturates within the critical care setting. Although useful for assessing sedation, BIS monitoring was not designed or validated for detecting ischaemic cerebral injury even though decreasing BIS values can correlate with severity of brain injury and brain death (Vivien *et al.*, 2002).

Evidence-based care

On the ward round, changes are initiated to Mark's current treatment. These are made in light of Mark's deterioration; his CPP is not optimised, his blood gases are not within recommended limits and his ICP has become elevated. He also has a low-grade pyrexia and is showing signs of cardiovascular compromise as he is tachycardic and hypotensive as well as having a low CVP. He is showing some signs of dehydration in view of his sodium measurement and haematocrit (HCT).

The changes made are largely to further control the influences on ICP and CPP which can contribute to alterations in CBF. By making CBF the focus of care management, the influences on CBF can be manipulated (Box 7.2).

Additionally, cerebral metabolic demands can be reduced if neuronal activity is suppressed. Reducing temperature and optimising sedation help to achieve this.

These influences have all been identified by the critical care team when they reviewed Mark.

Mechanical ventilation

Key considerations

What is the rationale for this mode of ventilation?
How would the changes in his blood gases be contributing to the situation?

Box 7.2 Influences on CBF

CPP: MAP and ICP

Blood vessel diameter: Respiratory gases; cerebral vasodilation/constriction

Viscosity of blood: HCT and fluid status

Mode of ventilation

The team change Mark's mode of ventilation from SIMV (VC) and PS to PRVC. His airway pressures on SIMV (VC) and PS are 28 cm H_2O. This pressure could be adversely affecting both his cardiac output and ICP. Therefore, a pressure-regulated volume-cycled mode of ventilation is useful, as the minute volume can still be controlled as well as the intrathoracic pressures (McLeod, 2006). Both of these features are desirable in Mark's situation.

Respiratory gases

Both Mark's pO_2 and pCO_2 are contributing to the increase in his ICP as both will be vasodilating his cerebral vasculature. The set aims in view of Mark's respiratory gases are in line with the BTF (2007) guidelines. As his F_1O_2 is only 0.3, it is likely that an increase in this will improve his pO_2. At this moment it would be preferable to increase the F_1O_2 to support his pO_2 rather than setting a higher PEEP to avoid further cardiovascular compromise. His preset respiratory rate on the ventilator is 12 BPM, so this could be increased to 14 BPM. The subsequent augmentation of his minute volume may be sufficient to reduce his pCO_2 to the target range.

Cardiovascular support

Key considerations

What fluid management should Mark receive?
How should his blood pressure be supported?

Normovolaemia

The team decide that Mark's MAP needs additional support in order to maintain a CPP > 60 mmHg. This again is in line with recommendations. As he appears to be hypovolaemic, initially he will require fluids to support his intravascular volume so that his CVP can be increased. Normovolaemia is aimed for and this can be assessed against the response of CVP measurements to fluid boluses. In view of fluid resuscitation, there is no evidence to support the use of colloids over crystalloids. However, the choice of maintenance fluids should allow for normal osmolality. Glucose-containing solutions are not recommended as they contain free water, which can exacerbate cerebral oedema. Therefore, 0.9% sodium chloride or Hartmann's solution can be used to achieve normovolaemia (Mestecky, 2007).

Mark's DI is significantly contributing to his hypovolaemia. In mild polyuria (3 ml/kg/hr) as in Mark's case, it is best to carefully observe plasma and urine osmolality and to replace hourly output. If the polyuria continues for more than 24 hours or is severe (>7 ml/kg/hr), then ADH replacement may be required. Usually desamino-D-arginine vasopressin (DDAVP) (desmopressin), which is a long-acting ADH analogue, is given to control the polyuria.

Haematocrit

Mark appears to be haemoconcentrated in view of both his Hb and HCT. Myburgh (2003) recommends that the optimal HCT for cerebral circulation is approximately 30%. This level should allow for oxygen delivery to be maintained as the velocity of blood flow will be increased as blood becomes more dilute. In view of the HCT, the use of colloids to enable a reduction in viscosity as well as to support his intravascular volume is clinically indicated.

Vasoactive agents

Once Mark appears to be adequately fluid resuscitated, if his MAP is still not adequate to achieve a CPP > 60 mmHg, vasoactive agents will be required. The choice of drug will depend on local preference: generally a vasopressor will be preferable rather than an inotrope unless the patient is demonstrating signs of reduced myocardial contractility. Therefore, an α_1 agonist such as adrenaline, noradrenaline or dopamine can be used and are equally effective in improving CPP (Myburgh, 2003). It is unclear to what degree these drugs affect the cerebral circulation, although there is some evidence that dopamine does have a direct effect, leading to an increase in ICP and cerebral oxygen utilisation, as well as hyperaemia (Myburgh *et al.*, 1998). In comparison, ICP, CBF and cerebral oxygen utilisation remain constant with the use of adrenaline and noradrenaline. Initially, the drug of choice may be adrenaline; however, this drug is associated with side effects such as hyperlactataemia and hyperglycaemia, both of which are undesirable in this patient group. Therefore, often noradrenaline is regarded by many as the preferred drug and is the most commonly used vasopressor (Johnstone *et al.*, 2004). The dose required will depend on the patient's CPP and it should be titrated against the haemodynamic response of the drug as well as possibly assessment of CBF, if available.

Changes in sedation

Key consideration

What are the rationales for the changes in his sedation?

Mark is currently receiving propofol and midazolam in conjunction with fentanyl. This quantity of sedation will make neurological assessment difficult; however, the nursing staff also need to avoid creating deleterious rises in Mark's ICP through stimulation. In this situation, as a variety of different drugs are being used (or considered for use), it is useful for the critical care team to carefully consider each drug in turn and their usage.

Propofol

Propofol is widely used in neurosurgical critical care. As stressed previously, it has a rapid onset and is short acting. It has also been shown to be neuroprotective as it depresses neuronal metabolism and oxygen consumption. Kelly *et al.* (1999) found that high dose propofol (total dose >100 mg/kg for >24 hours) was associated with a significant improvement in neurological outcome even though there was no difference in ICP/CPP as compared to patients who received low-dose propofol. However, there are safety issues to consider with this dose of propofol. Propofol infusion syndrome was first identified in children but can occur in adults also. Common features of this syndrome include hyperkalaemia, metabolic acidosis, rhabdomyolysis, renal failure and lipemia. Therefore, it is recommended to be very cautious if using a dose >5mg/kg/hr or if propofol is required for more than 48 hours (BTF, 2007).

Opioids

Morphine sulphate is widely used in the critical care setting. It is largely accepted as being safe to use and offers a high level of analgesia; however, its sedatory qualities are minimal and tachyphylaxis can occur. There can be a rebound effect on ICP and CPP once the infusion has been discontinued.

Fentanyl and sufentanyl are being used more often now in critical care. Studies, though, have demonstrated that ICP can increase when these drugs are used (Sperry *et al.*, 1992; Albanese *et al.*, 1993). Significant decreases in MAP and rises in ICP have been shown to occur when fentanyl is given as a bolus (2 μg/kg) (de Nadal *et al.*, 1998); however, slow continuous administration of these drugs can minimise the ICP elevations associated with these drugs (Laver *et al.*, 1997).

Benzodiazepines

Traditionally, benzodiazepines have been avoided in this patient group because of their neurosuppressive qualities and duration of effect. Midazolam, though, is becoming increasingly popular especially to control ventilator-associated agitation. It can, though, cause decreases in MAP and therefore CPP, especially if the ICP increases as a result of the drop in MAP.

Barbiturates

Barbiturates reduce cerebral metabolic rate and therefore requirements for nutrients. However, results from trials do not support its use as it fails to improve outcome and these drugs can cause significant haemodynamic compromise. The decrease in MAP offsets any decrease in ICP that may result; therefore, CPP is not enhanced. Therefore, the BTF (2007) suggests that barbiturates should only be used when other interventions have not been successful in controlling ICP.

Muscle relaxants

Muscle relaxants are not recommended for use unless coughing or straining (valsalva manoeuvre) puts the patient at risk of prolonged rises of ICP. Hsiang *et al.* (1994) found that early use of muscle relaxants did not improve patient outcome and may actually be detrimental due to prolonged mechanical ventilation and associated risks. However, they also conclude that the use of muscle relaxants should be reserved for situations of intracranial hypertension, which requires escalation of interventions. Prolonged use of non-depolarising muscle relaxants also predisposes the patient to developing polyneuropathies such as critical illness neuropathy.

In Mark's situation, despite increasing his sedation, his ICP is not being controlled and he is still coughing. In view of the undesirable consequences of barbiturates and muscle relaxants, the introduction of these drugs into his management will need to be carefully considered, controlled, monitored and discontinued as soon as possible.

Induced therapeutic hypothermia

Key consideration

What is the rationale for cooling Mark?

Induced hypothermia reduces metabolic demand and therefore cerebral metabolic requirements. During experiments, ICP was reduced when hypothermia was immediately induced following injury (Clifton, 2000), but these results have not been replicated during clinical trials (Clifton *et al.*, 2001). Despite the lack of consistent and statistically significant reductions of mortality in trials, patients treated with hypothermia are more likely to have a favourable neurological outcome. Initial findings suggest that a reduction in mortality is likely if patients are treated with hypothermia for more than 48 hours (BTF, 2007). Induced hypothermia places the patient at risk of prolonged ventilation (and associated complications), which could be detrimental. Currently, induced hypothermia (temperatures 30–33°C) is not recommended; however, Patel *et al.* (2002) feel that reduction of temperature to 35°C can sometimes be used if a patient has not responded to other ICP-controlling interventions.

Mark currently has a temperature of 37.3°C. Despite the lack of evidence to induce a hypothermia, Mestecky (2007) does recommend treating temperatures >37°C. An increase in temperature of 1°C increases cerebral metabolic requirements by 10%. Therefore, cooling methods such as paracetamol and the use of cooling blankets should be initiated to reduce any temperature >37°C (Gründe, 2006).

Planning of nursing activities

Key consideration

How should the nursing staff plan their interventions?

Potentially, nursing interventions such as repositioning, chest care and essential nursing care can cause increases in ICP. If carried out in succession, these activities can have a cumulative effect on ICP, increasing it higher for longer periods of time. Conversely, if the activities are spread out, the ICP may repeatedly rise without a reasonable period of time for recovery. If an ICP monitor is in situ, nursing staff can carefully observe for individual responses to the interventions and modify the timing of the interventions accordingly. Family voices and visits have not been shown to adversely affect ICP (Hendrickson, 1987). Conversations unrelated to the patient has been shown to reduce ICP, whereas conversations about the patients' condition do not have a similar effect (Johnson *et al.*, 1989). Level of consciousness will influence whether the patient is able to respond to family stimulation; but even so, family presence may create a feeling of comfort in the patient.

Nutrition and normoglycaemia

Key considerations

Why is nutrition important following a traumatic brain injury?
Why do blood sugars need to be controlled?

Following traumatic brain injury, studies have shown that there is hypermetabolism and nitrogen wasting, with an average increase of 140% of expected metabolic expenditure. Even when muscle relaxants are used, there is a 20–30% increase in expenditure in some patients (BTF, 2007). The BTF recommends that full feeding is in place within 7 days of admission, which requires nutrition to be commenced within 72 hours of admission. Taylor *et al.* (1999) found that when feeding was commenced on day 1, there was less risk of infection and complications.

Hyperglycaemia has been shown to worsen ischaemic injury and therefore patient outcome. Blood sugars must be maintained within normal limits with avoidance of both hypo- and hyperglycaemia.

Other strategies

> **Key consideration**
>
> What else could be included in Mark's care?

The critical care team may consider either or both of the following in Mark's situation as clinically indicated.

Mannitol and hypertonic solution

If Mark's CT scan indicates that cerebral oedema has formed around his contusion and is causing his ICP to rise, the team may decide to administer either mannitol or another hypertonic solution such as 3% saline. Both of these fluids increase the osmolality of blood, thereby creating an osmotic gradient. Water is drawn from the brain into blood as a consequence of the change in osmolality, which not only reduces ICP but also reduces the viscosity of blood, thereby increasing CBF. A risk of administering mannitol is that it can dehydrate the patient, leading to hypotension and acute renal failure. Therefore, repeated doses should be avoided and close monitoring of osmolality is required, with an upper limit set at 320 mmol/l (Mestecky, 2007). Hypertonic solutions may preserve haemodynamic parameters (BTF, 2007); however, currently there is not enough evidence to recommend a certain concentration of hypertonic solution or to recommend such solutions over mannitol.

Decompressive craniectomy

Surgical evacuation of a lesion or infarcted tissue may be undertaken. A decision to remove a portion of the skull (bone flap) may be made if a patient does not respond to medical management or has gross cerebral oedema. Therefore, the critical care team may decide to undertake this procedure in Mark if he does not respond to the additional interventions identified. Early studies into the prophylactic use of decompressive craniectomy had unacceptably high mortality and morbidity rates but more recent studies have demonstrated good results in relation to ICP control and patient outcome (Aarabi *et al.*, 2006; Timofeev *et al.*, 2006).

Conclusion

Traumatic head injuries can be devastating; however, if CBF and, therefore, perfusion are maintained, patient outcome is improved. Strategies to promote perfusion must be introduced and any factors which may decrease perfusion must be controlled. This involves careful manipulation of respiratory gases, haemodynamics and cerebral metabolic rate to ensure that perfusion meets the neuronal requirements. If secondary brain injury is controlled, patient prognosis is brighter.

References

Aarabi B, Hesdorffer D, Ahn E, Aresco C, Scalea TM and Eisenberg HM (2006) Outcome following decompressive craniectomy for malignant swelling due to severe head injury. *Journal of Neurosurgery* 104 (4) 469–479.

Albanese J, Durbec G, Viviand X, Potie F, Alliez B and Martin C (1993) Sufentanyl increases intracranial pressure in patients with head trauma. *Anesthesiology* 79 (3) 493–497.

Bouma GJ, Muizelaar JP, Stringer WA, Choi SC, Fatouros P and Young HF (1992) Ultra-early evaluation of regional cerebral blood flow in severely head injured patients using xenon-enhanced computerized tomography. *Journal of Neurosurgery* 77 (3) 360–368.

Brain Trauma Foundation (2007) *Guidelines for the Management of Severe Traumatic Brain Injury.* 3rd Edition, Mary Ann Liebert, Inc, New York.

Brunker C (2006) Assessment of sedated head-injured patients using the Glasgow Coma Scale: an audit. *British Journal of Neuroscience Nursing* 2 (6) 276–280.

Chesnut RM, Marshall LF, Klauber MR, *et al.* (1993) The role of secondary brain injury in determining outcome from severe head injury. *Journal of Trauma* 34 (2) 216–222.

Clayton TJ, Nelson RJ and Manara AR (2004) Reduction in mortality from severe head injury following introduction of a protocol for intensive care management. *British Journal of Anaesthesia* 93 (6) 761–767.

Clifton G (2000) Hypothermia and severe brain injury. *Journal of Neurosurgery* 93 718–719.

Clifton GL, Miller ER, Choi SC, *et al.* (2001) Lack of effect of induction of hypothermia after acute brain injury. *New England Journal of Medicine* 344 (8) 556–563.

Ghajar J, Hariri RJ, Narayan RK, Iacono LA, Firlik K and Patterson RH (1995) Survey of critical care management of comatose, head-injured patients in the United States. *Critical Care Medicine* 23 (3) 560–567.

Graham DI, Lawrence AE, Adams JH, Doyle D and McLellan DR (1988) Brain damage in fatal non-missile head injury without high intracranial pressure. *Journal of Clinical Pathology* 41 (1) 34–37.

Grände PO (2006) The "Lund Concept" for the treatment of severe head trauma – physiological principles and clinical application. *Intensive Care Medicine* 32 (10) 1475–1484.

Hayes M (2003) Cerebral protection. Chapter 43 in Bersten AD and Soni N (Eds) *Oh's Intensive Care Manual.* 5th Edition, Butterworth Heinemann, Edinburgh.

Hendrickson S (1987) Intracranial pressure changes and family presence. *Journal of Neuroscience Nursing* 19 (1) 14–17.

Hsiang JK, Chesnut RM, Crisp CB, *et al.* (1994) Early, routine paralysis for intracranial pressure control in severe head injury: is it necessary? *Critical Care Medicine* 22 (9) 1471–1476.

Johnson SM, Omery A and Nikas D (1989) Effects of conversation on intracranial pressure in comatose patients. *Heart and Lung* 18 (1) 56–63.

Johnstone AJ, Steiner LA, Chatfield DA, *et al.* (2004) Effect of cerebral perfusion pressure augmentation with dopamine and norepinephrine on global and focal brain oxygenation after traumatic brain injury. *Intensive Care Medicine* 30 (5) 791–797.

Kelly PF, Goodale DB, Williams J, *et al.* (1999) Propofol in the treatment of moderate and severe head injury: a randomized, prospective double-blinded pilot trial. *Journal of Neurosurgery* 90 (6) 1042–1057.

Laver KK, Connolly LA and Schmeling WT (1997) Opioid sedation does not alter intracranial pressure in head-injured patients. *Canadian Journal of Anaesthesiology* 44 (9) 929–933.

Lu J, Marmarou A, Choi S, Maas A, Murray G and Steyerberg EW, Impact and Abic Study Group (2005) Mortality from traumatic brain injury. *Acta Neurochirurgica* 95 (Suppl) 281–285.

Marion DW, Darby J and Yonas H (1991) Acute regional cerebral blood flow changes caused by severe head injuries. *Journal of Neurosurgery* 74 (3) 407–414.

Marshall LF, Barba D, Toole BM and Bowers SA (1983) The oval pupil: clinical significance and relationship to intracranial hypertension. *Journal of Neurosurgery* 58 (4) 566–568.

McLaughlin MR and Marion DW (1996) Cerebral blood flow and vasoresponsivity within and around cerebral contusions. *Journal of Neurosurgery* 85 (5) 871–876.

McLeod A (2004) Traumatic injuries to the head and spine 2: nursing considerations. *British Journal of Nursing* 13 (17) 1041–1049.

McLeod A (2006) Mechanical ventilation for raised intracranial pressure in the patient with a cerebral insult. *British Journal of Neuroscience Nursing* 2 (7) 338–344.

Mestecky A-M (2007) Management of severe traumatic brain injury: the need for the knowledgeable nurse. *British Journal of Neuroscience Nursing* 3 (1) 7–13.

Muizelaar JP, Marmarou A, Ward JD, *et al.* (1991) Adverse effects of prolonged hyperventilation in patients with severe head injury: a randomized clinical trial. *Journal of Neurosurgery* 75 (5) 731–739.

Myburgh JA (2003) Severe head injury. Chapter 65 in Bersten AD and Soni N (Eds) *Oh's Intensive Care Manual*. 5th Edition, Butterworth Heinemann, Edinburgh.

Myburgh JA, Upton RN, Grant C and Martinez A (1998) A comparison of the effects of norepinephrine, epinephrine, and dopamine on cerebral blood flow and oxygen utilisation. *Acta Neurochirurgica Supplement (Wien)* 71 19–21.

de Nadal M, Ausina A, Sahuquillo J, Pedraza S, Garnacho A and Gancedo VA (1998) Effects on intracranial pressure of fentanyl in severe head injury patients. *Acta Neurochirurgica* 71 10–12.

Narayan R, Kishore P, Becker D, *et al.* (1982) Intracranial pressure: to monitor or not to monitor? A review of our experience with head injury. *Journal of Neurosurgery* 56 (5) 650–659.

National Institute for Health and Clinical Excellence (2007) *Head Injury: Triage, Assessment, Investigation and Early Management of Head Injury in Infants, Children and Adults*. NICE, London.

Patel H, Menon DK, Tebbs S, Hawker R, Hutchinson PJ and Kirkpatrick PJ (2002) Specialist neurocritical care and outcome for head injury. *Intensive Care Medicine* 28 (5) 547–553.

Price T, Miller L and de Scossa M (2000) The Glasgow Coma Scale in intensive care: a study. *Nursing in Critical Care* 5 (4) 170–173.

Procaccio F, Polo A, Lanteri P and Sale F (2001) Electrophysiologic monitoring in neurointensive care. *Current Opinion in Critical Care* 7 (2) 74–80.

Ross DT, Graham DI and Adams JH (1993) Selective loss of neurons from the thalamic reticular nucleus following severe human head injury. *Journal of Neurotrauma* 10 (2) 151–165.

Salvant JB Jr and Muizelaar JP (1993) Changes in cerebral blood flow and metabolism related to the presence of subdural hematoma. *Neurosurgery* 33 (3) 387–393.

Saul TG and Ducker TB (1982) Effects of intracranial pressure monitoring and aggressive treatment on mortality in severe head injury. *Journal of Neurosurgery* 56 (4) 498–503.

Sioutos PJ, Orozco JA, Carter LP, Weinand ME, Hamilton AJ and Williams FC (1995) Continuous regional cerebral cortical blood flow monitoring in head-injured patients. *Neurosurgery* 36 (5) 943–949.

Sperry RT, Bailey PL, Reichman MV, Peterson JC, Petersen PB and Pace NL (1992) Fentanyl and sufentanyl increase intracranial pressure in head trauma patients. *Anesthesiology* 77 (3) 416–420.

Stocchetti N, Canavesi K, Magnoni S, *et al.* (2004) Arterio-jugular difference of oxygen content and outcome after head injury. *Anesthesia and Analgesia* 99 (1) 230–234.

Stocchetti N, Furlan A and Volta F (1996) Hypoxemia and arterial hypotension at the accident scene in head injury. *Journal of Trauma* 40 (5) 764–767.

Taylor SJ, Fettes SB, Jewkes C, *et al.* (1999) Prospective, randomized, controlled trial to determine the effect of early enhanced enteral nutrition on clinical outcome in mechanically ventilated patients suffering head injury. *Critical Care Medicine* 27 (11) 2525–2531.

Timofeev I, Kirkpatrick P, Corteen E, *et al.* (2006) Decompressive craniectomy in traumatic brain injury: outcome following protocol-driven therapy. *Acta Neurochirurgica (Suppl)* 96 11–16.

Vivien B, Paqueron X, Le Cosquer P, Langeron O, Coriat P and Riou B (2002) Detection of brain death onset using the bispectral index in severely comatose patients. *Intensive Care Medicine* 28 (4) 419–425.

Chapter 8

The patient with a traumatic injury

Elaine Cole and Anne McLeod

Introduction

Traumatic injury is the leading cause of death and disability in people aged between 1 and 40 years in the developed world (Davies and Lockey, 2005) and after heart disease and cancer, a common cause of death in the older population (Cole and McGinley, 2005). In November 2007, the National Confidential Enquiry into Patient Outcome and Death (NCEPOD) launched 'Trauma: Who Cares?' This study has reported that nearly 50% of severely injured patients in the United Kingdom did not receive effective quality care. Deficiencies in organisational and clinical aspects of trauma care were identified and NCEPOD have called for significant improvements in pre-hospital and in-hospital trauma care (Findlay *et al.*, 2007). To optimise recovery and minimise morbidity and mortality, it is essential that a seamless clinical journey is provided for the patient with a traumatic injury, from pre-hospital care through to discharge and rehabilitation. This journey starts as soon as the injury has occurred.

Patient scenario

Richard was a 30-year-old man who was involved in a road traffic accident. He was riding a motorbike at speed, when he lost control on a tight bend in the road. He was thrown off from the bike and slid on the road for approximately 50 m. He was wearing a motorcycle helmet and did not lose consciousness. The emergency department (ED) received a phone call from the ambulance service informing them of his impending arrival.

The reported clinical situation at the scene was as follows:

RR   24
SaO$_2$ 94% (15 l/min O$_2$ via a non-rebreathe mask)
HR   117
BP   120/90 mmHg (MAP = 100)
GCS   14 (E4, V4, M6)
Pupil size 3 and reactive

He looked pale, was complaining of abdominal and leg pain and had an obvious degloving injury to his right foot.

Mechanisms of injury

Key considerations

(1) What are the different mechanisms of traumatic injury?
(2) What injuries may Richard have sustained in relation to the mechanism of injury?

Following a traumatic event, information about the mechanism of injury can help identify up to 90% of a patient's injuries (American College of Surgeons, 2004a).

Classification of mechanisms of injury

Mechanisms of injury can be classified into four main groups (Greaves *et al.*, 2008a).

- Blunt – such as a road traffic accident or fall
- Penetrating – such as a stab wound or impalement
- Blast – caused by an explosive element, which may be intentional or accidental
- Thermal – caused by extreme heat such as a fire, or extreme cold such as frostbite

In general, 98% of the trauma in the United Kingdom is blunt, caused by injury, and other mechanisms make up the rest; however, this picture is changing in the urban settings, with an increase in penetrating injury becoming more prevalent. Blunt trauma is sustained through the following types of incidents:

- Road traffic collisions with the patient in the vehicle
- Road traffic collisions involving pedestrian impact
- Cycle and motorcycle incidents
- Assaults
- Falls

Blunt trauma causes injury as a result of energy transfer leading to tissue compression and disruption (Eaton, 2005). Common injuries include crushing, rupturing or shearing of organs or tissues, fractures (open and closed) and traumatic amputations.

Transmission of energy

The injury that a patient sustains is dependent on several factors; however, the most important consideration is the amount of *energy transmission* that has taken place. The transmission of energy is sometimes known as *velocity* or *impact energy* and can be considered as a shock wave that moves at various speeds. Energy is carried at the front of the wave and is concentrated in a small space (American College of Surgeons, 2004a). However, energy cannot suddenly disappear; it has to decrease, usually by being absorbed by something else, such as tissues, organs and bones.

Other factors impacting on this will be the size of the surface area involved, the tissue elasticity and the pre-existing state of the patient (such as a coexisting lung disease or known coagulopathy). In traumatic events involving high speed (such as a road traffic accident or fall from a great height), deceleration, which can be defined as a decrease in speed or velocity, has an effect on the severity of injury sustained. If deceleration takes place slowly, such as over a longer distance, injuries can be less severe. However, deceleration forces, and therefore significant injury, can be much greater if the vehicle or victim comes to a sudden stop (Eaton, 2005). This is because the energy level or velocity exceeds the tolerance level of the tissues.

It should be remembered that injuries caused as a result of energy exchange do not always manifest themselves immediately. Therefore, it is important that the patient's assessment is ongoing in both the emergency and definitive care settings so that injuries that may appear more slowly can be anticipated and dealt with (Middlehurst, 2008).

Motorcycle-related trauma

The main cause of major injuries involving motorcycles is the ejection of the motorcyclist (and their passenger) on to the road. This is due to the inherent instability of motorcycles, especially in poor weather conditions, and the high speeds that they can be driven at (Eaton, 2005). Despite protective clothing such as helmets and leather suits, many motorcyclists sustain head and lower limb injuries; however, every area of the body is susceptible to injury. Motorcycle injuries may also be caused by impact with another vehicle, for example, being hit by a car, or colliding with the back of another vehicle or by the motorcycle falling over, crushing the rider's lower limbs.

Richard was thrown off from his speeding motorbike, and his vital signs suggest that he was haemodynamically unstable, which indicated the potential for serious traumatic injury. When a motorcyclist is ejected from the speeding vehicle, being thrown forward can cause the pelvis and lower limbs to impact with the handlebars, causing significant injury (American College of Surgeons, 2004a). Once ejected, the victim will continue to travel through the air until he or she hits the ground. The force of the impact will be transmitted through the part of the body that hits the ground first (in this case the pelvis), causing the initial injury, with the speed of the ejection and the surface that the victim lands on determining the severity of injury (Eaton, 2005). If the victim then slides along the road surface at speed, burns, soft tissue injuries and fractures (open or closed) can be sustained. Ejection from the motorcycle may also lead to the patient being involved in a further incident with another vehicle (Middlehurst, 2008).

Assessment and diagnosis

> **Key consideration**
>
> What is the purpose of the primary and secondary surveys and how will Richard be assessed when he arrives at the ED?

At the scene of the traumatic incident, it is hoped that information about the mechanism of injury can be gained from the patient (where appropriate), from witnesses or from the emergency services. However, although determining the mechanism of injury is an integral part of the initial patient assessment, if the information is not available, this must not delay the assessment and the detection of life-threatening injuries (Middlehurst, 2008).

The American College of Surgeons Committee on Trauma (2004b) describes a trimodal death distribution, where death from trauma occurs in one out of three time periods:

- First – within seconds or minutes of the injury
- Second – within minutes to hours following the injury
- Third – several days or weeks following the injury

'Front-end' trauma care, that is, pre-hospital settings and EDs, focuses on the patient assessment and resuscitation during the first and second time periods. In these phases, injuries that cause hypoxia, hypovolaemia or a rapidly accumulating brain haemorrhage need prompt recognition and treatment. This is important not only in relation to patient survival in the ED but also survival in the third phase of care. Delayed treatment of hypoxia or haemorrhage may result in complex problems such as multisystem organ dysfunction syndrome (MODS) and coagulopathy (Cottingham, 2006), when the patient is in the intensive care unit (ICU).

In order to recognise life-threatening problems and initiate prompt treatment, a systematic approach to assessment is necessary. This is known as the *primary survey* (American College of Surgeons Committee on Trauma, 2004b). In many EDs, prior warning of the patient's arrival by pre-hospital personnel will result in the activation of a multidisciplinary trauma team made up of staff who have the prerequisite knowledge and skills to conduct the primary survey (Brohi, 2008; Cole, 2008).

Primary and secondary surveys

Assessment of the trauma patient is usually performed in two stages: first, the primary and later the secondary surveys (Cole and McGinley, 2005; Greaves *et al.*, 2008b).

Primary survey

The initial assessment, the primary survey, has five components A, B, C, D and E:

- Airway with cervical spine control
- Breathing and ventilation
- Circulation and haemorrhage control
- Disability and dysfunction
- Exposure and environmental control

Airway with cervical spine control

The first step of assessment is to ascertain airway patency. The airway can become obstructed because of structural damage, for example, bleeding or swelling of the face, mouth or oropharynx, a reduced level of consciousness (LOC) or vomiting and aspiration. Richard was talking on his arrival at the ED; therefore, it could be assumed that his airway was patent. Talking to the patient not only helps to keep evaluating airway patency, but also establishes psychological support (Greaves *et al.*, 2008b). Richard was complaining of pain in his abdomen, pelvis and hips; therefore, early on in his primary survey, intravenous analgesia such as morphine, with an antiemetic, were administered, titrated to pain.

Cervical spine immobilisation
A cervical spine injury must be suspected in any patient with multisystem trauma, especially with an altered LOC or blunt injury above the clavicles (American College of Surgeons Committee on Trauma, 2004b). Richard did not appear to have sustained a head injury; however, he was at risk of spinal injury due to the mechanism of injury. Richard had a semi-rigid collar, head blocks and tape applied to ensure spinal immobilisation until the following:

- He is fully alert with a GCS of 15.
- A senior clinician has examined the bony spine and soft tissues of the neck.
- Cervical spine imaging has been completed and reported as normal.

Breathing and ventilation

Assessment of Richard's respiratory status should involve *inspection, auscultation* and *palpation*. On inspection, he was tachypnoeic with a respiratory rate of 26, his oxygen saturation levels were 96% and no obvious chest injuries were noted. Auscultation and percussion are performed to clinically rule out any life-threatening chest injuries such as a haemothorax or a tension pneumothorax. Richard had bilateral air entry with normal lung sounds; however, it is standard practice to undertake a chest X-ray in all cases of major trauma to ensure that life-threatening injuries have not been missed (American College of Surgeons Committee on Trauma, 2004c).

Circulation and haemorrhage control

Here, the clinical priorities are assessing Richard's haemodynamic status and finding and arresting any haemorrhage (Cole and McGinley, 2005). Many trauma patients will develop hypovolaemic shock and may present with haemodynamic instability and an altered clotting picture (Brohi *et al.*, 2003). Haemodynamic status is initially assessed by measuring HR, BP, the patient's LOC (if haemorrhage is present, cerebral perfusion will be impaired) and skin colour.

Disability and dysfunction

Assessment of the LOC should be carried out in all trauma patients. Altered LOC in trauma is predominantly due to hypoxia, hypovolaemia or an intracranial injury. Assessment is carried out using the GCS (Teasdale and Jennett, 1974). The patient's eye opening, verbal response and motor function are assessed and given a numerical rating between 3 (the worst score) and 15 (the best score). Richard's initial GCS was 14 (he lost 1 point for being agitated/confused) and although he did not appear to have sustained a head injury, a reduced GCS and his high speed mechanism of injury mandated an urgent computerised tomographic (CT) scan to rule out an intracranial lesion (NICE, 2007).

Exposure and environmental control

If not already done, the remainder of Richard's clothes will be removed to allow for a full examination, ensuring that his dignity is maintained and that he is kept warm. At this stage, Richard's cervical spine could not be cleared; therefore, a log roll, keeping the spine in alignment, was necessary to allow the back to be examined. While being logrolled, Richard had a rectal examination to assess sphincter tone and to detect bony fragments or a high riding prostate gland, which may indicate a pelvic fracture (American College of Surgeons, 2004a).

Diagnostic investigations

Initial diagnostics aimed at finding haemorrhage will also include a pelvic X-ray and a focused assessment with sonography in trauma (FAST) scan. FAST involves ultrasound assessment of four regions of the torso: the perihepatic area, the perisplenic area, the pericardial area and the pelvis. The benefits of FAST include the ability to rapidly assess potential intra-abdominal bleeding and that it can be reliably carried out by non-radiologists who have had training in the use of the machine (Brooks *et al.*, 2005).

Underlying physiology and pathophysiology

Key consideration

What physiological mechanisms have been triggered?

Richard had an altered LOC and was tachycardic. This indicates hypovolaemic shock, despite his BP being within normal parameters, suggesting that compensatory mechanisms had been activated.

Table 8.1 Estimated blood loss and initial patient presentation (adult values)

	Class I shock	Class II shock	Class III shock	Class IV shock
Blood loss (ml)	Up to 750	750–1500	1500–2000	>2000
Respiratory rate	14–20	20–30	30–35	>35
Heart rate	<100	>100	>120	>140
BP	Normal range	Normal range	Decreased	Decreased
Pulse pressure (mmHg)	Normal	Decreased	Decreased	Decreased
Level of consciousness	Normal or slightly anxious	Mildly anxious/ agitated	Agitated/ confused	Very confused or lethargic

Shock compensatory mechanisms

A reduction in preload due to diminished circulating blood volume (as little as >10% total blood volume) causes a response from the carotid and aortic baroreceptors and the carotid artery chemoreceptors. This response stimulates an increased sympathetic activity by the vasomotor centre in the medulla. The increased sympathetic activity triggers the release of circulating β-adrenergic catecholamines (adrenaline and noradrenaline) in an attempt to increase cardiac contractility (McQuillan *et al.*, 2008). This is seen clinically with increased HR. The catecholamines also cause peripheral vasoconstriction to shunt blood to the heart and brain and trigger the release of corticosteroids from the adrenal gland. Plasma cortisol levels rise between 2 and 6 hours following the traumatic injury. Cortisol has a 'permissive action' helping to further increase the vasoconstrictive effect of catecholamines (Bongard *et al.*, 2008).

Antidiuretic hormone (ADH), a hormone stored in the pituitary gland, is released in response to decreased circulating volume and increased osmolarity. ADH inhibits diuresis by encouraging water reabsorption through the tubules of the kidneys (Bongard *et al.*, 2008). In addition, reduced blood flow initiates the stimulation of the juxtaglomerulus apparatus which produces renin. This enzyme reacts with angiotensinogen to form angiotensin I in the liver. This then converts to angiotensin II, a powerful vasoconstrictor, in the lungs (McQuillan *et al.*, 2008). In addition, angiotensin II stimulates the secretion of aldosterone from the adrenal cortex. Aldosterone helps to improve blood volume by retaining sodium and water through the kidneys.

Pulse pressure is the difference between the systolic and diastolic BP. A narrowing or decrease in this measurement is usually seen with a rise in the diastolic BP because of circulating catecholamines, increased vascular tone and systemic vasoconstriction (American College of Surgeons Committee on Trauma, 2004b; Cottingham, 2006).

The degree of shock is dependent on the volume and speed of blood lost and, to some extent, the age and pre-existing state of the patient (Edwards, 2005). *Early* signs and pathophysiology of hypovolaemic shock are demonstrated in Table 8.1 (American College of Surgeons Committee on Trauma, 2004b), from which it is evident that Richard was already in class II hypovolaemic shock.

Evidence-based care

> **Key considerations**
>
> How will Richard's care be clinically prioritised?
> What management strategies are clinically indicated?

Patient care interventions should be prioritised against the ABCDE process; in this initial stage of the patient scenario, ABC will be focused on.

Airway

Richard was maintaining a patent airway. However, should Richard's airway deteriorate while in the ED, anaesthetic help should be sought immediately. ED staff must be able to maintain airway patency using simple manoeuvres such as application of a jaw thrust and insertion of an oropharyngeal airway while awaiting expert anaesthetic help.

In the ED, serious traumatic injury may result in the need for a definitive airway (endotracheal intubation) to be secured. Indications for a definitive airway include the following (American College of Surgeons Committee on Trauma, 2004c; Cole, 2008):

- Apnoea
- Inability to maintain the patient's airway
- The need to protect the lungs from aspiration
- Potential airway compromise, for example, following burns and facial fractures
- GCS < 8
- Inability to maintain adequate oxygenation using a facemask

Breathing and ventilation

A trauma patient like Richard is at risk of hypoxia due to lung injury and/or haemorrhage. Diminished blood flow reduces the delivery of oxygen. This causes a mismatch between oxygen supply (e.g. reduced due to bleeding or lung injury) and tissue demand (McQuillan *et al.*, 2008). Cellular metabolism stores energy derived from normal oxygenation (aerobic metabolism) in the form of adenosine triphosphate (ATP). When there is impaired oxygen delivery, ATP is still produced but at concentrations lower than normal, and as a result of anaerobic metabolism. Prolonged hypo-oxygenation and hypoventilation can result in profound hypoxia and metabolic acidosis (Matthews and Bentley, 2005) where there is a concomitant rise in lactate levels. Therefore, *all trauma patients need early supplemental oxygen*. In the self-ventilating patient, this is administered as 15 l/min via a non-rebreathe mask with a reservoir bag (Cole, 2008). If the patient's oxygen supply is restored within minutes of the injury occurring, ATP synthesis and tissue function are supported and the risk of metabolic acidosis is reduced (McQuillan *et al.*, 2008).

Circulation and haemorrhage control

Richard had two large bore (14–16 g) cannulae sited in upper limb veins and had blood taken for cross-matching, full blood count, urea and electrolytes assessment and clotting and a venous or arterial blood gas analysis (according to local policy). Because Richard was in class II shock, intravenous crystalloid was started until cross-matched blood was available. Traditionally, the standard approach to the unstable trauma patient has been to infuse large volumes of intravenous fluid (Rizoli, 2002). The aim was to restore and maintain a normal BP and was based on controlled animal experiments (Stern, 2001). However, contemporary fluid resuscitation is changing, because most of the traumatic haemorrhages are *uncontrolled* rather than controlled. Evidence from both human and animal studies now recommends a more cautious approach to fluid administration (Revell *et al.*, 2003).

Permissive hypotension following traumatic injury

The premise of *permissive hypotension* or *low volume–fluid resuscitation* is that by restoring the BP to 'normal' parameters, clots that may have formed will be dislodged by the fluid causing the patient to start to bleed. Large volumes of fluid may also cause dilutional coagulopathy. Therefore, small volumes of fluid should be given, for example, 250–500 ml boli in adults (Brohi, 2008), and the patient's haemodynamic status should be assessed to see whether they:

- respond to the fluid and improve – *responders* – these patients are unlikely to be actively bleeding;
- respond to the fluid temporarily and then deteriorate again – *transient responders*;
- do not respond to the fluid – *non-responders*.

Transient or non-responders are unstable, high risk patients and as such need blood and clotting factors rather than crystalloid.

Choice of fluids in trauma

Use of crystalloids versus colloids in early trauma fluid replacement is an ongoing source of discussion and controversy (Cottingham, 2006). Criticism of intravenous crystalloids suggests that they are distributed or 'leaked' from the intravascular space, possibly causing the need for more fluids. Because colloids remain within the intravascular space for longer, it would seem logical that these would be recommended over crystalloids; however, evidence suggests that in early trauma care, colloids cause clot instability and alteration of platelet function. The consensus in the literature is that there is no role for colloids in the pre-hospital and initial assessment stages of early trauma resuscitation (Rizoli, 2002; Brohi *et al.*, 2003; Moore *et al.*, 2004; Criddle *et al.*, 2005; Perel and Roberts, 2007).

Given that Richard was haemodynamically unstable, as previously mentioned, he was given intravenous crystalloid in small boli (NICE, 2004; Brohi, 2008) with close monitoring of his physiological response. If he continues to lose blood, he may require a blood transfusion. Pelvic injuries can cause overwhelming hypovolaemia and a massive transfusion may be necessary. Massive transfusion is defined as the replacement of a patient's total blood volume in less than 24 hours or as the acute administration of more than half the patient's estimated blood volume per hour (Brohi, 2006). The aim of this is the rapid and effective restoration of an adequate blood volume and to maintain blood composition within safe limits in relation to haemostasis, oxygen carrying capacity, oncotic pressure and biochemistry (Brohi, 2006).

However, in the haemodynamically unstable patient, focus should be placed on finding the source of bleeding and accessing expert help to stop the haemorrhage early. This mandates clinical examination of the chest, abdomen, pelvis and long bones, which are all areas of potential bleeding.

Soft tissue injury

Significant soft tissue injury can cause severe haemorrhage, overwhelming infection and loss of limb function due to nerve damage or ischaemia. Unfortunately, because of wearing training shoes rather than protective footwear, Richard had sustained a degloving injury (Figure 8.1). However, there is no obvious haemorrhage from this site; therefore, direct pressure is not needed. Degloving injuries cause the skin and underlying soft tissue to be peeled back over the bones (Davies, 2002) and although these can be visually distracting, they are rarely immediately life-threatening; therefore, the team must not focus on this more than on other resuscitation priorities. The wound should be irrigated thoroughly and covered with a sterile drape until such time that a senior clinician can determine whether surgical debridement of devitalised tissue and exploration of underlying structures will be necessary. Intravenous antibiotics will be commenced in the ED according to local antibiotic policy.

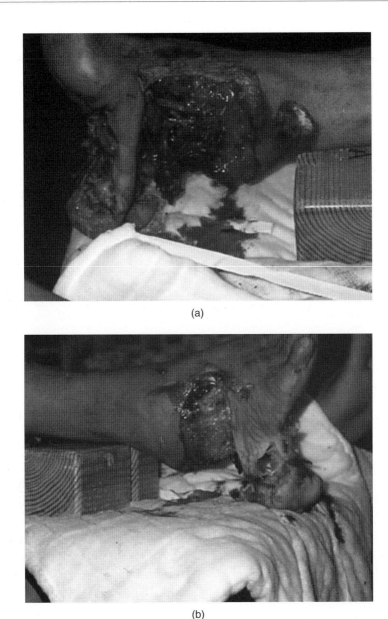

(a)

(b)

Figure 8.1 Degloving injury.

Continuing patient scenario

Richard had been in the ED for approximately 20 minutes. His primary survey shows the following:

RR   26
SaO$_2$ 96% (15 l/min O$_2$ via a non-rebreathe mask)
HR   120 (SR)

BP   115/68 mmHg (MAP = 83)
GCS   13 (E = 3, V = 4, M = 6)
Pupil size is 3 and reactive
His chest X-ray was normal.
No spinal levels are displaced or painful on examination of the bony spine and soft
   tissues of the neck.
His pelvic X-ray shows that he has an anterior–posterior pelvic fracture.
He has a degloving injury to his right foot.

Assessment: secondary survey

Key consideration

What further assessments will be undertaken in the ED?

The secondary survey is a head-to-toe evaluation of the patient. This includes ongoing assessment of Richard's vital signs, a full physical examination and, if possible, a patient history. The mnemonic AMPLE is useful when taking a history from the trauma patient because seemingly innocuous yet important information may be overlooked (Cole and McGinley, 2005).

A   Allergies
M   Medications currently used
P   Past medical history (including tetanus status)
L   Last meal
E   Events or environment related to the injury

Where the skin has been breached, the patient's tetanus immunity should be established because a tetanus toxoid booster may be required. However, Richard had a large area of devitalised tissue, which may be considered a tetanus-prone wound and tetanus immunoglobulin administration may be necessary (DH, 2006).

The full secondary survey may not be completed if the patient needs to be transferred urgently for imaging or operative management. A pelvic binder will be applied to splint the pelvis and reduce bleeding from the bone ends. Importantly, the binder should provide fracture stability to allow clots to form at the site of vascular injury; however, it will not control arterial bleeding (Brohi, 2008). Richard had maintained his BP following 2 × boli of 500 ml crystalloid; however, he remained tachypnoeic and tachycardic. O rhesus positive blood were made available, while awaiting his group and cross-match reports. It was essential that movement, logrolls, etc. were kept to a minimum to avoid clot displacement and further bleeding from the injury site (Cole, 2008).

Evidence-based care

Key considerations

(1) Given the nature of Richard's injuries, what are the priorities and next steps in his treatment?
(2) Which is the most appropriate area of definitive care to send Richard to: A ward? A high dependency unit? The intensive care unit?

Pelvic injuries

Richard had an anterior–posterior fracture of his pelvis. Fractures of the pelvis can be stable or unstable; however, haemorrhage-related mortality associated with pelvic injuries continues to be a challenge for contemporary trauma care (Verbeek *et al.*, 2008). An unstable pelvic fracture suggests that the patient has sustained a high-energy injury, which can often result in arterial and vascular disruption causing major haemorrhage (Brohi, 2008). The direction and type of force that the patient has been exposed to will cause a specific type of injury, although these can be combined.

A number of systems have been used for describing pelvic fractures (Young *et al.*, 1986; Tile, 1988); however, these injuries can be broadly classified into three types:

Anterior–posterior (AP) compression fractures

This type of injury is sometimes called an *open-book fracture* due to the damage to the sacroiliac ligaments and widening of the pelvic ring (Figure 8.2). This can render the pelvis horizontally unstable and disruption of the sacroiliac joints can cause vascular injury and therefore haemorrhage.

Lateral compression injury

Lateral compression fractures are caused by an impact from the side (Figure 8.3). The force causes internal rotation or compression of one side (or both) of the hemi-pelvis (Smith, 2005). There is a risk of haemorrhage from the anterior branches of the internal iliac artery (Brohi, 2008) and structural damage to underlying organs such as the bladder, urethra and uterus.

Vertical shear injury

The high-energy shearing force associated with this injury causes major vertical disruption to the bony pelvic ring (Figure 8.4). This leads to severe vertical pelvic instability and commonly life-threatening haemorrhage. Patients with pelvic injuries who present in hypovolaemic shock have a mortality rate of 30–50% (Brohi, 2008).

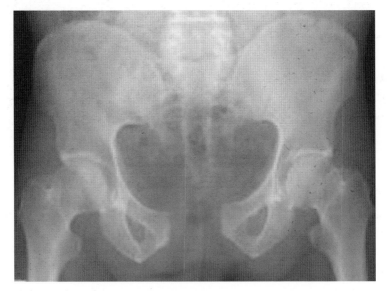

Figure 8.2   Anteroposterior compression pelvic injury. (Reproduced with permission from D Dean Thornton, 'Pelvic Ring Fractures: Imaging', http://emedicine.medscape.com/article/394515-imaging.)

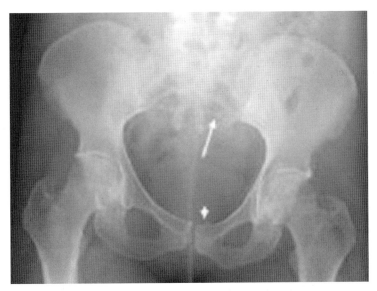

Figure 8.3   Lateral compression pelvic injury. (Reproduced with permission from D Dean Thornton, 'Pelvic Ring Fractures: Imaging', http://emedicine.medscape.com/article/394515-imaging.)

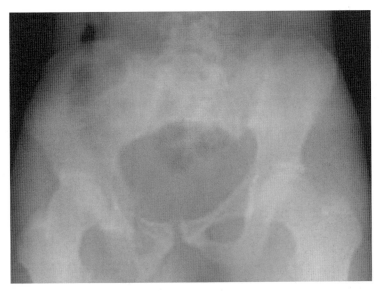

Figure 8.4   Vertical shear pelvic injury. (Reproduced with permission from D Dean Thornton, 'Pelvic Ring Fractures: Imaging', http://emedicine.medscape.com/article/394515-imaging.)

Complex pattern injury

The complex pattern of injuries does not fit into other classifications neatly. These injuries result from a combination of the aforementioned types of injuries.

Management of the pelvic injury

Treatment of pelvic injuries includes external and internal fixation, packing and damage control surgery and angioembolisation (Balogh *et al.*, 2005; Cothren *et al.*, 2007).

Treatment is often dependent on the fracture type, the haemodynamic status of the patient and the resources available at the receiving institution. A pelvic injury that is causing haemodynamic instability should be considered as a vascular injury (Balogh *et al.*, 2005; Brohi, 2008). Initial management should be based on the patient's haemodynamic status and whether arterial injury is suspected. It is the volume deficit and resulting hypovolaemia that will have an earlier detrimental effect on the patient, rather than the bony injury!

Continuing management within the Emergency Department

Richard remained tachycardic and a decision needed to be made as to whether he was stable enough to go for a CT scan of the head and pelvis (to define the type and severity of pelvic fracture). The haemodynamically unstable patient with a pelvic injury may not be suitable to go for a CT scan (due to the risk of deterioration and cardiac arrest) and may need immediate angiography or surgery. If the decision is made to take such a patient for a CT scan, they should be accompanied by the entire trauma team and blood products must be immediately available.

Haemorrhage from internal iliac arteries is best controlled by angiographic embolisation (Brohi, 2008) and Richard may need to be taken to the angio suite (if available) for endovascular control prior to being admitted to definitive care. This is a high-risk transfer and the patient must be closely monitored to detect increasing instability and haemodynamic deterioration.

Ongoing patient scenario

It is 6 hours since Richard arrived at the ED. He has just been transferred to the intensive care setting from the ward in a state of cardiovascular collapse. The nurse says that Richard has tried to get out of bed because he was in pain. Following that, his condition deteriorates. On assessment, the following are found:

HR	145 BPM SR
BP	80/35 mmHg (MAP = 50)
CVP	2
RR	32 BPM
SaO_2	98% on a non-rebreather system
Capillary refill	4 seconds
UO	10 ml for last hour
AVPU	V
Temp (core)	36.5°C

Blood gases:

pH	7.2
pO_2	12 kPa
pCO_2	4.2 kPa
HCO_3	18 mmol/l
BE	−5
Lactate	4
Hb	6 g/dl

His pulses feel thready and his peripheries are cool.
His abdomen feels tense.

Richard is assessed by the ICU team and the following decisions are made:

(1) To intubate and mechanically ventilate him
(2) To reassess his abdomen and pelvic injury

(3) To assess his state of haemostasis
(4) To treat any coagulapathies as clinically indicated
(5) To assess his intra-abdominal pressures (IAP)
(6) To maintain his MAP > 65 mmHg
(7) To increase his Hb > 8 g/dl

Key considerations

(1) What stage of shock is he now in?
(2) What are the potential complications in relation to his abdomen?

Progressing pathophysiology

Richard is now showing signs of considerable cardiovascular collapse. Previously, he was in the compensatory stage of shock, but now he is in the progressive stage. The human body cannot tolerate acute blood loss, with an acute loss of 40% of the blood volume being fatal. If blood loss is <15% of blood volume, the body's response to this has been described in the following three steps:

Stage 1: This stage, which occurs a few hours after the onset of blood loss, is characterised by the movement of interstitial fluid into the capillaries. This movement is known as *transcapillary refill* and helps to maintain blood volume but leaves a resultant interstitial fluid deficit.

Stage 2: The renin–angiotensin–aldosterone system becomes activated by the fluid loss, leading to the replenishment of the interstitial fluid deficit.

Stage 3: Within a few hours after the onset of the blood loss, the bone marrow increases the production of erythrocytes. However, as this is a gradual response, complete replacement of erythrocytes can take up to 2 months.

Richard must have lost more than 15% of his blood volume as he is demonstrating signs of shock. The above occurs in mild haemorrhage and normally does not require fluid resuscitation. Hypovolaemia may not produce any clinical signs until the volume loss is greater than 30% of the blood volume. In view of his clinical presentation, he appears to be in Class III haemorrhage, based on Table 8.1, and has therefore lost 30–40% of his total blood volume.

Progressive stage of shock

The progressive stage of shock comprises of a number of positive feedback systems, which further depress cardiac output, thus causing the shock to become 'progressive'.

Cardiac depression

Cardiac depression occurs when the arterial BP is too low to maintain the metabolic requirements of the myocardium. This will decrease the contractile function of the myocardium, thereby reducing cardiac output further. Deterioration in myocardial function is the key contributor to the progression of shock and largely causes the other positive feedback systems that are involved in shock.

Vasomotor failure

The sympathetic response that is seen in the compensated stage of shock helps to delay the depression of cardiac output and helps to prevent a decrease in arterial pressure. However, if the cause of the shock is not resolved, eventually the vasomotor centre in the brain stem will become less active (and ultimately inactive) as the blood flow to it reduces. When this happens, the sympathetic response to a reduced cardiac output will also cease.

Blockage of minute vessels

Sluggish blood flow in the microvessels will lead to blockage of these vessels and also causes the shock to progress. Despite the low blood flow, tissue metabolism occurs, but this will lead to blood acidosis as lactic acid and carbonic acid are produced and released into the blood vessels. This will cause local blood agglutination, leading to minute clots and plugs in the blood vessels. Even if the blood vessels do not become plugged, there is a tendency for the blood cells to stick together, which makes it difficult for blood to flow easily through the blood vessels, leading to sluggish blood flow.

Increased capillary permeability

There is an increase in capillary permeability as a consequence of hypoxia and lack of nutrients to the tissues. Large quantities of fluid transduce into the tissues, which will further reduce intravascular volume and cardiac output.

Release of toxins from ischaemic tissues

Histamine and serotonin, for example, can be released from ischaemic tissues, which can cause further circulatory system alterations. Increased capillary permeability and cardiac depression can result, again exacerbating the shock cycle.

Generalised tissue deterioration

As shock continues, signs of generalised tissue deterioration may be seen. The liver is especially vulnerable due to its high metabolic requirements and that it has an increased exposure to blood-borne toxins due to the large proportion of the cardiac output that it receives.
    The cellular effects of continuing shock are detailed in Box 8.1.

Acidosis

Poor delivery of oxygen to cells will lead to the production of cellular energy through anaerobic processes. Not only does this produce less energy than through aerobic processes but large quantities of lactic acid also. In addition, carbon dioxide cannot be removed from

---

Box 8.1 Cellular effects of continuing shock

- Accumulation of intracellular sodium and chloride accompanied by an efflux of potassium. There is dysfunction of the sodium/potassium pump due to a lack of cellular energy.
- Cellular swelling will occur as water will accompany the movement of sodium into the cell.
- Mitochondrial activity becomes depressed.
- Lysosomes will rupture leading to the intracellular release of hydrolases, which will further injure the cells.

tissues due to the lack of blood. This will worsen the acidosis as the carbon dioxide will react with water to form intracellular carbonic acid.

Abdominal haemorrhage

Richard's abdomen appears tense and in view of the marked decrease in his haemoglobin, he seems to be bleeding into his abdomen, which would account for the shock he is demonstrating. The retroperitoneum can hold up to 4 l of blood and this haemorrhage may not be clinically obvious, as in Richard's situation prior to his cardiovascular collapse. He could be developing abdominal compartment syndrome due to the haemorrhage and subsequent increase in IAP. The pathophysiological effect of this originates from hypoperfusion of the intestines caused by the reduction in blood flow due to the increased pressures and any shock mechanisms. The ensuing tissue hypoxia leads to the following:

(1) The release of cytokines, which will lead to vasodilation and an increase in capillary permeability
(2) The production of oxygen-derived free radicals
(3) A decrease in ATP production due to anaerobic respiration and thus derangements in cellular ion balance

(Walker and Criddle, 2003)

The increase in the IAP will also be contributing to Richard's overall presentation of reduced cardiac output, respiratory failure and reduced urine output.

Reduced cardiac output

Reduced cardiac output occurs as a consequence of decreased venous return as the vena cava is compressed. Also, the pressures will increase afterload, which will impair ventricular ejection.

Respiratory failure

Respiratory failure occurs due to diaphragm contraction becoming impaired. This will reduce functional residual capacity and worsen the oxygen debt (Lozen, 1999). The plan is for Richard to be intubated and ventilated: if a volume-cycled mode is used, his peak airway pressures may be elevated and if a pressure-cycled mode is used, a decrease in tidal volume may be noted.

Reduced urine output

Reducing urine output and renal function develops as a result of pre-renal (sometimes also referred to as *fluid responsive renal failure*) renal failure due to the renal arteries being compressed. Even when BP is normal, raised IAP can compress the renal veins and collecting ducts again leading to oliguria (Nebelkopt, 1999). The renin–angiotension–aldosterone system will also be activated, which will lead to a reduction in urine output.

Ongoing assessment

Key considerations

(1) How is the post-traumatic injury patient assessed in the ICU setting?
(2) What assessment strategies are used to assess bleeding?

Richard had been stabilised in the ED prior to transfer; however, he tried to get out of bed. This is likely to have lead to the movement of any clots that had formed over bleeding points on the pelvic ring. Richard has signs of abdominal haemorrhage: along with signs of cardiovascular compromise, his Hb has significantly decreased from when he was first admitted and his abdomen appears tense. As his condition has significantly deteriorated, he should be reassessed using an ABCDE process so that care can be prioritised.

Tertiary assessment

Although Richard has already had a primary and secondary survey, the intensive care team will want to undertake a tertiary assessment. This will be to largely confirm previous findings and to ensure that all injuries have been identified. This should be undertaken systematically, with the patient's back and front being examined. It will be important for the team to assess for any abdominal organ injury, such as a liver laceration or spleen damage, which may have not been obvious in the secondary assessment.

In addition, any haematuria should be noted because this could indicate kidney or bladder injury; gastric aspirate should also be tested for blood.

Diagnostic tools

There are a number of diagnostic tools that can be used in the intensive care setting to confirm the abdominal haemorrhage.

Diagnostic peritoneal lavage

Diagnostic peritoneal lavage (DPL) can be used to diagnose intra-abdominal haemorrhage when the patient is shocked and there are no plans to proceed to a laparotomy. It can also be used when there is no shock but when repeated physical examination is not possible if, for example, the patient is sedated. If 10 ml of frank blood is aspirated, then immediate laparotomy is indicated (Judson, 2003). Otherwise, the lavage fluid specimen should be examined for red and white blood cell count and for amylase.

However, DPL has been shown to be inaccurate (DiGiacomo *et al.*, 2001) because the movement of red blood cells across the peritonium give a high percentage of false positive results. DiGiacomo *et al.* (2001) suggest, however, that a supraumbilical diagnostic tap is a sufficiently accurate assessment tool.

CT abdomen

If the patient is stable, then CT abdomen is useful. This would be difficult in Richard's case in view of the degree of cardiovascular compromise which is displayed; however, once he has been adequately resuscitated, abdominal CT is useful to assess the retroperitoneum and pelvic injury.

Abdominal ultrasound

Although user dependent, abdominal ultrasound can give fast information in situations when the patient is unstable as DPL can then be avoided. Intra-abdominal bleeding can be identified, but bleeding in the pelvis is difficult to visualise and there can be false positive results.

Assessment of haemostasis

Dilutional coagulopathy can occur following resuscitation with fluids that do not contain haemostatic factors. Routine clotting tests give useful information in relation to haemostasis.

Prothrombin time

The prothrombin time (PT) indicates whether the extrinsic system of the clotting cascade is sufficient and can become prolonged when there is factor VII deficiency, liver disease, vitamin K deficiency or if the person is taking oral anticoagulants.

Activated partial thromboplastin time

The activated partial thromboplastin time (APTT) relates to the intrinsic system. An isolated prolongation of APTT can occur with a deficiency of factor VIII or IX.

Prolongation of both PT and APTT can occur when there are deficiency factors X, V or II because then the common pathway will be affected.

Thrombin clotting time

The thrombin clotting time (TCT) indicates fibrinogen conversion and will be prolonged if there is a lack of fibrinogen or if heparin has been given.

D-dimer assay

This assay measures breakdown products from fibrin lysis and can become elevated postoperatively, following trauma or in renal impairment, sepsis or venous thrombosis. High levels suggest excessive fibrinolysis.

Bedside tests such as activated clotting time (ACT) and thromboelastography® (TEG®) (Haemoscope corporation) can also offer useful information.

Activated clotting time

ACT measures the duration of time it takes for a clot to form but does not differentiate between intrinsic/extrinsic pathways. It is largely useful in situations when heparin is or had been used, for example, during/after cardiopulmonary bypass, during haemodialysis or following angioplasty. Although Richard has not had any heparin, measuring his ACT could give useful information about his state of coagulation and whether the haemorrhage is largely due to a coagulapathy. In Richard's case, a low ACT would indicate the hypercoagulability that is initially found in major trauma; whereas, a prolonged ACT would suggest that he has a coagulapathy and that haemostatic mechanisms are becoming exhausted (Aucar *et al.*, 2003).

Thromboelastography®

TEG® (Haemoscope corporation) is a bedside test that can give information about the speed and strength of clot formation. The speed of clot formation offers information on the adequacy of quantitative factors required for clot formation, whereas the strength and stability of the clot is useful in determining the ability of the clot to create haemostasis. A typical cigar-shaped figure is obtained, which can be analysed to determine, for example, the duration of time taken for clot formation to commence, how quickly the clot starts to break down and the strength of the clot (Wenker *et al.*, 1997) (Figure 8.5). Changes in the

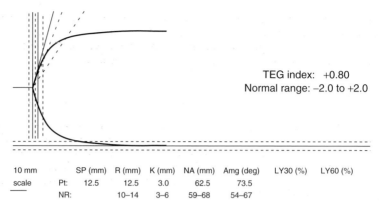

TEG index: +0.80
Normal range: –2.0 to +2.0

10 mm		SP (mm)	R (mm)	K (mm)	NA (mm)	Amg (deg)	LY30 (%)	LY60 (%)
scale	Pt:	12.5	12.5	3.0	62.5	73.5		
	NR:		10–14	3–6	59–68	54–67		

Figure 8.5 Thromboelastography (TEG) normal waveform. (Image of the hemostatis tracing generated by the TEG® 5000 Thromboelastograph® Hemostasis Analyser is used by permission of Haemoscope Corporation.)

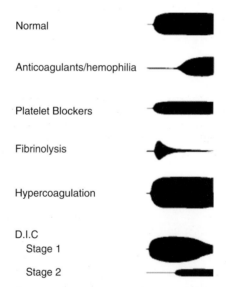

Normal

Anticoagulants/hemophilia

Platelet Blockers

Fibrinolysis

Hypercoagulation

D.I.C
  Stage 1

  Stage 2

Figure 8.6 Thromboelastography (TEG) alterations in waveform. (Image of the hemostatis tracing generated by the TEG® 5000 Thromboelastograph® Hemostasis Analyser is used by permission of Haemoscope Corporation.)

obtained figure occur when there is, for example, platelet dysfunction, hyperfibrinolysis, disseminated intravascular coagulation and hypercoagulation (Figure 8.6). Appropriate treatment strategies can then be identified to resolve the alterations in haemostasis or if the profile is normal but the patient is still bleeding, then a surgical solution may be required if the patient is postoperative.

Assessment of intra-abdominal pressures

As Richard's abdomen appears distended, it is important to assess his IAP. IAP can easily be measured through measuring intravesical pressure and is normally less than 10 mmHg (Streat, 2003). Abdominal compartment syndrome can occur following abdominal trauma (or surgery for trauma) or during sepsis. Consequences of IAP >12 mmHg include reduced cardiac output due to reduced preload and increased afterload, pre-renal renal failure and splanchic impairment due to hypoperfusion (Saggi *et al.*, 1998). However, it is unclear when decompression should occur, with Joynt *et al.* (2001) suggesting that in acute increases >20–25 mmHg, urgent decompression should be considered especially if accompanied by severe cardiorespiratory compromise or impending acute renal failure.

Evidence-based care

Richard requires fluid resuscitation and management of his haemorrhage. Because Richard's blood loss is >25% of his blood volume and oxygen delivery is impaired (as indicated by his lactate), homologous blood transfusion is indicated. He will also require crystalloids because his interstitial fluid as well as his circulating blood volume will be depleted. Specific blood component replacement might also be required to aid haemostasis or if a dilutional coagulopathy has developed following his initial resuscitation in the ED.

Key considerations

(1) What are the possible complications of massive blood transfusion?
(2) What interventions are indicated to enable coagulation?

Blood transfusion

Richard may require a substantial volume of blood to maintain his Hb and circulating volume until the source of the haemorrhage is identified and controlled. There are a number of complications of large (or massive) blood transfusion, but usually those people requiring a large quantity of blood will be seriously ill and have multiple problems. Therefore, it can be difficult to define any complications caused or exacerbated by blood transfusion.

Citrate toxicity

Citrate is present within stored blood to stop it from clotting; however, when transfused, ionised calcium is mobilised. Although, the healthy adult liver can metabolise the amount of citrate within each unit of blood every 5 minutes, citrate toxicity and hypocalcaemia can occur if transfusion rates are greater than 1 unit every 5 minutes or if the liver function is impaired. There is no apparent effect on coagulation because of the hypocalcaemia but patients may show signs of tetany and hypotension. Toxicity can be potentiated by alkalosis, hypothermia, cardiac disease and hyperkalaemia. Metabolism of citrate is impaired by hypotension, hypothermia, hypovolaemia and liver disease. Many critically ill patients will have these complications and therefore hypocalcaemia needs to be observed for. However, calcium should only be given if there is biochemical, clinical or electrocardiographic evidence of hypocalcaemia.

Acid–base alterations

Stored blood contains citric acid in its anticoagulant and when transfused in large amounts can exacerbate a pre-existing acidosis or cause an acidosis. In addition to citric acid, stored blood can also contain lactic acid, which has been generated by the red blood cells during storage. Therefore, a metabolic acidosis can develop or be exacerbated.

Potassium levels

Stored blood can have high potassium levels, but it is unlikely to have pathological effects (Isbister, 2003). However, hypokalaemia can create problems during the 24 hours following massive blood transfusion. This is due to the infused cells correcting their electrolyte balance and potassium shifting into the cells. Therefore, initially a patient may have a hyperkalaemia and acidosis following massive blood transfusion, this is then followed by delayed hypokalaemia and alkalosis.

Sodium levels

Stored blood and fresh frozen plasma (FFP) both have a higher sodium level than normal blood because of quantities of sodium citrate, which is within these products. This can create problems if the patient has cardiac, renal or liver disease all of which can lead to disordered sodium/water handling.

Jaundice

Jaundice is a common consequence of massive blood transfusion. Around 30% of the stored cells do not survive, which will lead to an increased bilirubin load as they are broken down by the liver. This will be demonstrated as hyperbilirubinaemia and therefore jaundice. This can be exacerbated by hepatic hypoperfusion and therefore impaired liver function since an important rate-limiting step in bilirubin transport is the energy-dependent transportation of conjugated bilurubin into the hepatic cannaliculus for removal of the bilirubin in bile. If there is reduced hepatic perfusion (as can occur in shock), then this process will be restricted by a reduction in ATP production. Thus, conjugated hyperbilirubinaemia occurs.

Hypothermia

If cold blood is transfused, 1255 kJ (300 kcal) is required to warm it from 4°C to 37°C. This is equivalent to an hour of muscular activity. In addition, the hypothermia that can result if large volume of cold blood is transfused will impair citrate and lactate metabolism, shift the oxygen disassociation curve to the left, increase intracellular potassium release and delay drug metabolism. Clinically, the patient may have cardiac arrthymias, a reduced cardiac output and demonstrate signs of altered haemostasis (Isbister, 2003). To avoid these, blood warmers should be used if the patient requires the rapid transfusion of more than two units of blood.

Transfusion-related acute lung injury

This is a complication of blood transfusion which presents as acute respiratory distress. Unlike acute respiratory distress syndrome or acute lung injury, recovery from transfusion-related acute lung injury (TRALI) usually occurs within 48 hours. It is thought to occur when there are leukoagglutinins in the donor plasma. If these are present, complement is activated leading to neutrophil aggregation in the pulmonary vasculature. Consequently, the endothelium of the blood vessels will be damaged, allowing for pulmonary oedema to develop (Isbister, 2003).

Although TRALI can occur after any blood transfusion, the greater the volume of the transfusion, the greater is the potential for TRALI to develop.

Blood product transfusion

In addition to packed red cells, Richard may also require blood products once his platelet levels and clotting studies have been measured.

Box 8.2 Indications for platelet transfusion

Diffuse microvascular bleeding when the platelet count is <100 × 10⁹/l
In any bleeding patient, when thrombocytopenia is secondary to bone marrow failure
Prophylactically when there is bone marrow failure and the platelet count is <10 × 10⁹/l
    without risk factors for bleeding or <20 × 10⁹/l with risk factors
Before surgery or invasive procedures when the platelet count is <50 × 10⁹/l

(Isbister, 2003)

Platelets

In situations of platelet deficiency or defect, platelet transfusion may be required. Because Richard is bleeding, platelet transfusion would be appropriate if his platelet count is <50 × 10⁹/l (Spahn *et al.*, 2007). Other situations when platelet transfusion may be indicated are detailed in Box 8.2.

Platelets are not required if:

(1) there is thrombocytopenia due to immune-mediated destruction and
(2) there is thrombotic thrombocytopenia pupura and haemolytic uraemia.

Fresh frozen plasma

FFP contains the clotting factors and therefore is clinically indicated when the coagulation studies are prolonged (PT or APTT more than 1.5 times control) (Spahn *et al.*, 2007). Therefore, situations when FFP can be used include the following:

(1) Single factor deficiencies
(2) When there is bleeding and abnormal clotting following bypass surgery, massive blood transfusion or liver dysfunction
(3) Acute disseminated intravascular coagulation
(4) Bleeding due to warfarin-induced anticoagulation, in conjunction with vitamin K

Cryoprecipitate

Cryoprecipitate is prepared from FFP and contains fibrinogen and factor VIII. Cryoprecipitate is used to treat coagulation defects including massive haemorrhage and disseminated intravascular coagulation if the fibrinogen level is <0.5 g/l; however, Spahn *et al.* (2007) suggest that it can be given in trauma patients if the fibrinogen level is <1 g/l and there is significant bleeding. Cryoprecipitate can also be used as an alternative to the administration of factor VIII in the treatment of inherited disorders such as deficiencies of von Willebrand factor, factor VIII and factor XIII. In Richard's case, he may require cryoprecipitate if his fibrinogen levels are significantly decreased due to haemorrhage.

Individual factors

Administration of factor VIII and IX is established in the treatment of haemophilia and in cases of antithrombin III (AT III) deficiency, AT III concentrates can be given.

Recombinant activated factor VII

Increased interest in the use of recombinant haemostatic proteins and inhibits has occurred in the past few years. Recombinant activated factor VII (rFVIIa), although originally developed for haemophilic patients with coagulation factor inhibitors, is now also used for a wide range of haemostatic disorders such as liver disease, following massive blood transfusion and platelet disorders. rFVIIa initiates the extrinsic clotting pathway when complexed with tissue factor at the site of injury. It therefore bypasses the intrinsic pathway. Boffard *et al.* (2005) found that patients who received rFVIIa after requiring eight units of blood following blunt or penetrating trauma had reduced requirements for blood transfusion in the next 48 hours than the control group that received placebo. Therefore, they conclude that rFVIIa is safe to administer in situations of severe traumatic injury. Levi *et al.* (2005) agree with the use of rFVIIa when there is life-threatening haemorrhage but conclude that further studies are required before rFVIIa can be recommended for use in patients with no pre-existing clotting problems, who have severe bleeding. Spahn *et al.* (2007) recommend the use of rFVIIa if major bleeding persists despite attempts to control bleeding and blood products have been administered.

Pharmacological agents

Depending on Richard's coagulation studies, there are some drugs that could be considered to reduce his bleeding.

Tranexamic acid

This is an antifibrinolytic drug that is a competitive inhibitor of plasmin and plasminogen. Spahn *et al.* (2007) suggest that it should be considered in the treatment of patients such as Richard, with rate of administration of 1–5 mg/kg/hr. However, they also acknowledge that the evidence to support its use is limited to the elective surgical patient and therefore, within their recommendations, have transferred the previous research findings to the trauma patient.

Aprotinin

Aprotinin is a serine protease inhibitor and a powerful antiplasmin agent. Similar to tranexamic acid, aprotinin has been used extensively in elective surgery and in particular in cardiac surgery. Its efficacy has not been proven in the trauma patient, but Spahn *et al.* (2007) again suggest that the evidence for its use in the elective surgical patient can be transferred to the trauma patient. Aprotinin, however, has been linked to an increased risk of renal dysfunction as well as increased risk of myocardial infarction and stroke when used in cardiac surgery (Karkouti *et al.*, 2006; Mangano *et al.*, 2006). Therefore, it is used with caution.

Protamine

Protamine reverses the action of heparin by binding with it and therefore inhibiting the anticoagulation effect of heparin. Richard did not have any heparin, so protamine would not be clinically indicated.

Vitamin K

Clotting factors II, VII, IX and X all require vitamin K for their action. In liver dysfunction, there may be deficiency of these factors or of vitamin K, which can contribute to a coagulopathy. Drugs such as warfarin are vitamin K antagonists, thereby creating anticoagulation effects. Richard does not have liver failure and is not on warfarin, so vitamin K would not be clinically indicated for him.

Management of his pelvic injury

> **Key considerations**
>
> (1) Rationalise management strategies in relation to the pelvic injury.
> (2) Rationalise management strategies in relation to the limb injury.

Although blood can be given to increase Richard's circulating volume, and blood products can be given to resolve any coagulopathy, it is essential that any bleeding points are identified and treated. About 90% of haemorrhage associated with pelvic fractures is due to venous bleeding from the fractured bone surfaces (Frakes and Evans, 2004), with the fracture site itself acting as the primary source of bleeding in about 86% of injuries. If there is injury to the large vessels, there is a high mortality rate (up to 85%), thus necessitating control of Richard's haemorrhage.

There are a number of treatment options that Richard could have for the management of his pelvic fracture and bleeding. Trauma management protocols recommend early pelvic stabilisation if the patient is hypotensive with an unstable pelvic fracture (Shackford, 2000; DiGiacomo *et al.*, 2001). Depending on the results of abdominal assessment, he may require a laparotomy and surgical control of bleeding; if the pelvis is unstable, external fixation should precede the surgery. Anterior fixation reduces bleeding by realigning the fractures (and therefore bony ends) and preventing clot disruption. Anterior external fixation is achieved by attaching a frame to each iliac crest with pins.

The C-clamp is another form of external fixation that can create greater compression of the posterior portion of the pelvic ring. Two pins are placed on the posterior part of the ileum, near the sacroiliac joint. Buckle *et al.* (1994) found that when the C-clamp was used in hypotensive patients, their requirement for blood products was reduced and their BP improved.

Surgery to control bleeding is usually only indicated when there is injury to large vessels. However, depending on Richard's IAP, he may require a laparotomy with the wound remaining open and not surgically closed to reduce the risk of abdominal compartment syndrome. De Waele *et al.* (2006) found, however, that although IAPs are lower following laparotomy, mortality remains high. Packs may be left in situ to compress any bleeding points.

The degloving injury

The plastic surgeons will need to review Richard's degloving injury; care will need to be taken to avoid it becoming infected and also it could be a source of bleeding, if coagulopathy develops. Perfusion to the tissue must be maintained, but this may become compromised if vasopressors such as noradrenaline are used. He may require skin grafts in the future. Both Wong *et al.* (2006) and Josty *et al.* (2001) report using vacuum-assisted closure in cases of lower limb degloving injuries in conjunction with grafts to achieve successful granulation of the injury.

Other considerations

Blood pressure control

Spahn *et al.* (2007) recommend that a systolic BP of 80–100 mmHg is aimed for until the bleeding is controlled, unless a head injury is also present. Although aggressive fluid management will help to restore tissue perfusion, there is a risk that

(1) blood clots could be displaced;
(2) coagulation factors will become diluted;
(3) the patient could cool down.

Therefore, until Richard's bleeding is controlled, a slightly lower than normal BP (permissive hypotension) that still allows for tissue perfusion will be aimed for.

Avoid hypothermia

Richard's temperature is currently within a normal range and it would be desirable to maintain his normothermia. Hypothermia (temperature <35°C) is associated with acidosis, hypotension and coagulation derangements with altered platelet and clotting factor function. Patients who are hypothermic require more blood products and there is a higher mortality rate (Spahn *et al.*, 2007). Therefore, should Richard's temperature drop any further, strategies to increase his temperature back to normal (such as forced air warming) would be indicated.

Conclusion

This chapter has illustrated complications and treatment strategies that the trauma patient may experience and require. Their care demands a coordinated and collaborative approach from the out-of-hospital care into the ED and then onward into critical care, whether that is the assessment/admission ward, the high-dependency unit or intensive care. Treatment strategies are focused on patient stabilisation, the promotion of perfusion through fluids and control of haemorrhage as well as avoiding complications. This requires careful haemodynamic management and ongoing assessment.

References

American College of Surgeons (2004a) Biomechanics of injury. In *Advanced Trauma Life Support for Doctors. Student Course Manual.* 7th Edition, American College of Surgeons, Chicago, pp. 315–335.

American College of Surgeons Committee on Trauma (2004b) Initial assessment and management. In *Advanced Trauma Life Support for Doctors. Student Course Manual.* 7th Edition, American College of Surgeons, Chicago, pp. 11–32.

American College of Surgeons Committee on Trauma (2004c) Airway and ventilatory management. In *Advanced Trauma Life Support.* 7th Edition, American College of Surgeons, Chicago, pp. 41–52.

Aucar JA, Norman P, Whitten E, *et al.* (2003) Intraoperative detection of traumatic coagulopathy using the activated coagulation time. *Shock* 19 (5) 404–407.

Balogh Z, Cladwell E, Heetveld M, *et al.* (2005) Institutional practice guidelines on management of pelvic fracture-related hemodynamic instability: do they make a difference? *Journal of Trauma, Injury, Infection and Critical Care* 58 (4) 778–782.

Boffard KD, Riou B, Warren B, *et al.* (2005) Recombinant factor VIIa as adjunctive therapy for bleeding control in severely injured trauma patients: two parallel randomized, placebo-controlled, double-blind clinical trials. *The Journal of Trauma: Injury, Infection, and Critical Care* 59 (1) 8–18.

Bongard FS, Sue DY and Vintch JR (2008) *Current Diagnosis and Treatment: Critical Care.* 3rd Edition, McGraw-Hill Medical, Maidenhead.

Brohi K (2006) Massive Transfusion for Blood Loss [online]. Available from: http://www.trauma. org/index.php/main/article/376/ [Accessed 30th November 2008].

Brohi K (2008) Management of Exsanguinating Pelvic Trauma [online]. Availaible from: http://www.trauma.org/index.php/main/article/668 [Accessed 30th November 2008].

Brohi K, Singh J, Heron M and Coats T (2003) Acute traumatic coagulopathy. *Journal of Trauma, Injury, Infection and Critical Care* 54 (6) 1127–1130.

Brooks A, Paynter A and Phillips E (2005) Abdominal trauma. Chapter 27 in O'Shea R (Ed) *Principles and Practice of Trauma Nursing.* Elsevier limited, Edinburgh, pp. 443–455.

Buckle R, Browner BD and Morandi M (1994) Emergency reduction for pelvic ring disruption and control of associated haemorrhage using the pelvic stabiliser. *Techniques in Orthopaedics* 9 (4) 258–266.

Cole E (2008) Initial assessment and resuscitation of the trauma patient. Chapter 2 in Cole E (Ed) *Trauma Care: Initial Assessment and Management in the Emergency Department*. Wiley Blackwell, Oxford, pp. 24–52.

Cole E and McGinley A (2005) A structured approach to caring for the trauma patient. Chapter 4 in O'Shea R (Ed) *Principles and Practice of Trauma Nursing*. Elsevier Limited, Edinburgh, pp. 37–60.

Cothren CC, Osborn PM, Moore EE, Morgan SJ, Johnson JL and Smith WR (2007) Preperitoneal pelvic packing for haemodynamically unstable pelvic fractures: a paradigm shift. *Journal of Trauma, Injury, Infection and Critical Care* 63 (2) 453–454.

Cottingham C (2006) Resuscitation of traumatic shock: a hemodynamic review. *AACN Advanced Critical Care* 17 (3) 317–326.

Criddle L, Eldredge D and Walker J (2005) Variables predicting trauma patient survival following massive transfusion. *Journal of Emergency Nursing* 31 (3) 236–242.

Davies KA (2002) Soft tissue trauma. In Peitzman AB, Rhodes M, Schwab CW, Yealy DM and Fabian TC (Eds) *The Trauma Manual*. 2nd Edition, Lippincott Williams & Wilkins, Philadelphia, pp. 352–355.

Davies G and Lockey D (2005) Prehospital care in trauma patients. Chapter 7 in Galley H (Ed) *Critical Care Focus 11: Trauma*. Blackwell Publishing, Oxford, pp. 76–83.

Department of Health (2006) Immunisation against infectious disease. The Green Book. Chapter 30 in *Tetanus*. http://www.dh.gov.uk/en/Policyandguidance/Healthandsocialcaretopics/Greenbook/DH_4097254.

De Waele JD, Hoster EAJ and Malbrain MLNG (2006) Decompressive laparotomy for abdominal compartment syndrome – a critical analysis. *Critical Care* 10 (2) R51.

DiGiacomo JC, Bonadies JA, Cole FC, *et al.* (2001) *Practice Management Guidelines for Haemorrhage in Pelvic Fracture*. Eastern Association for the Surgery of Trauma, Winston-Salem, NC. [online] Available from: http://www.east.org/tpg/pelvis.pdf. [Accessed 14th March 2009].

Eaton J (2005) Kinetics and mechanics of injury. Chapter 3 in O'Shea R (Ed) *Principles and Practice of Trauma Nursing*. Elsevier limited, Edinburgh, pp. 15–35.

Edwards S (2005) Pathophysiological mechanisms of shock. Chapter 14 in O'Shea R (Ed) *Principles and Practice of Trauma Nursing*. Elsevier Limited, Edinburgh, pp. 181–192.

Findlay G, Martin IC, Carter S, Smith N, Weyman D and Mason M (2007) *Trauma: Who Cares? A Report on the National Confidential Enquiry into Patient Outcome and Death (NCEPOD)*. NCEPOD, London, pp. 10–14.

Frakes MA and Evans T (2004) Major pelvic fractures. *Critical Care Nurse* 24 (2) 18–30.

Greaves I, Porter KM, Ryan JM and Garner J (Eds) (2008a) Mechanism of injury. In *Trauma Care Manual*. 2nd Edition, Arnold, London.

Greaves I, Porter KM, Ryan JM and Garner J (Eds) (2008b) Patient assessment. In *Trauma Care Manual*. 2nd Edition, Arnold, London.

Isbister JP (2003) Blood transfusion. Chapter 86 in Bersten AD and Soni N (Eds) *Oh's Intensive Care Manual*. 5th Edition, Butterworth Heinemann, Edinburgh.

Josty IC, Ramaswamy R and Laing JH (2001) Vacuum assisted closure: an alternative strategy in the management of degloving injuries of the foot. *British Journal of Plastic Surgery* 54 (4) 363–365.

Joynt GM, Ramsay SJ and Buckley TA (2001) Intra-abdominal hypertension – implications for the intensive care physician. *Annals of the Academy of Medicine, Singapore* 30 (3) 310–319.

Judson JA (2003) Severe and multiple trauma. Chapter 64 in Bersten AD and Soni N (Eds) *Oh's Intensive Care Manual*. 5th Edition, Butterworth Heinemann, Edinburgh.

Karkouti K, Beattie WS, Dattilo KM, *et al.* (2006) A propensity score case-control comparison of aprotinin and tranexamic acid in high-transfusion-risk cardiac surgery. *Transfusion* 46 (3) 327–338.

Levi M, Peters M and Büller H (2005) Efficacy and safety of recombinant factor VIIa for treatment of severe bleeding: a systematic review. *Critical Care Medicine* 33 (4) 883–890.

Lozen Y (1999) Intraabdominal hypertension and abdominal compartment syndrome in trauma: pathophysiology and intervention. *AACN Clinical Issues* 10 (1) 104–112.

Mangano DT, Tudor IC and Dietzel C (2006) The risk associated with aprotinin in cardiac surgery. *New England Journal of Medicine* 354 (4) 353–365.

Matthews W and Bentley P (2005) Applied biochemistry pertaining to the trauma patient. Chapter 9 in O'Shea R (Ed) *Principles and Practice of Trauma Nursing*. Elsevier Limited, Edinburgh, pp. 119–128.

McQuillan K, Flynn Macik MB and Whalen E (2008) *Trauma Nursing: From Resuscitation through Rehabilitation*. 4th Edition, Saunders, Philadelphia.

Middlehurst T (2008) Mechanism of Injury. Chapter 1 in Cole E (Ed) *Trauma Care: Initial Assessment and Management in the Emergency Department*. Wiley Blackwell, Oxford, pp. 1–23.

Moore FA, McKinley BA and Moore EE (2004) The next generation in shock resuscitation. *Lancet* 363 (9425) 1988–1996.

National Institute for Clinical Excellence (2004) Trauma–Fluid Replacement Therapy [online]. Available from: http://www.nice.org.uk/Guidance/TA74 [Accessed 15th October 2008].

National Institute for Clinical Excellence (2007) Head Injury. Triage, Assessment, Investigation and Early Management of Head Injury in Infants, Children and Adults. Clinical Guideline 56 [online]. Available from: http://www.nice.org.uk/nicemedia/pdf/word/CG56NICEguidelineword.doc [Accessed 15th October 2008].

Nebelkopt H (1999) Abdominal compartment syndrome. *American Journal of Nursing* 99 (11) 53–59.

Perel P and Roberts I (2007) Colloids vs. crystalloids for fluid resuscitation in critically ill patients. *Cochrane Database of Systematic Reviews* (3). Art. No.: CD000567. DOI: 10.1002/14651858.CD000567.pub3.

Revell M, Greaves I and Porter K (2003) Endpoints for fluid resuscitation in hemorrhagic shock. *Journal of Trauma, Injury, Infection and Critical Care* 54 (5) S63–S67.

Rizoli S (2002) Crystalloids and colloids in trauma resuscitation: a brief overview of the current debate. *Journal of Trauma, Injury, Infection and Critical Care* 54 (5) S82–S88.

Saggi BH, Sugarman HJ, Ivatury RR and Bloomfield GL (1998) Abdominal compartment syndrome. *Journal of Trauma* 45 (3) 597–609.

Shackford SR (recorder) (2000) Pelvic injury symposium. Presented at: OTA-AAST combined Annual Meeting October 12, 2000 San Antonio Texas [online]. Available from: http://www.hwbf.org/ota/s2k/ [Accessed 14th March 2009].

Smith M (2005) Orthopaedic trauma. Chapter 25 in O'Shea R (Ed) *Principles and Practice of Trauma Nursing*. Elsevier Limited, Edinburgh, pp. 379–419.

Spahn DR, Cerny V, Coats TJ, *et al.* (2007) Management of bleeding following major trauma: a European guideline. *Critical Care* 11 (1) R17.

Stern S (2001) Low volume fluid resuscitation for presumed haemorrhagic shock: helpful or harmful? *Current Opinion in Critical Care* 7 (6) 422–430.

Streat SJ (2003) Abdominal surgical catastrophes. Chapter 37 in Bersten AD and Soni N (Eds) *Oh's Intensive Care Manual*. 5th Edition, Butterworth Heinemann, Edinburgh.

Teasdale G and Jennett B (1974) Assessment of coma and impaired consciousness. A practical scale. *Lancet* 2 (7872) 81–84.

Tile M (1988) Pelvic ring fractures: should they be fixed? *Journal of Bone and Joint Surgery* 70 (1) 1–12.

Verbeek D, Sugrue M, Balogh Z, *et al.* (2008) Acute management of haemodynamically unstable pelvic trauma patients: time for a change? Multicenter review of recent practice. *World Journal of Surgery* 32 (8) 1874–1882.

Walker J and Criddle LM (2003) Pathophysiology and management of abdominal compartment syndrome. *American Journal of Critical Care* 12 (4) 367–371.

Wenker OC, Wojciechowski Z, Sheinbaum R and Zisman E (1997) Thrombelastography. *The Internet Journal of Anesthesiology* 1 (3) [online]. Available from: http://www.ispub.com/journal/the_internet_journal_of_anesthesiology/volume_1_number_3_1/article/thrombelastography.html. [Accessed 5th March 2009].

Wong LK, Nesbit RD, Turner LA and Sargent LA (2006) Management of a circumferential lower extremity degloving injury with the use of vacuum-assisted closure. *Southern Medical Journal* 99 (6) 628–630.

Young JW, Burgess AR, Brumback RJ and Poka A (1986) Pelvic fractures: value of plain radiography in early assessment and management. *Radiology* 160 (2) 445–451.

Chapter 9

The patient with a diabetic emergency

Sarah McGloin

Introduction

Diabetes mellitus is a prevalent lifelong condition, with an estimated 300 million people likely to be affected worldwide by the year 2025 (Zimmet *et al.*, 2001). Diabetes UK (2009) estimates that more than two-and-a-half million people are diagnosed with the condition while a further 500,000 individuals remain undiagnosed. Such statistics drove the development of the *National Service Framework for Diabetes* (DH, 2003), which set out a vision for the delivery of diabetic service within England by 2013.

Patient scenario

Gary Williams, a 20-year-old, was admitted to the Emergency Department with a 5-day history of nausea and vomiting. Gary reported that he had also been experiencing difficulty passing urine and it stung when he did manage to pass urine. His urine was concentrated and smelt offensive. However, despite this, he had also experienced frequency of passing urine and an extreme thirst for the past 2 weeks. Gary also complained of a temperature and a dry cough for the past couple of days.

Gary's past medical history is that he was diagnosed with type I diabetes since the age of seven. His diabetes has been well controlled with subcutaneous insulin injections twice a day.

Gary has recently left home and started university where he is studying art and design. He lives in a student house and is having to manage his money for the first time. It is now towards the end of the term and he does not have a lot of money left to buy food. He also enjoys socialising with his friends.

On admission to Emergency Department, Gary was drowsy, lethargic and only rousable to pain.

Gary's observations were as follows:

Blood pressure	125/80 mmHg
Heart rate	127 beats per minute
Respiratory rate	28 breaths per minute
Temperature	35.9°C

Gary's blood results were as follows:

WBC	24,400/μl
Haemaglobin	14.5 g/dl
HCT	60%
Cl^-	95 mmol/l
Creatinine	175 mmol/l
Urea	12 μmol/l
Calcium	8.8 mmol/l
Glucose	30 mmol/l
Phosphorous	6.8 mg/l
Acetone	Moderate
Na^+	126 mmol/l
AST	248 U/l
K^+	5.5 mmol/l
Creatinine kinase (CK)	34/35 U/l
Lactate dehydrogenase (LDH)	38 U/l
Alkaline phosphate	132 U/l

Arterial blood gas results were as follows:

pH	7.14
pCO_2	2.6 kPa
pO_2	12.5 kPa
SaO_2	94%
HCO_3^-	6 mmol/l
Base excess	−10

Urinalysis results were as follows:

Specific gravity	1015
Glucose	+++
Ketones	+++
Protein	+++
Haemoglobin	+++

Ketones were measured in the urine and found to be 150 mg/dl
Glucose was measured in the urine to be 314 mg/dl

A chest x-ray was clear.
On the basis of Gary's past medical history and his clinical presentation, a diagnosis of diabetic ketoacidosis (DKA) was made.

Underlying physiology and pathophysiology

Key consideration

How are blood sugar levels normally controlled?

Control of normal blood sugar levels

The blood glucose of a healthy individual is maintained within the narrow range of between 4 and 7 mmol/l (Wallymahmed, 2006). This tight range is maintained through the action of the endocrine portion of the pancreas.

As has previously been discussed, the pancreas has both the endocrine and exocrine functions (Chapter 4). Situated throughout the exocrine portion are 1–2 million clusters of tissues referred to as *islets of Langerhans* (Totora and Derrickson, 2009). Seventeen percent of the islets of Langerhans are alpha cells responsible for secreting the hormone glucagon, while 70% of the islets of Langerhans are beta cells responsible for secreting the hormone insulin. Delta cells make up 7% of the pancreatic islet cells and secrete the hormone somatostatin, while the remainder are F cells, which secrete pancreatic polypeptide.

Insulin is responsible for lowering the blood glucose levels, while glucagon is responsible for increasing the blood glucose levels. In contrast, somatostatin is responsible for inhibiting the local release of either insulin or glucagon. Somatostatin also slows the absorption of nutrients from the gastrointestinal tract. Pancreatic polypeptide prevents the secretion of somatostatin, while also reducing gall bladder contraction and the secretion of pancreatic juices (Totora and Derrickson, 2009).

The secretion of glucagon and insulin and hence the consistent level of blood glucose are maintained through a negative feedback system.

While blood sugar levels are the main determinate for insulin and glucagon secretion, a number of hormones and neurotransmitters are also involved with regulation of blood glucose levels (Totora and Derrickson, 2009).

The neurotransmitter acetylcholine is released by the vagus nerve of the parasympathetic nervous system (McArdle, 2000). This serves to stimulate the islets of Langerhans to secrete insulin. Increased levels of amino acids such as arginine and leucine also stimulate the secretion of insulin, while glucose-dependent insulin tropic peptide (GIP), which is a hormone secreted by the small intestine, also promotes the secretion of insulin.

In contrast, glucagon is secreted following the innervation of the sympathetic nervous system, particularly during exercise. Glucagon secretion is also stimulated by a rise in amino acids if the blood glucose level is too low.

Glucagon can also directly stimulate insulin secretion, while insulin suppresses glucagon. As blood glucose levels fall, less insulin is secreted. Insulin normally suppresses the alpha cells; so with lower levels of insulin, there is less suppression of the alpha cells and more glucagon are secreted. Human growth hormone (GH) and adrenocorticotropic hormone (ACTH) all increase insulin secretion, as they aim to increase blood glucose levels (Totora and Derrickson, 2009).

Underlying pathophysiology

> **Key considerations**
>
> (1) What are the pathophysiological processes associated with DKA?
> (2) What are the implications for the patient?

Diabetes is a condition which is responsible for significant morbidity (Wallymahmed, 2006). It damages both the microvasculature and the macrovasculature that can affect the quality of life.

Type I diabetes

Type I diabetes is a chronic disease worldwide affecting 10% of the population with diabetes, with the majority of those affected being the young (Zimmet *et al.*, 2001). Type I diabetes – the type Gary has – is the result of the autoimmune destruction of the beta cells. This results in an insulin deficiency, which must be managed with insulin injections (Wallymahmed, 2006). Mortality due to cardiovascular or cerebrovascular disease is common (Soedamah-Muthu *et al.*, 2006). However, Laing *et al.* (1999) have found DKA to be the greatest cause of death among the patients with diabetes who are less than 30 years old.

Type II diabetes

In contrast to type I diabetes, the majority of people with diabetes are those experiencing type II diabetes. Type II diabetes is the result of insufficient insulin production or insulin resistance where the body develops resistance to the effects of insulin. This is a progressive condition, which is the result of increasing hyperglycaemia along with a slow loss of the beta cell function (Wallymahmed, 2006). Type II diabetes is normally treated with lifestyle changes, which progress on to oral hypoglycaemic therapy (Lowey, 2005). Winocour (2002) found that 50% of patients with type II diabetes progress to require insulin therapy. Cardiovascular disease is the main cause of death in this group of patients (Morrish *et al.*, 2001).

Diabetic ketoacidosis

Regarded to be a life-threatening emergency, DKA is a serious complication of diabetes. Mainly associated with type I diabetes, the condition can still be apparent in patients with type II diabetes (Welch and Zibb, 2004).

Trigger factors

Marinac and Mesa (2000) found DKA to be the most common cause of death in patients with diabetes who are 20 years old or younger. Kearney and Dang (2007) and Kitabchi *et al.* (2004) pointed out that infection is the most common cause of DKA. Infection alone results in a lack of insulin being produced and this in itself is the main cause of DKA (Jones and Huether, 2002).

Gary has reduced bladder emptying and is experiencing a stinging sensation upon urination and there is protein, blood and glucose present in his urine. The urine that is produced smells strongly. All this would indicate that Gary has a urinary tract infection (UTI), which could be contributing to his DKA.

Stressful conditions such as cerebral vascular accident, myocardial infarction and trauma have all been seen to precipitate DKA (Kitabchi *et al.*, 2004). Some drugs can also contribute to DKA including atypical antipsychotic agents, corticosteroids, interferon and salbutamol, dobutamine and dopamine (Mofredj *et al.*, 2002; Wilson *et al.*, 2003). However, poor compliance to insulin therapy has been seen to be a further major cause of DKA (Kearney and Dang, 2007).

Features of DKA

Palmer (2004) identifies three concurrent features associated with DKA. These are as follows:

- Hyperglycaemia, which is the result of a hyperosmolar hyperglycaemic state
- Hyperketonaemia, which can result from poor nutrition associated with starvation and alcoholism
- Metabolic acidosis, which is the result of lactic acidosis

A concise diagnostic criteria is put forward by Palmer (2004) who postulates that DKA can be diagnosed from a blood glucose level of equal to or less than 12 mmol/l (or 216 mg/dl), ketonuria and a pH equal to or less than 7.35.

Pathophysiology of DKA

Insulin deficiency is the primary event resulting in DKA (Wolfsdorf *et al.*, 2006). Insulin deficiency can be seen to be the result of poor compliance with therapy, beta cell failure, and the ineffectiveness of insulin in responding to triggers such as stress or infection or the counter-regulatory hormone excesses. The excess of counter-regulatory hormone promotes glucose production from glycogenolysis (increased hepatic glucose production from glycogen) and gluconeogenesis (increased glucose production from amino acids) while simultaneously limiting the use of this glucose (Wolfsdorf *et al.*, 2006). This has the overall result of an increased blood sugar level.

As the blood sugar levels rise, there is an increased urine output, which is referred to as *osmotic diuresis*. As the counter-regulatory hormones break down fats into fatty acids, the oxidation of these fatty acids results in the formation of ketones. Lewis (2000) observed that the ketones then deplete the body's buffer supplies, which results in an overwhelming metabolic acidotic state.

There are a variety of counter-regulatory hormones, which include catecholamines, cortisol, glucagon and GH. Clark (2002) observed that such hormones work as an antagonist against insulin by simply increasing the glucose production.

Piano and Huether (2002) found that glucagon exacerbate the development of DKA through the initiation of lipolysis – the breakdown of fat stored in the adipose tissue as triglycerides. During lipolysis, glucocorticoids stimulate the breakdown of triglycerides into free fatty acids, which are then released into the circulation. Lipolysis also has a ketogenic effect when fatty acids are broken down in the liver resulting in the secretion of ketones, which can then be used for producing energy. This can result in the evolution of a metabolic acidosis, which requires further investigation.

Catecholamines

The catecholamines, adrenaline and nonadrenaline are secreted by the adrenal medulla and the adrenergic nerve fibres. Adrenaline and nonadrenaline play an essential role in the mobilisation of stored energy (Piano and Huether, 2002). Adrenaline and nonadrenaline release the lipid from the adipose tissue and glucose from sources outside the liver. Along with glucagon, the catecholamines assist in the synthesis of glucose. They do this by enhancing the release of fatty acids, stimulating gluconeogenesis and inhibiting the oxidation of fatty acids. Gluconeogenesis is the conversion of a substance other than glycogen or other monosacharides into glucose. Importantly, the catecholamines are responsible for the fright, fight, flight mechanism in response to stress. This inherently needs to mobilise glucose for energy.

Adrenaline and nonadrenaline also inhibit insulin secretion through stimulating the beta adrenergic receptors. Jones and Huether (2002) found that adrenaline, nonadrenaline and glucagon actually oppose the anabolic effect of insulin, that is, the increased uptake of amino acids by the tissues, while simultaneously activating the enzyme systems for lipolysis and glycogenolysis. Glycogenolysis involves the formation of glycogen from glucose and ensures that the central nervous system continues to receive adequate supplies of glucose to continue to function in times of hypoglycaemia. Adrenaline and nonadrenaline also support the gluconeogenesis of amino acids. Thus, if there is little or no insulin, the catecholamines and glucagon will intrinsically increase blood glucose levels through increasing lipolysis and ketogenesis.

Glucocorticoids

In contrast, glucocorticoids are produced by the adrenal cortex. Glucocorticoid production is stimulated by the ACTH. ACTH is produced by the anterior pituitary gland. Cortisol is the main glucocorticoid. During states such as starvation, significant amounts of ACTH are secreted. Cortisol then works on the body's stores of fat as a suitable energy source. As fat becomes depleted, protein becomes the next available energy source.

Insulin normally tempers the effects of all these mechanisms to maintain adequate blood glucose levels. However, if there is infection or poor compliance to therapy, these diabetogenic mechanisms continue unchecked.

It is Gary's first time away from home and he is near the end of his first term at the university. He is starting to run low on money and in an attempt to make his income last until the end of term, Gary has started to skip meals. Thus, his probable UTI, coupled with a reduced dietary intake, is likely to exacerbate his DKA.

Growth hormone

GH is also secreted by the anterior pituitary gland. GH is also thought to increase blood glucose levels by increasing liver glycogenolysis and fat mobilisation. GH is also thought to indirectly increase insulin secretion. GH also reduces glucose uptake by the peripheral tissues by somehow reducing the effect of insulin at the peripheries (Piano and Huether, 2002). GH also inhibits gluconeogenesis. Importantly, the higher the circulating levels of GH, higher is the increased insulin resistance and glucose intolerance.

Triidothyronine and thyroxine

Triidothyronine (T3) and thyroxine (T4) also affect the body's use of glucose. The main function of T3 is to control respiratory oxygen consumption. It accomplishes this by promoting the movement of sodium ions out of the cell. In low concentrations, T3 supports growth, lipogenesis and protein synthesis. However, at higher concentrations, T3 becomes catabolic, resulting in increased heat production, adenosine triphosphate (ATP) and reduced energy within the cells. T3 raises blood glucose levels through gluconeogenesis and glycogenolysis. T3 also stimulates lipolysis, which results in raised blood glucose levels when insulin is not available to temper the effects.

Such factors may also result in insulin resistance. High levels of free fatty acids along with high concentrations of the counter-regulatory hormones, acidosis and hydrogen can all contribute to insulin resistance. In particular, acidosis affects the hormone receptor site as well as inhibiting glycolysis (Gill, 2000).

Insulin

Insulin is secreted by the beta cells of the islets of Langerhans, from its precursor form proinsulin. Insulin is responsible for the uptake of glucose by the cells. In order to do this, insulin binds to its receptor within the cell, this receptor being tyrosine kinase (RTK) receptor. A series of reactions activates proteins, especially glucose transporter 4 (GLUT4). As this GLUT4 translocates, 10–20 times more insulin is taken up by the cells.

Insulin promotes the synthesis of protein, carbohydrate, lipids and nucleic acids. It also increases the uptake of amino acids by the tissues and also the generation of protein by the liver.

Once in the liver, insulin stimulates the uptake of glucose as well as the synthesis of glycogen and fatty acids. It simultaneously suppresses gluconeogenesis, glycogenolysis and ketogenesis. In the tissues, it inhibits fat and protein breakdown, while stimulating protein synthesis and cellular metabolism.

In DKA, it is the lack of insulin, for whatever reason, which leads to the disease condition. The lack of insulin, whether due to infection, poor compliance to therapy or poorly controlled counter-regulatory hormones, results in reduced insulin levels, which in turn results in DKA if left untreated.

Signs and symptoms of DKA

> **Key considerations**
>
> What are the signs and symptoms of DKA?
> What are the complications associated with DKA?

DKA is rapidly occurring, and patients with DKA will present with polyuria, and polydipsia secondary to the osmotic diuresis, polyphagia, weakness and weight loss due to tissue catabolism and dehydration and Kussmauls (deep and rapid breathing) breathing (Trachtenbarg, 2006). The patient may have abdominal pain, along with nausea and vomiting, which may at times have coffee ground appearance. The patient's body temperature will be normal or low as they compensate for an infective state. The mucous membranes will appear dry, there will be an elevated heart rate associated with the dehydration and the blood pressure will be low. The patient will also excrete ketones via the respiratory system, resulting in ketotic or 'pear drop' breath (Palmer, 2004). The patient may either be alert, confused, fatigued or even comatose (Williams and Pickup, 2004).

To summarise, the overwhelming manifestations of DKA include hyperglycaemia, ketonaemia, ketonuria, acidosis, dehydration and electrolyte imbalance (Chiasson *et al.*, 2003).

Complications associated with DKA

The complications associated with DKA include cerebral oedema. This is fatal in 50% of cases. Cerebral oedema occurs within 2 hours following the start of treatment for DKA and is associated with headache, confusion, lethargy and hyperpyrexia (Trachtenbarg, 2006). The exact mechanism for the onset of cerebral oedema is poorly understood (Park, 2006). However, the patients with newly diagnosed diabetes and those who have been in a DKA state for a protracted time are at greater risk of developing cerebral oedema. Rapid fluid replacement, rapid correction of blood glucose levels and bicarbonate replacement have all been associated with cerebral oedema and as such Kitabchi *et al.* (2004) suggest preventing over-hydration and rapid reduction in blood glucose levels.

An osmotic diuresis is also associated with DKA. This is the result of an increased osmotic pressure within the kidney tubule. The increased osmotic pressure is due to the high levels of glucose in the filtrate, which is present within the kidney tubule. As a result, fluid is retained by this high osmotic pressure within the kidney tubule rather than being reabsorbed back into the circulation. The patient then produces a high volume of very dilute urine, while the cardiovascular system becomes hypovolaemic and blood pressure is then affected. Palmer (2004) found that patients may also experience acute respiratory distress syndrome (ARDS), thromboembolism, gastric stasis and mediastinal surgical emphysema.

Assessment and diagnosis

> **Key considerations**
>
> What strategies should be used to assess Gary?
> What diagnostic studies should be taken?

Upon admission to the Emergency Department, a thorough physical assessment took place using the A, B, C, D, E taxonomy.

Airway: Gary was assessed as having a patent airway, which he was able to protect himself.

Breathing and ventilation: His respiratory rate was elevated and he was demonstrating Kussmaul. His breath did have a fruity odour. Gary's oxygen saturation was 94%. A chest X-ray was taken to assess for signs of ARDS (Palmer, 2004).

Circulation: Considering Gary's circulation, his pulse should be monitored for rate, strength and regularity. While his blood pressure remained acceptable, he was tachycardic. It would be necessary to insert an arterial line in order to continuously monitor Gary's blood pressure and intermittently monitor his arterial blood gases. Gary's arterial blood gases were showing a severe uncompensated metabolic acidosis. Gary was trying to compensate for this through his respiratory system, which manifested itself as very low pCO_2 levels. In view of his significant electrolyte imbalance, a 12-lead electrocardiogram (ECG) was taken. Wiggamm *et al.* (1997) found that ECGs are a useful way of determining a baseline potassium level prior to receiving blood results. Gary was then commenced on continuous cardiac monitoring. No arrhythmias were detected.

Gary had vomited a number of times. His capillary refill time was 5 seconds and his peripheries looked cold and clammy. Gary had reduced skin turgor.

Gary's urine output remained poor although he did have a palpable bladder. A urinary catheter was inserted, and 1.5 l of very dilute but cloudy urine was passed. A catheter stream urine sample was sent for microbiology. There were ketones present in his urine. Blood and throat cultures were also sent for examination.

Disability: Gary had an AVPU (Alert, Verbal, Painful, Unresponsive) score of P. He was extremely drowsy and lethargic. His blood sugar was 30 mmol/l. Gary's Glasgow Coma Score was 10, indicated by Gary opening his eyes and localising to pain, while at the same time making incomprehensible sounds. Gary was not complaining of a headache and his pupils were equal and reacting to light size 4.

Exposure: Being young, Gary's pressure areas were intact. A university friend had arrived with Gary and was able to provide a limited history that Gary was an insulin-controlled patient with diabetes. The friend gave details of Gary's general practitioner (GP). The GP was contacted for a full history.

Diagnostic studies

Blood samples should be taken to measure the serum or plasma glucose levels (Wolfsdorf *et al.*, 2006). Electrolytes should also be measured, including blood urea nitrogen (BUN) levels, creatinine, pH, osmolarity, haemoglobin, haematocrit, full blood count, calcium, phosphorous, magnesium concentrations, HbA1C and blood β-hydroxybutyrate concentration (Wiggamm *et al.*, 1997).

The anion gap

The anion gap is a useful tool that can be used to diagnose the presence and severity of a metabolic acidosis. The test can also be used to measure the response of such an acidosis to treatment.

The anion gap itself is the concentration of all unmeasured plasma ions. During metabolic acidosis, acid anions are produced. Such anions include lactate and sulphate, anions that are not normally measured by usual biochemistry tests. Hence these anions are referred to as *unmeasured.*

During an acidotic state, hydrogen ions are produced. These react with bicarbonate ions, and carbon dioxide is also excreted by the lungs as a means of compensating for the increased hydrogen ions. All of these result in a decrease in the measured anions and an increase in the unmeasured anions. Consequently, the anion gap increases. The normal range is 8–16 mmol/l.

The anion gap is calculated by the simple formula:

$$Na^+ - (Cl^- + HCO_3^-)$$

Therefore in Gary's case his anion gap can be calculated as:

$$126 - (95 + 6) = 25 \text{ mmol/l}$$

Therefore, Gary has a metabolic acidosis.

It was felt that a central venous pressure (CVP) line would be useful to guide Gary's fluid management. CVP lines have also been seen to enhance venous access (Jevon and Ewens, 2007).

Evidence-based care

Key considerations

How should Gary's fluid be managed?
How should his blood sugars be controlled?
How should his electrolytes be managed and controlled?

Kitabchi *et al.* (2004) argue that those with mild DKA can actually be managed in the primary care setting. However, as Gary had a blood glucose level of 30 mmol/l along with a metabolic acidosis and ketonuria, this would be inappropriate and the decision was made to admit him to an acute medical ward for management of his condition. Indeed Park (2006), Trachtenbarg (2006) and Xue (2007) argue that those with severe DKA should be admitted to critical care settings.

The primary aims of the treatment of DKA are to replace fluid losses, lower the blood glucose level, correct the electrolyte imbalance and treat the underlying cause of the crisis (Xue, 2007).

Fluids

Xue (2007) found that fluid depletion for patients with DKA is seen to be between 5 and 8 l with Kitabchi *et al.* (2004) finding it to be 100 ml/kg of body weight. As far back as 1983, Schade and Eaton (1983) have seen that 80% of declines in blood glucose levels are the result of fluid therapy.

If the patient is in hypovolaemic shock, rapid fluid replacement is required. Kitabchi *et al.* (2004) and Xue (2007) recommend the administration of intravenous, isotonic saline solution between 1 and 1.5 l/hr until the hypovolaemia is reversed. The aim is to restore renal perfusion. Simply by administering the fluid, plasma osmolarity will be lowered and blood glucose levels reduced. If the patient is normotensive as Gary is, Kitabchi *et al.* (2004) recommend that serum sodium levels be obtained. If the serum sodium levels are low, they suggest giving normal saline between 4 and 14 ml/kg/hr depending on the hydration, whereas if the sodium levels are high, they suggest giving 0.45% normal saline at 4–14 ml/kg/hr. However, Park (2006) argues against the use of 0.45% saline, finding that there is no evidence to support its use for the treatment of DKA. If the patient has cardiogenic shock, it is advised to administer fluid determined upon haemodynamic monitoring results. Should the blood glucose level fall below 14 mmol/l 10% dextrose may be added at a rate of 100 ml/hour.

All patients should be commenced on a strict fluid balance chart (Park, 2006). Patients who are able to drink should be allowed to do so. This should be included into their fluid balance. Importantly, as the serum osmolarity reduces, so will the diuresis, as the osmotic effect on diuresis will be reduced. The rate of serum osmolarity should not be reduced by any value greater than 3 mOsm/hr. If the rate of osmolarity changes too fast, it can result in cerebral oedema (Kearney and Dang, 2007).

As soon as the blood glucose level drops below 250 mg/dl, dextrose saline should be administered to prevent further ketosis developing.

A nasogastric tube should be inserted if the patient is experiencing long periods of nausea and vomiting (Park, 2006).

Insulin therapy

Insulin therapy reduces glycogenolysis while increasing the volume of glucose taken up by the peripheral tissues. Consequently, blood glucose levels are also reduced. A continuous intravenous infusion of moderate doses of insulin is the standard delivery for patient with DKA (Lee *et al.*, 2004; Park, 2006). The rate is 0.1 unit/kg/hr or 6 units/hr (Trachtenbarg, 2006). This enables a steady fall in blood glucose levels. If there is too rapid a fall in blood sugar levels greater than 5 mmol/hr, there is an increased risk of cerebral oedema (Park, 2006).

If the blood sugar levels remain stubbornly high, refusing to fall by 50–70 mg/dl/hr, then insulin should be doubled until the glucose level falls by 50–70 mg/dl. When the serum glucose returns to 2250 mg/dl or less, the infusion should be reduced to 0.05–0.10 unit/kg/hr to maintain a serum glucose level between 150 and 200 mg/dl, until the metabolic profile improves. Interestingly, Umpierrez *et al.* (2004) found that despite lowering the blood glucose level quicker, intravenous insulin had no effect on mortality or morbidity rates.

Insulin therapy also assists the acid–base balance. Because insulin reduces the number of free fatty acids which are released there are fewer ketones that are synthesised. With a lower ketone level, the level of acid produced also falls and homeostasis is returned.

Potassium

Metabolic acidosis will increase the potassium levels, as the hydrogen ions have a greater affinity with the intracellular fluid than the potassium ions. A treatment for increased potassium levels is to administer glucose with insulin (Trachtenbarg, 2006). However, this should only be commenced if the patient is passing urine (Park, 2006). As soon as the potassium levels fall below 5 mmol/l, potassium should be replaced through the maintenance fluids at 20–30 mmol/l. If the potassium level drops to below 3.3 mmol/l, Kitabchi *et al.* (2004) recommend that the potassium be replaced and the insulin infusion halted until the potassium level returns to normal.

Bicarbonate

There is no empirical evidence to suggest that bicarbonate replacement is beneficial in patients with a pH of 6.9 or above (Park, 2006; Trachtenbarg, 2006). Indeed, Viallon *et al.* (1999) found that bicarbonate therapy may actually be harmful by delaying the correction of the metabolic acidosis. Park (2006) argues that bicarbonate may also be associated with hypoxia, hypokalaemia and an increase in cerebral spinal fluid acidosis. Trachtenbarg (2006) does advise giving bicarbonate if the pH is below 6.9, while Park (2006) only recommends its use in patients with cardiogenic shock or other conditions resulting in raised lactic acid.

Phosphate

It is argued that phosphate replacement fails to improve outcomes in those with DKA and can actually result in hypocalcaemia (Kitabchi *et al*. 2004). If the phosphate level remains low, Trachtenbarg (2006) suggests administering phosphate in the form of potassium phosphate; however, the calcium level will need to be closely monitored (Kitabchi *et al*., 2004).

Magnesium

Often, with DKA the magnesium level is reduced. Trachtenbarg (2006) suggests replacing magnesium if the levels are below 0.50 mol/l and if the patient is experiencing symptoms such as parathesis, tremor, agitation and seizures.

Sodium

A raised sodium level will be the result of dehydration and will resolve with the rehydration therapy (Trachtenbarg, 2006).

Ongoing care

Having been admitted to the Emergency Department, Gary has an internal jugular CVP line inserted and is commenced on continuous cardiac monitoring. Gary also has an arterial line to monitor his arterial blood gases and his urea and electrolyte levels. Gary is catheterised and a nasogastric tube is inserted. He is commenced on a strict fluid balance chart. Gary's observations are recorded hourly and his Glasgow Coma Score also completed hourly to assess for signs of cerebral oedema. An Early Warning Score is also commenced.

Gary is commenced on intravenous fluid replacement of normal saline at 1000 ml/hr. A sliding scale of intravenous human sequence insulin (Actrapid) is also commenced at a rate of 6 IU/hr. Gary is then transferred to the High Dependency Unit (HDU).

On the HDU, the normal saline is continued at a rate of 1000 ml/hr for a further 2 hours. Gary's BUN and electrolyte levels are recorded after 2 hours. The normal saline is then reduced to 500 ml/hr for a further 2 hours after which further BUN and electrolyte levels are recorded. Gary's potassium levels then start to fall to 4.2 mmol/l and so 20 mmol of potassium is added to the saline infusion.

Gary remains on hourly blood glucose monitoring. As his blood glucose level start to fall below 9 mmol/l, the rate of his sliding scale is reduced to 3 IU/hr. This maintains his blood glucose levels at 9 mmol/l.

As Gary's metabolic acidosis improves and his blood glucose levels return to normal at 5 mmol/l, Gary's level of consciousness improves. As Gary continues on his intravenous insulin via a sliding scale, it is decided to commence 10% dextrose with 20 mmol of potassium at 100 ml/hr along with normal saline at 250 ml/hr. This is continued until Gary's bicarbonate level returns to normal and he is able to start to eat and drink. Gary's potassium levels return to normal as he starts to eat and drink and so the potassium replacement is also discontinued.

After 2 days of the sliding scale insulin infusion, Gary's blood glucose levels return to 8 mmol/l. It is decided to stop the intravenous insulin infusion and to recommence Gary's normal subcutaneous insulin injections. The fluids and intravenous insulin are discontinued

30 minutes after the subcutaneous injection was administered. This is to ensure that therapeutic insulin levels were maintained (Park, 2006).

Gary's DKA was precipitated by a urinary infection secondary to acute retention. The urology team review Gary for the cause of the retention. Gary is commenced on intravenous antibiotics. The DKA had also been exacerbated by Gary's poor diet and lifestyle changes since he started his life at the university. Following his discharge, Gary has regular follow-up appointments with the diabetic nurse specialist who monitors Gary's management of his diabetes.

Conclusion

DKA is a potentially life-threatening condition, which is predominately seen in patients with type I diabetes. This condition occurs as a result of a lack of insulin and a rapid rise in blood sugar levels. In order to obtain energy, the body breaks down fats, the by-product of which is the secretion of ketone bodies, resulting in metabolic acidosis. Depending on the severity of the DKA, the patient will require treatment with insulin and fluids and may also require other organ support including ventilation and haemofiltration, particularly to manage the acidosis. Upon discharge from critical care, it is essential that the reason for the lack of insulin is identified and addressed if necessary through appropriate patient support and education.

References

Chiasson JL, Aris-Jilwan N, Belanger R, Bertand S, Beauregard H and Ekoe JM (2003) Diagnosis and treatment of diabetic ketoacidosis and the hyperglycaemic hyperosmolar state. *Canadian Medical Association Journal* 168 (7) 859–866.

Clark JM (2002) Endocrine disorders and therapeutic management. Chapter 37 in Urden LD, Stacey KM and Lough ME (Eds) *Thelan's Critical Care Nursing: Diagnosis and Management.* 4th Edition, Mosby, St Louis, MO.

Department of Health (2003) *National Service Framework for Diabetes Delivery Strategy.* The Stationary Office, London.

Diabetes UK (2009) What is Diabetes? Website http://www.diabetes.org.uk/Guide-to-diabetes/Introduction-to-diabetes/What_is_diabetes/ [Accessed 19th May 2009].

Gill GN (2000) Endocrine diseases. In Goldman L and Bennett JC (Eds) *Cecil Textbook of Medicine.* 21st Edition, WB Saunders, Philadelphia.

Jevon B and Ewens P (2007) *Monitoring the Critically Ill Patient.* 2nd Edition, Wiley Blackwell, Oxford.

Jones RE and Huether SE (2002) Alterations of hormonal regulation. Part two; Chapter 2 in McCance KL and Huether SE (Eds) *Pathophysiology: The Biological Basis for Disease in Adults and Children.* 4th Edition, Mosby, St Louis, MO.

Kearney T and Dang C (2007) Diabetic and endocrine emergencies. *Postgraduate Medical Journal* 83 79–86.

Kitabchi AE, Umpirerrez GE, Murphy MB, Barrett EJ, Kreisberg RA and Malone JL (2004) Hyperglycaemic crises in diabetes. *Diabetic Care* 27 (Suppl. 1) S94–S102.

Laing SP, Swerdlow AJ and Slater SD (1999) The British Diabetic Society Cohort Study I: all cause mortality in patients with insulin treated diabetes mellitus. *Diabetes Medicine* 16 (6) 459–465.

Lee SW, Im R and Magbaul R (2004) Current perspectives on the use of continuous subcutaneous insulin infusion in the acute care setting and overview of therapy. *Critical Care Nursing Quarterly* 27 172–184.

Lewis R (2000) Diabetic emergencies: part 2. Hyperglycaemia. *Accident and Emergency Nursing* 8 (1) 24–30.

Lowey A (2005) Drug treatment of type 2 diabetes in adults. *Nursing Standard* 20 (11) 55–64.

Marinac J and Mesa L (2000) Using a severity scoring system to assess intensive care admissions for diabetic ketoacidosis. *Critical Care Medicine* 28 (7) 2238–2241.

McArdle J (2000) The biological and nursing implications of pancreatitis. *Nursing Standard* 14 (48) 46–53.

Mofredj A, Howaizi M, Grasset D, Licht H, Loison S and Devergie B (2002) Diabetes mellitus during interferon therapy for chronic viral hepatitis. *Digestive Diseases and Sciences* 47 (7) 1649–1654.

Morrish NJ, Wang S-L, Stevens LK, Fuller JH and Keen H (2001) Mortality and causes of death in the WHO Multinational Study of Vascular Disease. *Diabetologia* 44 (Suppl. 2) S14–S21.

Palmer R (2004) An overview of diabetic ketoacidosis. *Nursing Standard* 19 (10) 42–44.

Park C (2006) Diabetic ketoacidosis. *Journal of the Royal College of Physicians Edinburgh* 37 40–43.

Piano MR and Huether SE (2002) Mechanisms of hormonal regulation. Part two; Chapter 2 in McCance KL and Huether SE (Eds) *Pathophysiology: The Biological Basis for Disease in Adults and Children*. 4th Edition, Mosby, St Louis, MO.

Schade DS and Eaton PR (1983) Diabetic ketoacidosis – pathogenesis, prevention and therapy. *Clinical Endocrinology Metabolism* 12 (2) 321–338.

Soedamah-Muthu SS, Fuller J, Mulnier HE, Raleigh VS, Lawrenson RA and Colhoun MH (2006) High risk cardiovascular disease in patients with type 1 diabetes in the UK. *Diabetes Care* 29 (4) 798–804.

Totora GJ and Derrickson BH (2009) *Principles of Anatomy and Physiology*. 12th Edition, John Wiley & Sons, Hoboken , NJ.

Trachtenbarg DE (2006) Diabetic ketoacidosis. *American Family Physician* 71 (9) 1705–1714.

Umpierrez GE, Latif K, Stoever J, Cuervo R, Park L and Freire AX (2004) Efficacy of subcutaneous insulin lispro versus continuous intravenous regular insulin for the treatment of patients with diabetic ketoacidosis. *American Journal of Medicine* 117 (5) 291–296.

Viallon A, Zeni F, Lafond P, Venet C, Tardy B and Page Y (1999) Does bicarbonate therapy improve the management of severe diabetic ketoacidosis. *Critical Care Medicine* 27 (12) 2690–2693.

Wallymahmed M (2006) Insulin therapy in the management of type 1 and type 2 diabetes. *Nursing Standard* 21 (6) 50–56.

Welch BJ and Zibb I (2004) Case study: diabetic ketoacidosis in type 2 diabetes; "look under the sheets". *Clinical Diabetes* 22 (4) 198–200.

Wiggamm MI, O'Kane MJ, Harper R, *et al.* (1997) Treatment of diabetic ketoacidosis using normalization of blood 3-hydroxybutyrate concentration as the end point of emergency management: a randomized controlled study. *Diabetes Care* 20 (9) 1347–1352.

Williams G and Pickup J (2004) *Handbook of Diabetes*. 3rd Edition, Blackwell Science, Oxford.

Wilson DR, D'Souza L, Starker N, Newton M and Hammond C (2003) New onset diabetes and ketoacidosis with atypical antipsychotics. *Schizophrenia Review* 59 (1) 1–6.

Winocour PH (2002) Effective diabetes care: a need for realistic targets. *British Medical Journal* 324 (7353) 1577–1580.

Wolfsdorf J, Glaser N and Sperling MA (2006) Diabetic ketoacidosis in infants, children and adolescents. *Diabetes Care* 29 (5) 1150–1159.

Xue Y (2007) *Diabetic Ketoacidosis and Hyperglycaemia Hyperosmolar Nonketotic Syndrome: Clinical Information. Evidence Summaries*. The Joanna Briggs Institute, Adelaide , Australia.

Zimmet P, Alberti KG and Shaw J (2001) Global and societal implications of the diabetes epidemic. *Nature* 414 (6865) 782–787.

Chapter 10

The long-term patient in intensive care unit

Phillipa Tredant

Introduction

The intensive care unit (ICU) has a long history of being a frightening and traumatic environment, where a patient can suffer severe disorientation, pain, communication problems, sensory deprivation, amnesia and confusion (Maddox *et al.*, 2001; Bennun *et al.*, 2003). The aim of this chapter is to give an insight into what many of these issues are and how health-care professionals can provide intuition, understanding and empathy to their patients and their relatives.

Patient scenario

John is a 28-year-old man who was involved in a road traffic accident when he was riding his motorbike. He was hit by a car and sustained a T2-3 spinal cord contusion. He required mechanical ventilation due to ascending spinal oedema.

He had been in the ICU for 8 weeks and has now been weaned from the ventilator. He developed acute respiratory distress syndrome (ARDS) due to a chest wall injury at the time of the accident; however, he is now self-ventilating via a tracheostomy. He required muscle relaxants and sedation during the period of ARDS to maintain critical gas exchange.

He has power in his upper limbs; however, he has reduced motor and sensory function below the level of the injury. He has had a swallow assessment and can commence on thickened fluids.

He no longer requires level 3 care and is due to be transferred to the neurological ward when a bed is available and he is very anxious about this. Jane, his partner, and his family are also anxious about the transfer and John's ongoing psychological well-being.

Impact of being in the critical care environment

John's time in ICU will have affected him on many different levels from psychological through to physical, and some of these will be short-lasting while others will have a longer term effect upon his whole well-being. The psychological and physiological effects can be separated into individual categories (Tables 10.1 and 10.2), although it should be noted that these issues are ultimately interlinked and will often interface one another.

Table 10.1   Examples of psychological disorders

Delirium
Post-traumatic stress disorder (PTSD)
Flashbacks
Hallucinations
Nightmares
Fear of dying
Fear of family members dying
Panic attacks
Depression
Disorientation
Guilt
Paranoia
Bizarre bodily sensations
Fear that their lives will never be the same again
Abnormal sleep patterns
Agoraphobia

Table 10.2   Examples of physical disorders

Generalised weakness/tiredness/irritability
Severe muscle wastage
Critical illness neuropathy/peripheral neuropathy
Foot and wrist drop
Recovering organ failure/multiorgan failure
Reduced pulmonary and circulatory reserve
Appetite loss
Stiffness from not mobilising for a long period of time
Changes to sleep patterns
Tracheal stenosis from multiple intubations
Scarring from drains/invasive monitoring/tracheostomies
Altered body image
Sexual dysfunction/erectile dysfunction
Voice changes
Weight loss
Thirst
Skin irritation/rashes
Hair loss

Survival in ICU was once deemed successful if the patient was discharged to the ward, but now there is a different interpretation of what is meant by a 'successful outcome'. There is a greater emphasis on a more transitional approach adopted for success to be expressed in the broader sense of restoring these patients ideally back to their former health status – psychologically and physically. With recommendations from the Department of

Health's *Quality in Critical Care: Beyond Comprehensive Critical Care*, a report by the Critical Care Stakeholder Forum (2005), there is an ongoing need to improve the patient's experience and this has raised many issues within the ICU setting. The challenge for the multidisciplinary team (MDT) in the ICU environment is to continue to have a role in the care of the patient and relative beyond discharge from the ICU. Many patients continue to suffer significant physical and psychological problems following discharge from the intensive care environment (Culter *et al.*, 2003; Strahan *et al.*, 2003; Chaboyer *et al.*, 2005).

Psychological effects

Key considerations

(1) What are the psychological effects of being in the critical care environment for this length of time?
(2) How may these effects be displayed?

John identified with many of the psychological consequences outlined in Table 10.1. He found his psychological well-being to be of a cyclic nature (Figure 10.1). For example, if he had nightmares, he felt he had not slept and with that he felt more anxious, which made him prone to panic attacks. This, overall, made him feel more tired and so this had a direct impact on his physical well-being as he was then unable to carry out his physiotherapy. When he was unable to participate in his physiotherapy, this in turn made him feel more depressed as he felt he was not making any progress towards recovery. This would then make him fret about not sleeping properly and feel even more anxious, and hence the

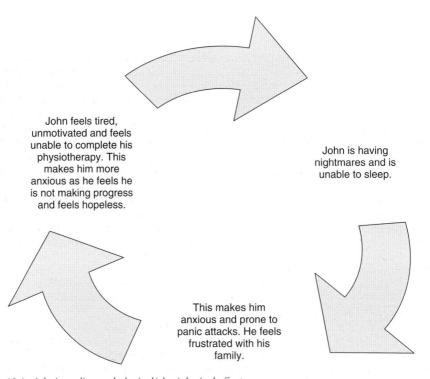

John feels tired, unmotivated and feels unable to complete his physiotherapy. This makes him more anxious as he feels he is not making progress and feels hopeless.

John is having nightmares and is unable to sleep.

This makes him anxious and prone to panic attacks. He feels frustrated with his family.

Figure 10.1 John's cyclic psychological/physiological effects.

cycle starts again. John also experienced altered sensory interpretation of stimuli, which he found frightening and difficult to comprehend. This was identified as lack of accurate recall of situations and cognitive alterations, which ultimately can be similar to post-traumatic stress disorder (PTSD).

Memories

Many of John's psychological issues and problems are related to his memory (and conversely, his lack of remembering) of ICU, which is not uncommon (Bennun *et al.*, 2003). Despite his lack of memory of his stay in ICU, he has reported a number of altered recollections, for example, flashbacks, hallucinations and nightmares. ICU, as an environment, has many metaphors but John described it as a bright white technical place, with unfamiliar voices and touch. At times, he said it could be very loud with shouting, which could also be incomprehensible and piercing beeps were described as coming from all directions.

Noise

Christensen (2007) suggested that extreme noise levels are a contributing feature towards developing ICU delirium. According to Christensen (2007), the World Health Organization (WHO) recommends that noise levels do not exceed 35 dB during the night and 40 dB during the day. However, in a small study within a nine-bedded ICU, Christensen (2007) found that the mean noise level was 56.42 decibels, with spikes up to 80 decibels. Noise levels such as these can have considerable deleterious effects such as excessive cardiovascular stimulation, pituitary/adrenal gland stimulation and immunocompromise due to immune suppression. Noise at this level can also cause psychological alterations by contributing to the development of ICU delirium and consequences of sleep deprivation.

Altered perception

John also reported that he felt wires were wrapped around him to hold him down, which at an instant turned into snakes. It is likely that he was probably referring to his arterial line, central venous catheter, which had numerous infusions running through, his pulse oximeter probe and indwelling catheter. The worrying factor is that John's lack of memory for actual events has been replaced by vivid hallucinations and nightmares, which can be of a persecutory/torturous nature (Rattray and Crocker, 2007) and furthermore can have a causative effect on psychological morbidity of ICU post discharge (Bennun *et al.*, 2003). This could account for the fear of dying some patients have been known to have post-ICU discharge and there have also been suggestions of patients having cognitive impairment following discharge (Maddox *et al.*, 2001).

Memories are related to the patient's emotions and emotional stability in ICU (Löf *et al.*, 2008). John felt secure when his partner Jane and immediate family members were visiting. He also felt safe with the nursing staff; however, his feelings of anxiety, pain and discomfort were related to painful scenarios such as invasive line insertion but also his lack of control over his body. At times, these feelings can be related to unreal experiences or false memories and also towards the feeling of impending death (Löf *et al.*, 2008).

Memories lessen with time, and Löf *et al.* (2008) noted that by 12 months these objectionable feelings reduced. However, they also reported that memories can intensify, with this being a precursor to developing PTSD.

For many patients, an opportunity to discuss the memories or lack of them with a health-care professional is vital in recovery as there is no set treatment for the memories or lack of them. Using follow-up services would be the most appropriate and then further referrals to counsellors can be made ensuring that the patients stay within the system and can be easily monitored.

Delirium/cognitive function

Cognitive function

John showed early signs of difficulty in concentrating. His ability to remember and follow conversations was also delayed and understandably this manifested into pure frustration and resentment. This would suggest that John was developing or showing signs of cognitive impairment/delirium, which is not uncommon (Maddox *et al.*, 2001). Angus and Carlet (2003) described cognitive function as a more generalised term, which also includes language and numerical skills and the ability to absorb information and respond.

Delirium

Historically, delirium was put under the large umbrella term of ICU psychosis/syndrome; however, with advances in research and the introduction of follow-up clinics this term has been narrowed down to the diagnosis of delirium.

Delirium is considered to be an acute, alternating state of mental well-being that can have fluctuating levels of consciousness and has been noted to affect 20–80% of the ICU population (Pandharipande *et al.*, 2005). The pathophysiological aspects of delirium and how it manifests itself appears to be related to systemic infections and injury of the brain and how this in turn produces an inflammatory reaction (Pandharipande *et al.*, 2005). This reaction creates cell damage and the production of cytokines and cell infiltration and this is considered to change the patterns of neuronal action, resulting in delirium (Pandharipande *et al.*, 2005). There are other common medical causes (Table 10.3). One of the other major contributing medical causes includes the use of sedation and analgesia, especially benzodiazepines, in the development of delirium (Pandharipande *et al.*, 2005). Predisposing factors include patients with a history of hypertension, smoking, alcohol abuse and recreational drug use, and have been predominately found in the older population (Ridley, 2005). According to Rattray and Crocker (2007) and Pandharipande *et al.* (2005), delirium is associated with increased mortality.

Delirium can be misdiagnosed, especially when a patient is intubated; it is difficult in these circumstances to appropriately assess if a patient has a fluctuating mental health status or is having difficulty processing information. Delirium can be associated with aggressiveness and hallucinations, which are not uncommon; however, patients can have delirium but be completely passive and lethargic with it (Granberg *et al.*, 1999).

Assessment of delirium

To aid the diagnosis, an assessment tool, with easily answerable criteria, is the most appropriate form of assessment. Pandharipande *et al.* (2005) and Ridley (2005) cite the confusion assessment method (CAM) as an appropriate tool. The use of this tool is

Table 10.3   Examples of medical causes of delirium

Tumour necrosis syndrome

Metabolic derangements

Electrolyte imbalance

Hypoxemia

Poor cerebral perfusion from shock/coagulopathy

Mechanical ventilation

(Adapted from Pandharipande *et al.* [2005] Delirium: acute cognitive dysfunction in the critically ill. *Current Opinion in Critical Care* 11 360–368; Ridley [2005]. *Critical Care Focus 12: The Psychological Challenges of Intensive Care*. Blackwell, London.)

meant to standardise the diagnoses of delirium and can be adjusted to the ICU setting. There is no set protocol for the treatment of delirium; however, early recognition is vital. Pharmacological agents are useful; however, benzodiazepines should be avoided and should only be used once all contributing pathophysiological factors are corrected as seen in Table 10.3 (Pandharipande *et al.*, 2005).

Care strategies

Simple strategies, such as regulating sleeping patterns, can be incorporated within patient care and can aid in the avoidance of ICU delirium. If necessary, pharmacological agents can be used but benzodiazepines should be avoided. 'Normalising the patient' within the ICU is important, for example, by removing invasive lines, monitoring and using catheters when appropriate. The patient should be appropriately cognitively stimulated and encouraged to interact with relatives and the MDT. Strategies such as these should allow the patient to feel secure within the ICU environment. Noise levels should be kept low and the patient orientated to time and place. Avoiding delirium is a far better outcome for the patient, especially in relation to the long-term psychological outcomes and is also more cost-effective for the ICU.

Post-traumatic stress disorder (PTSD)

John survived a highly traumatic injury and spent a long period of time in ICU. The long-term effects of these situations can act as a precursor to developing PTSD due to the unfamiliar, terrifying and at times painful environment and memories. It has been well-documented that patients can suffer signs and symptoms of PTSD in ICU and post discharge, with some patients experiencing PTSD for up to 10 years (Culter *et al.*, 2003; Chaboyer *et al.*, 2005; Granja *et al.*, 2005; Storli *et al.*, 2008).

There is varying statistics on the number of patients thought to have PTSD; however, Griffiths *et al.* (2008) noted that PTSD can occur in intensive care patients with an incidence rate as widespread as 5–64%. PTSD is a term used for a severe psychological disorder that is highly traumatic for the individual. It is an event that usual psychological defences are incapable of coping with. PTSD may be triggered by any number of external or internal factors (Table 10.4) but symptoms can include flashbacks, nightmares, intrusive thoughts and psychological numbing (Glendinning, 2001).

Historically, PTSD is a well-recognised disorder in survivors of accidents, war zones and disasters (Hall-Smith *et al.*, 1997). It is distinguished by a number of reactions to an unusual event experienced outside the norm of everyday human life. In the ICU, it is often the dreams/nightmares post discharge and during the patients' admission that exemplify their own experiences and are a constant reminder of how unwell they once were.

It is during the time of discharge that patients often rationalise how their own personal disaster has impacted upon their own life (Hall-Smith *et al.*, 1997). There is also no set

Table 10.4   Examples of internal and external factors of PTSD

Internal	External
Genetic vulnerability	The environment
Gender	Socio-economic stressors
Cortisol levels	General life ongoing stressors
Personality characteristics	Poor support network
Recent life stressors	How others react to oneself
Recent life change	

period when PTSD can occur; however, Perrins *et al.* (1998) emphasised that it may occur at less than 3 months, which would be considered acute. After that period, if the PTSD persists, it would be considered a chronic phase with delayed onset being not uncommon.

There appears to be no set protocol treatment for PTSD; however, early referrals to a mental health specialist and careful use of medication to improve sleep patterns and mood may well help the patient. At worst, if not recognised, a patient may have suicidal thought/tendencies and once in the home environment this can manifest as the patient's use of drugs and alcohol as coping mechanisms.

Sedation

Key consideration

What are the lasting effects of sedation and analgesics on psychological well-being?

During John's initial admission, he was mechanically ventilated and had invasive monitoring. To facilitate these interventions and to decrease any discomfort, pharmacological sedation was used along with analgesia. This increased comfort reduced the stress response and allowed diagnostic and therapeutic procedures to be carried out (Shelly, 1998; Samuelson *et al.*, 2007). The purpose of using two types of drugs together is to reduce the need for high doses of sedation, as analgesic drugs such as opioids have their own sedative effect if administered in large doses and can also induce anaesthetic properties (Samuelson *et al.*, 2007).

Alteration in memories due to sedation

One of the more noxious effects of oversedation is that when the brain is deprived of stimulation, it makes its own 'false memories'. These can be of a horrifying nature; for example, John had thought he had been locked in a room and been unable to escape and felt persecuted. Some drugs have been known to have a certain orientation; an example of this is propofol, which when administered has been known to cause dreams with a sexual nature to them (Brandner *et al.*, 1997). The extreme scenario of this is that some patients believe that they have been sexually interfered with; a simple explanation for this is that the patient was having catheter care. Shelly (1998) identified other such effects from oversedation, such as bradycardia, respiratory depression, deep vein thrombosis, ileus, renal and hepatic dysfunction, to name a few. The opposite effect of this is to undersedate a patient, during which time they can become tachycardic, hypertensive, clammy and tachypnoeic.

It is obvious to see how medical intervention can be misconstrued and false memories can take over a patient's perception of reality. This can exacerbate and contribute to further detrimental psychological effects such as delirium and PTSD, which can be long-lasting for the patient and have a devastating effect on their well-being.

Sedation hold/sedation holiday

In response to the recognition of the noxious effects of sedation, recently the use of sedation and analgesia has changed. In the 1980s, it was greatly preferred to ensure that patients were deeply sedated with the added use of muscle relaxants and awakened occasionally (Shelly, 1998). Over the years, this has changed to achieve a more arousable state where the patients are sedated but are regularly given sedation holidays to ensure comfort, and the use of muscle relaxants has become less popular (Shelly, 1998; Samuelson *et al.*, 2007). One of the reasons for this is that the long-term use of muscle relaxants has been associated with the development of critical illness polyneuropathy (CIP) (Walther *et al.*, 2002;

Fletcher *et al.*, 2003; Keaveney, 2004). Sedation holidays are given to avoid oversedating, which has been shown to prolong the recovery process and delay discharge.

Sedation scoring

Sedation scoring has been introduced to enable assessment of the effectiveness of sedation. Recent research from Herridge (2008) indicates a tendency towards having patients less sedated, thereby creating a more mobile patient, which will reduce muscle wastage and weakness allowing for greater physiotherapy. This in turn will decrease the amount of stay but also impact upon and improve psychological well-being (Herridge, 2008) along with reducing cost.

Underlying physiology and physiological effects

Key considerations

What are the physiological effects of being in the critical care environment for this length of time?
How may these effects be displayed?

There are a number of physiological effects of being in intensive care for a long period as seen in Table 10.2. John suffered from many of these and at times felt these issues were too big to overcome as seen in Figure 10.1.

Respiratory

One of the lasting effects of being mechanically ventilated for a prolonged period of time is breathlessness and it can be caused by a number of physiological and psychological factors (Broomhead and Brett, 2002). These can include issues such as depression, tiredness, severe weakness and reduced lung function. Patients often feel dependent on their ventilators and can become very anxious when the weaning process begins as they may feel unable to breathe and are therefore scared that they will not be able to breathe without mechanical support. The consequences of this is that anxiety then triggers other pathophysiological responses such as tachycardia, hypertension, tachypnoea, sweating and reduced tidal volume, which then impairs the patient's gas exchange, thus exacerbating the breathlessness and feelings of anxiety.

Angus and Carlet (2003) found that the lung function of patients who had survived ARDS took up to 1 year to return to normal, although further research has demonstrated that through computed tomography (CT) it is possible to see persisting physical damage, mostly with fibrotic changes, which reduce respiratory function in the long term. Ultimately, Griffiths and Jones (1999), Broomhead and Brett (2002) and Angus and Carlet (2003) all noted that reduced pulmonary reserve is a consequence of surviving ARDS and ICU. Exercise tolerance can be greatly reduced and may take some time to recover, with even a small task bringing on a period of breathlessness. This can heavily affect the patient's quality of life and his or her perceived health recovery, which can also be very damaging psychologically and make the patient fear that a regression of his or her illness is reoccurring.

Tracheostomy formation in the critically ill patient

John is now successfully self-ventilating through his tracheostomy, following a collaborative MDT weaning plan from the ventilator. Frequently, long-term ICU patients have a tracheostomy formed, which can be performed percutaneously or surgically. The advantage of receiving a tracheostomy is that it enables the patient to be ventilated without being on large quantities of sedation, therefore enabling him or her to wean off the ventilator. It also allows the patient to be awake and to start communicating, which often involves the nurses and family being able to lip-read. This at times can be frustrating for both parties involved, so the patient may need to write down what he or she requires or use picture boards but this can be very limiting, frustrating and also tiring for the patient. In relation to an endotracheal tube (ETT), the shorter length of the tracheostomy allows the patient to breathe more easily and with less resistance.

The disadvantages to having a tracheostomy include scarring, which can be so unsightly to some patients that some have required surgical revision of the site. Other issues include the formation of granulation tissue, tracheal stenosis, haemorrhaging through a tracheoinnominate artery fistula and tracheo-oesophageal fistula, which increases the risk of aspiration (Epstein, 2005).

Communication with a tracheostomy

For many patients communicating through lip-reading can be exceptionally frustrating. John was of no exception, so a phonation valve was introduced into his weaning plan once his swallow had been assessed. The aim of this was to help him communicate more effectively, which would help him to feel more 'normal' and therefore improve his quality of life. The phonation valve can have a very positive psychological effect on patients but from a physiological viewpoint it can help to assist the weaning process from mechanical ventilation.

The main role of the phonation valve is to improve communication, provided patients can tolerate having their tracheostomy cuff deflated for a period of time. The one-way valve in the phonation valve opens on inspiration and enables air to be breathed in through the tracheostomy; once inspiration is finished the valve closes, creating a positive airway pressure, which is similar to 'normal' breathing. The air on expiration flows out around the tracheostomy, up through the vocal cords, and voice is produced (Figure 10.2).

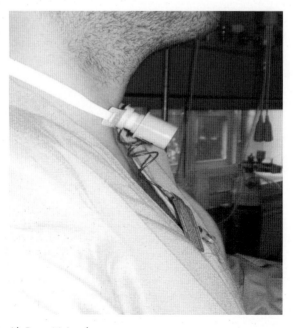

Figure 10.2   Patient with Passy-Muir valve.

Cardiovascular

Unless the patient has cardiac failure or has had a myocardial infarction, there are minimal effects on the cardiovascular system of being in ICU for a prolonged period of time (Broomhead and Brett, 2002). Therefore, it is unlikely that John would experience any cardiovascular dysfunction as a consequence of being in the ICU for 2 months. This would only be relevant to patients who have undergone cardiac surgery or who have a cardiac history, in which case there is an increased mortality associated with a prolonged ICU stay. This is despite many of these patients without a cardiac history having received large amounts of cardiovascular support either through inotropes or vasopressors during a shock or septic episode.

Critical illness polyneuropathy (CIP)

CIP is a syndrome of severe weakness that can take years to recover from and is often associated with patients who suffered from sepsis or systemic inflammatory response syndrome (SIRS), multiorgan failure (MOF) and the use of certain drugs (such as muscle relaxants) during their ICU stay; however, the reason why it occurs is unclear (Kane *et al.*, 2002). Walther *et al.* (2002) described it as part of a neurological manifestation of critical illness and can occur when a patient has been critically ill for more than a week.

Patients usually present with CIP when they have difficulty weaning from mechanical ventilation mostly due to the involvement of the phrenic nerve (Walther *et al.*, 2002) and have severe muscle wasting (de Letter *et al.*, 2001). Fletcher *et al.* (2003) commented that more than 90% of long-term patients can continue to suffer from CIP up to 5 years after discharge, resulting in years of rehabilitation. The histophysiological aspect of CIP is the axonal deterioration of motor and sensory fibres (Griffiths, 2007) leading to motor weakness and sensory alterations.

John was clearly having problems associated with severe weakness, above the level of his spinal injury. His spinal injury was at T2-3 level, so he should have been able to move his head, shoulders and arms. Innervation of his respiratory muscles should also have been unaffected. However, he was slow to wean from the ventilator and had difficulty moving his forearms and hands although he could shrug his shoulders. John was diagnosed as suffering from CIP, following the diagnostic approach of having an electromyography (EMG). Prior to completing any diagnostic tool for CIP, the following conditions need to be disqualified: Guillain-Barré syndrome, muscular dystrophy, electrolyte imbalance, rhabdomyolysis, myasthenia gravis and, as with John, spinal cord disorders (Griffiths, 2007). An EMG shows debilitated muscle strength and has two main functions.

(1) To separate primary muscle conditions from muscle weakness caused by neurological disorders and
(2) To distinguish between true weakness and lack of motivation or severe pain

The other forms of diagnosis of CIP are through a muscle biopsy, magnetic resonance imaging (MRI) and phrenic nerve studies; however, an EMG is the gold standard diagnostic tool.

Prevention of CIP involves several aspects of care, quick recognition and treatment of sepsis and multiorgan failure (Griffiths, 2007). Cautious use of corticosteroids and neuro-muscular blocking agents, if used, should be reviewed regularly along with tight glycaemic control (Walther *et al.*, 2002; Griffiths, 2007). Enteral feeding should be commenced early as it is a contributing factor in reducing CIP (de Letter *et al.*, 2001). Although there is no research to clarify this, passive movements on limbs may be helpful in avoiding CIP, as it is intensified by muscle wastage secondary to catabolism and immobility (Griffiths, 2007).

There is no specific treatment of CIP apart from treating the underlying illness and intense physiotherapy within a multidisciplinary approach; however, it is a long road to recovery. CIP is not only debilitating for the patient but is a draining resource on the ICU due to the increased length of stay, and it is one of the most frequent morbidities in ICU (Herridge, 2008).

Sexual dysfunction

For many patients sexual dysfunction is an issue once discharged home but still has relevance for the long-term in-patient in ICU. According to Broomhead and Brett (2002), estrangement of sexual intimacy can not only have a long-lasting effect on relationships but also on patient's physiological and psychological well-being. This can affect affection towards loved ones and can cause patients to withdraw from social and intimate contact. Further, during the recovery process patients can demonstrate anger towards their relatives, therefore, withdrawing themselves from their own social support network.

Once discharged, patients may feel unable to have or restart a sexual relationship due to shortness of breath, erectile dysfunction, weakness, tiredness, disfigurement and scarring. Broomhead and Brett (2002) even discussed that it may cause enough concern that a patient may consider it to trigger a regression of their illness.

For John, his main fear was of restarting a sexual relationship with his partner Jane, and this was related to his T2-3 spinal injury. The Spinal Cord Injury Information Network (2007) states that many men with spinal cord injuries are capable of getting and maintaining an erection. However, erectile dysfunction is common and medications such as the use of phosphodiesterase inhibitors can be helpful. The alternatives include surgical penile prosthesis, penile injection therapy, a vacuum pump or transuretheral therapy. Although interventions such as these will not be used in the critical care setting, critical care nurses need to be aware of these strategies should either the patient or their family wish to discuss the possibility of future sexual activity and procreation.

For many patients, there is often a period of adjustment that is required and it will take time for them to be comfortable with their bodies again and feel confident enough to engage again with loved ones. A relationship counsellor may help the individual or couples over this period.

Nutrition

Key consideration

How do nutrition and mobilisation contribute to the recovery of patients?

All ICU patients who have been sedated and ventilated will have had enteral or parenteral feeding during their admission. Enteral feeding has been linked to reducing ICU mortality and is the preferred route compared to the parenteral (Artinian *et al.*, 2006). Despite early enteral feeding, weight loss is often inevitable in the ICU and it has been noted that some patients can loose up to 2% lean body mass every day (Broomhead and Brett, 2002). Griffiths and Jones (1999) suggested that it can take up to 1 year to rebuild that muscle mass. Along with weight loss and lack of exercise due to lying in bed for a long period of time, patients also suffer from loss of muscle tone. Considering all these issues, patients can have a massive deficiency of calories and proteins, which can hinder their improvement. This is often due to patient's enteral feeding being stopped for procedures, which sometimes can happen on consecutive days. In addition, the increase in basal metabolic rate that is seen during critical illness and which is further increased by, for example, pyrexia and sepsis, will demand an increased calorific intake, which may be difficult to deliver, especially if there is any dysfunction of the gastrointestinal system.

If a patient has been orally intubated for a long period of time and then has a tracheostomy formed, the mechanical aspects of swallowing can be difficult. Bruising and oedema of the trachea can make swallowing sore and food quite often can taste differently.

Other physiological and psychological issues, such as severe weakness due to CIP, scarring of the trachea, vocal cord paralysis, depression, breathlessness and poor swallowing, can put a patient at risk of aspiration. Other problems such as loose teeth or ill-fitting dentures due to weight loss can all impact and decrease a patient's appetite. Therefore, the recovery process is slowed, reducing the patient's quality of life.

Mobility

From the MDT perspective, early mobilisation is paramount to successful rehabilitation for all long-term patients (Bailey *et al.*, 2007). Physiotherapy management of a patient encompasses several dimensions and involves some form of mobilisation. These include the following:

- Improving ventilation/perfusion mismatch
- Restoring fluid compartment shifts
- Increasing lung capacity
- Preserving/recovering function/fitness
- Reducing the effects of immobility

(Stiller *et al.*, 2004)

Both the loss of muscle tone and the severe weakness in CIP make mobilisation very difficult: patients can be grossly stiff and can be in overall body discomfort and pain. The patients can be so weak that even sitting on the side of the bed can be laborious and demanding. Sitting out can cause postural hypotension and dizziness, which is not uncommon. Once in a chair, careful positioning is important to ensure that limbs are correctly flexed/extended and well supported (Figure 10.3).

John found his mobilisation particularly tiring and painful; his pain control medications had to be readdressed and he often slept for an hour post mobilisation. Motivational

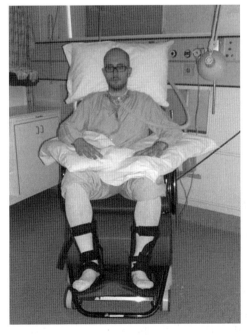

Figure 10.3   Correct patient positioning.

issues were also prominent at this point, with him being uninterested and listless in his manner. This improved with time, but the question of motivation only came when he saw improvement in himself. Long-term patients can often feel depressed along with having motivational issues and if the patient's psychological well-being is not improving with positive input it may be beneficial to consider a pharmacological aid. However, it is worth remembering that medication is not helpful in all cases as side effects can make a patient feel worse.

Motivational techniques or setting achievable goals within the ICU may be helpful. Making the ICU environment a positive area where patients feel valued and secure promotes patient empowerment (Wahlin and Idvall, 2006). This links in with Maslow's hierarchy of needs, encompassing the basic needs to self-actualisation.

- Physiological need
- Safety need
- Social need
- Self-esteem
- Self-actualisation

Each need has to be met; however, because John has been so unwell, he will initially be focusing on the physiological aspect – breathing, sleeping, food, excretion and sex. Once he has felt satisfied he will move on from this and concentrate on his own safety needs and the impact his accident has had over his life. Financial worries may also come into play. The next level is social and this will be difficult for him when thinking about intimacy and how this will affect his relationship with Jane, his partner. At this level, John feels accepted within the ICU environment and he has a good social network, with plenty of friends visiting him, and a loving family. The esteem level concentrates on John's need to be respected, respect of others and to have self-respect. Empowering John will give him the self-respect of himself and others and his desire to be accepted within society. This is particularly relevant as John will feel this need to be important when considering how he will be perceived by society and how he will be accepted in society along with his sense of belonging. When John has finally satisfied all the levels he will be able to realise his own maximum potential and this is the need for self-actualisation.

Quality of life

> **Key consideration**
>
> How is quality of life addressed within the ICU environment?

Following a critical illness with long-term intensive care intervention, reduction in quality of life or perceived quality of one's own life is not uncommon; this is especially understandable with the large physiological and psychological effects. Success in intensive care should be measured by whether a patient returns to their former health status and continues their old social and life-pattern (Maddox *et al.*, 2001). While this is important to the individual patient, it also has relevance on how ICUs are managed as a whole and could provide information for better care during and after admission.

For many patients, quality of life can be measured in so many different ways, as it is a very individualised question that really is only significant to that patient. Health-related quality of life (HRQL) questionnaires are a form of measurement and an excellent way of obtaining information (Chaboyer and Elliot, 2000). An example is the SF-36 measurement model, which is a good form of measurement taking on two main themes, physical and mental health, which can be divided into the following:

Physical health	Mental health
Physical functioning	Vitality
Physical role	Social functioning
Bodily pain	Emotional role
General health	Mental health

The disadvantage with some of the HRQL questionnaires is that they can be quite long and comprehensive and some patients may have difficulty with this in view of their cognitive and concentration abilities. However, the HRQL questionnaires have highlighted that patients' perception of their quality of life is poor up to a 12-month period (Chaboyer and Elliot, 2000). Recommendations for further research in this area would include HRQL questionnaires over a 10-year period. This would truly identify how patients perceive their own quality of life post ICU and the true recovery period.

Rehabilitation process

> **Key considerations**
>
> What is the nurse's role in providing a smooth transition from level 3 to level 2 or level 1 care? How can critical care follow-up aid patient recovery?

The rehabilitation process begins in the ICU and will last long till the patient's transfer home. Nurses and members of the MDT within the ICU are excellent at the critical care phase, caring for patients with multiorgan failure who are often sedated and ventilated. However, once over this phase, nurses and the MDT need to give the patients empowerment, control over their bodies and involvement in the decision-making process.

Historically and within nursing culture today, patients and relatives can easily become institutionalised. ICU as an environment is very structured; with rigorous times set for documentation of observations and generalised care it could almost be described as quite sterile. With this in mind, it can be difficult to pull away from this and encourage the patient who is now awake to engage in his or her own care and make choices and decisions. Simple choices such as patients wanting to wear their own clothes or deciding when to have a wash can impact heavily on their psychological well-being and therefore their rehabilitation.

Maddox *et al.* (2001) described the recovery process as a long procedure which is influenced by many different factors from individual temperaments, life experiences, spiritual/religious view points, support from family and friends and the actual experience of intensive care and post intensive care. These areas will then be re-influenced and the patient will have a different outcome past the acute intensive care phase. Those who have developed coping strategies for other areas in their lives will often do better than those who have not (Maddox *et al.*, 2001). The most frustrating area is often that patients find it difficult to return to their former health status and do the things that are considered 'normal', such as emptying the dishwasher. Maddox *et al.* (2001) went further and felt that patients will often gauge their physical well-being more importantly than psychological as they will want to regain their independence and normality.

Patient diaries

For some relatives a therapeutic way of coping with their family member in ICU is to write a diary of daily events. These diaries can contain anything from what the weather is like to how many friends visited the patient on a daily basis. Nurses can also add to the diary, provided it has no medical notes in it. There are legal and ethical issues relating to the use of patient diaries and they are considered to be quite confusing (Egerod *et al.*, 2006). However, if clear guidelines and protocols are put in place, which includes auditing of the diaries and how to destroy them in case a patient does not want it, then these issues should diminish.

A diary may help patients to piece together their time in ICU and enable them to work through the traumatic experience, almost similar to being in a type of therapy. Bergbom *et al.* (1999) stated that the use of the diaries enhanced the patients' understanding of their time in ICU. Diaries helped them to recall memories of both the positive and the negative aspects and they put perspective and reality on their admission (Bergbom *et al.*, 1999). The diaries belongs to the patient and should be kept with the patients at all times. It should be given to the patients once they are in the rehabilitation phase and are well enough to read it. Box 10.1 is an example from John's diary.

Social adjustment

Along with physical and psychological issues there is also the social adjustment during the recovery period, which can continue well into the patient's discharge home (Maddox *et al.*, 2001). Interestingly, Perrins *et al.* (1998) concluded that some patients had low self-esteem and PTSD up to 1 year post ICU discharge. This of course may well have relevance to the fact that many of these patients, at some point during their admission, were close to death, and it could make patients question their own mortality. It will take time for patients to socially adjust to their illness on top of the physiological and psychological aspects and for some they may never wish to speak about how ill they were or even if they almost died. It may be beneficial to consider community care and help once the patient is discharged and this can come in several forms to help aid overall recovery and may even benefit the next of kin. This can be anything from meals on wheels to the local priest visiting once a week.

Transitional care

McKinney and Deeny (2002) and Hall-Smith *et al.* (1997) referred to the discharge from the ICU as an occurrence similar to a 'relocation stress'. Patients and relatives often find this transition hard as they are leaving a one-to-one nursing scenario, which could change to up to one nurse and nine patients. They also often feel reassured with the presence of the technology surrounding them, along with the detailed explanations they receive from nursing staff and the MDT.

Box 10.1 John's diary

23/3/08. Today was the first day that Jane and the nurses (Sam and Nicola) took you out of the unit and on to the balcony. We wheeled you out in the trauma chair. It was really warm and spring finally looks like it has arrived. You really enjoyed being outside as we worked out; it was the first time in 6 weeks. Jane brought in some photos of you on your last birthday – we have put the lovely photo of the two of you on the left side of your safety rails on your bed so that you can look at it before you go to sleep as you prefer sleeping on that side. Tottenham won 3–2 against Manchester United last night.

John felt secure in a one-to-one nursing environment and felt anxious at the prospect of leaving this protected environment. Many patients are often aware that returning to the ward may leave them feeling vulnerable and uncared for compared to what they have become accustomed to (Chaboyer *et al.*, 2005). All professionals within the MDT can help to ensure that this transition has no negative effects upon the patient and family and this should include the whole discharge from planning to after the actual transfer to the new ward area.

A poor transition can lead to a number of drawbacks that can be detrimental to the patient's well-being; this can result in a readmission to ICU and at the very worst increase the patient's mortality (Chaboyer *et al.*, 2005). This can build poor relationships between nursing staff on the wards and patients/families as readmissions at times can bring resentment and negativity from the patients and relatives. This can redefine their fears of returning to a ward, which they will feel is very much justified due to their own experiences. It can then be quite challenging to gain their cooperation and acceptance of the need to be transferred back to the ward for a second time once their condition has improved again.

From the nursing perspective it is vital to prepare the patient and family for this 'horizontal transition'; this can be done in a systematic way to provide support and structure to all of those involved. The actual process should start early with standardised discharge policies and care plans. The patient should, at the point of transfer, be nursed in a high-dependency/step-down area with an increased ratio of two patients to one nurse, and all technological monitoring should be reduced appropriately. All members of the MDT should be aware of the transfer. An appropriate plan should be in place to continue ongoing rehabilitation that is structured and realistic with the patient and family. It is important to provide reachable goals that are both pragmatic and rational, to provide a sense of achievement that will drive the patient and relative to continue and to give them further incentive. Patient notes should be provided that describe clearly the events that have taken place prior to and during the ICU admission. If resources allow it, a discharge liaison nurse can negotiate and plan the transfer solely with the patient and family, providing extra emotional support. A visit to the transferring ward prior to discharge may help to alleviate any anxieties and also give the patient and family some familiar faces to see on the actual day of transfer. This would provide an excellent opportunity to show the patient who would be looking after them and also where they would be nursed. This should be in a close observation area that is near the nurse's station and provides a reduced number of patients to one nurse. Strategies such as this should be in place until the patient is at an optimum stage where the ratio can be stepped down again to a higher number of patients per nurse. This should provide a greater continuity of care that will also be preventative in reducing the number of readmissions.

An out-of-hospital transfer can be obviously more terrifying to the patient and family; it is in these situations that appropriate communication and documentation to the accepting ward is imperative. Clear goals and outcomes should be documented in the rehabilitation process and all members of the MDT should ensure that they have also clearly handed over their fields of expertise to their appropriate counterparts in the receiving hospital.

The National Institute for Health and Clinical Excellence (NICE) has recently released a clinical guideline focused on rehabilitation after critical illness (NICE, 2009). This emphasises five phases of assessment and support:

- During the critical care stay
- Prior to discharge from critical care
- During ward-based care
- Prior to discharge home or into the community
- Two to three months post discharge from critical care

NICE (2009) suggests that one health-care professional oversees the rehabilitation programme. The guideline intends to promote the concept of optimisation of recovery as the therapeutic goal rather than survival from a critical illness. With this shift in focus, continuing health and social care needs can be identified and addressed.

Support services for patients and staff

Services such as the patient at risk team (PART)/outreach team should help to bridge some of the anxieties; they provide a system of support where patients deemed most at risk of deteriorating and requiring a higher level of care are monitored on a ward level. One of the additional roles that the PART may offer is a counselling service to the patient and family, where they can give information and explanations over their time in ICU. They also ensure that the patient's rehabilitation process continues, by giving the staff on the ward leadership on scenarios such as continuing the patient's weaning programme on continuous positive airway pressure (CPAP) with a tracheostomy.

Follow-up clinics

ICU follow-up clinics are a relatively new concept and were developed when it was noted that for some patients it can take up to 9 months to recover and return to their former health status (Glendinning, 2001; Chaboyer *et al.*, 2005). Maddox *et al.* (2001) went on to claim that although physical recovery takes up to 6 months, psychological recovery could take far longer. For many critical care units, ICU follow-up is still a neglected area (Sawdon *et al.*, 1995; Hall-Smith *et al.*, 1997; Glendinning, 2001) and is an obvious implication for practice. With the latest government initiatives and improving the patient experience, it would indicate that all ICUs should be providing the highest quality care that is in line with national standards supported by robust clinical governance.

It is through follow-up clinics that it has been possible to examine the patients' experience in ICU and explore their perceived quality of life (Hall-Smith *et al.*, 1997). Without a follow-up clinic, it is almost as if the ICU patients are abandoned following intensive medical care and left to convalesce in a period of possible physical and psychological strain (Perrins *et al.*, 1998).

In John's situation, he was initially dubious at going to the follow-up clinic but Jane felt it could help to piece together some of the main events for John and herself. John's main worry was his lack of memory; he remembers snippets such as conversations he heard – someone talking about clothes they bought – but his main memory was of setting off that day on his motorbike prior to the accident. He later remembers days of light sleep and then of feeling unable to move. He recalls faces but is unable to name anyone and feels embarrassed; prior to his accident he worked as a freelance photographer and was good at putting names to faces. Pain was not really an issue. Even so, John still did not recognise himself in the mirror; in total, he had lost 9 kg and he avoided looking at his tracheostomy.

Jane was feeling hyperanxious and still could not believe what had happened and how much their lives had changed. Her main anxiety was related to how close she came to losing John and it was during the clinic stay when she felt most able to discuss this. There is the obvious emotional pressure that relatives are exposed to during the patient's stay in ICU (Perrins *et al.*, 1998) and also later on through discharges to the ward and further on home. Frequently, relatives become the patient's support network and as such often carry the emotional burden of knowing and understanding just how unwell their relative once was. They are also the people closest to the patient and at times can be the ones that the patients will take out all their frustrations and worries on. They can also become overprotective and have unrealistic expectations of the patient's progress.

John and Jane's fears, anxieties and concerns could be discussed in the follow-up clinic. The follow-up clinic allows for physical and psychological health to be monitored and assessed, ensuring that they are receiving the best health care and support. From another angle, the clinic provides feedback from the patients in the form of interviews and questionnaires, and this is fundamental in helping to change/improve practice and aids all the members of the MDT.

Conclusion

Surviving a critical illness in itself can be a mountainous passage as intensive care can leave a long-lasting damaging effect on the long-term patient both from the psychological and physiological perspective. It is vital to ensure that patients' recovery to their former health status is a continuous transition especially after so much time, effort and money has been put into keeping them alive and supporting the family.

Health-care professionals play one of the most vital roles within the patient's and the family's journey from the onset of being admitted through the critical illness to the discharge to the ward, but the most rewarding is the achievement of the patient going home. Follow-up clinics and support networks can only aid this and it also provides a base for continuous research through data collection where change in practice can be easily influenced. It is only through greater understanding, empathy and research that health-care professionals can truly appreciate and change practice to ensure that the whole process of admission through to discharge is as smooth as possible.

References

Angus D and Carlet J (2003) *Surviving Intensive Care. Update in Intensive Care and Emergency Medicine 39*. Springer-Verlag, Berlin, Heidelberg, New York.

Artinian V, Krayem H and Di Giovine B (2006) Effects of early feeding outcome of critically ill mechanically ventilated medical patients. *Chest* 129 (4) 960–967.

Bailey P, Thomsen G, Spuhler V, *et al.* (2007) Early activity is feasible and safe in respiratory failure patients. *Critical Care Medicine* 35 (1) 139–145.

Bennun I, Wright M, Ingram D and Ley A (2003) An investigation of patient memories in intensive care. *Care of the Critically Ill* 19 (2) 49–52.

Bergbom I, Svensson C, Berggren E and Kamsula M (1999) Patients' and relatives' opinions and feelings about diaries kept by nurses in an intensive care unit: pilot study. *Intensive and Critical Care Nursing* 15 (4) 185–191.

Brandner B, Blagrove M, McCallum G and Bromley LM (1997) Dreams, images and emotions associated with propofol anaesthesia. *Anaesthesia* 52 (8) 750–755.

Broomhead LR and Brett SJ (2002) Clinical review: intensive care follow-up – what has it told us? *Critical Care* 6 (5) 411–417.

Chaboyer W and Elliot D (2000) Health-related quality of life of ICU survivors: review of the literature. *Intensive and Critical Care Nursing* 16 (2) 88–97.

Chaboyer W, James H and Kendall M (2005) Transitional care after the intensive care unit. Current trends and future directions. *Critical Care Nurse* 25 (3) 16–29.

Christensen M (2007) Noise levels in a general intensive care unit: a descriptive study. *Nursing in Critical Care* 12 (4) 188–197.

Critical Care Stakeholder Forum (2005) *Quality Critical Care: Beyond 'Comprehensive Critical Care': A Report by the Critical Stakeholder Forum*. Department of Health, London.

Culter L, Brightmore K, Colqhoun V, Dunstan J and Gay M (2003) Developing and evaluating critical care follow-up. *Nursing in Critical Care* 8 (3) 116–124.

Egerod I, Schwartz-Nielsen KH, Hansen G and Laerkner E (2006) The extent and application of patient diaries in Danish ICUs in 2006. *Nursing in Critical Care* 12 (3) 159–167.

Epstein S (2005) Late complications of tracheostomy. *Respiratory Care* 50 (4) 542–549.

Fletcher S, Kennedy D, Ghosh I, *et al.* (2003) Persistent neuromuscular and neurophysiologic abnormalities in long-term survivors of prolonged critical illness. *Critical Care Medicine* 31 (4) 1012–1015.

Glendinning A (2001) Intensive care follow-up: setting up a new practice area. *Nursing in Critical Care* 6 (3) 128–132.

Granberg A, Engberg I and Lundberg D (1999) Acute confusion and unreal experiences in intensive care patients in relation to the ICU syndrome. Part II. *Intensive and Critical Care Nursing* 15 (1) 19–33.

Granja C, Lopes A, Moreira S, Dias C, Costa-Pereira A and Carneiro A (2005) Patients' recollections of experiences in the intensive care unit may affect their quality of life. *Critical Care* 9 (2) 1–14.

Griffiths J (2007) Critical Illness Polyneuropathy. *Anaesthesia UK* [online]. Available from: http://www.frca.co.uk/article.aspx?articleid=100908 [Accessed March 2009].

Griffiths R and Jones C (1999) ABC of intensive care: recovery from intensive care. *British Medical Journal* 319 (7207) 427–429.

Griffiths J, Morgan K, Barber V and Duncan Young J (2008) Study protocol: the intensive care outcome (ICON) *BMC Health Services Research* 8 132. http://www.biomedcentral.com/1472-6963/8/132. [Accessed February 2009].

Hall-Smith J, Ball C and Coakley J (1997) Follow-up services and the development of a clinical nurse specialist in intensive care. *Intensive and Critical Care Nursing* 13 (5) 243–248.

Herridge MS (2008) Mobile, awake and critically ill. *Canadian Medical Association Journal* 178 (6) 725–726.

Kane S, Pharm D and Dasta J (2002) Clinical outcomes of critical illness polyneuropathy. *Pharmacotherapy* 22 (3) 373–379.

Keaveney M (2004) Critical illness polyneuropathy in adults after cardiac surgery: a case study. *American Journal of Critical Care* 13 (4) 421–424.

de Letter M, Schmitz P, Visser L, Schellens R, Op de Coul D and Van der Meche F (2001) Risk factors for the development of polyneuropathy and myopathy in the critically ill patients. *Critical Care Medicine* 29 (12) 2281–2286.

Löf L, Berggren L and Ahlström G (2008) ICU patients' recall of emotional reactions in the trajectory from falling critically ill to hospital discharge: follow-ups after 3 and 12 months. *Intensive and Critical Care Nursing* 24 (2) 108–121.

Maddox M, Dunn S and Pretty L (2001) Psychosocial recovery following ICU: experiences and influences upon discharge to the community. *Intensive and Critical Care Nursing* 17 (1) 6–15.

McKinney A and Deeny P (2002) Leaving the intensive care unit: a phenomenological study of the patients' experience. *Intensive and Critical Care Nursing* 18 (6) 320–331

National Institute for Health and Clinical Excellence (NICE) (2009) *Rehabilitation after Critical Illness*. NICE, London.

Pandharipande P, Jackson J and Ely EW (2005) Delirium: acute cognitive dysfunction in the critically ill. *Current Opinion in Critical Care* 11 360–368.

Perrins J, King N and Collings J (1998) Assessment of the long-term psychological well-being following intensive care. *Intensive and Critical Care Nursing* 14 (3) 108–116.

Rattray J and Crocker C (2007) The intensive care follow-up clinic: current provision and future direction? *Nursing in Critical Care* 12 (1) 1–3.

Ridley S (2005) *Critical Care Focus 12: The Psychological Challenges of Intensive Care*. Blackwell, London.

Samuelson K, Lundberg D and Fridlund B (2007) Stressful experiences in relation to depth of sedation in mechanically ventilated patient. *Nursing in Critical Care* 12 (2) 93–104.

Sawdon V, Woods I and Proctor M (1995) Post-intensive care interviews: implications for future practice. *Intensive and Critical Care Nursing* 11 (6) 329–332.

Shelly M (1998) Sedation in the ICU. *Care of the Critically Ill* 14 (3) 85–88.

Spinal Cord Injury Information Network (2007) Available from: http://www.spinalcord.uab.edu/show.asp?durki=22405. [Accessed March 2009].

Stiller K, Phillips A and Lambert P (2004) The safety of mobilisation and its effect on haemodynamic and respiratory status of intensive care. *Physiotherapy Theory and Practice* 20 (3) 175–185.

Storli S, Lindseth A and Asplund K (2008) A journey in quest of meaning: a hermeneutic-phenomenological study on living with memories from intensive care. *Nursing in Critical Care* 13 (2) 86–96.

Strahan E, McCormick J, Uprichard E, Nixon S and Lavery G (2003) Immediate follow-up after ICU discharge: establishment of a service and initial experiences. *Nursing in Critical Care* 8 (2) 49–55.

Wahlin I and Idvall E (2006) Patient empowerment in intensive care – an interview study. *Intensive and Critical Care Nursing* 22 (6) 370–377.

Walther N, Van-Mook M, Riquette P and Hulsewe-Evans M (2002) Critical illness polyneuropathy. *Current Opinion in Critical Care* 8 (4) 302–310.

Chapter 11

Ethical considerations in critical care

Anne McLeod

Introduction

Ethical principles form the basis of decision-making within critical care and guide care provision. Situations that can create an ethical dilemma can arise and may make health-care professionals question as to how decisions are made. These situations may also make health-care professionals question their own feelings and beliefs. The aim of this chapter is to clarify the principles upon which decisions are made with the use of a developing clinical scenario, which is familiar to critical care practitioners.

Patient scenario

Ethel is a 68-year-old lady who had a perforated duodenal ulcer. This has been previously oversown; however, she had developed an anastomosis leak and possible ischaemic bowel. She is due to go to theatre and will require intensive care management following the surgery. She appears to be septic and has precipitating renal failure. The ward nurses have asked the outreach team for support. The intensivist assesses her in view of her impending intensive care unit (ICU) admission. She normally enjoys a good quality of life and is independent. It is likely that she will require a stoma following the surgery.

Admission to critical care

Within the United Kingdom, admission to the ICU is appropriate for the following types of patients:

(1) Patients who require or are likely to require advanced respiratory support alone (e.g. intermittent positive-pressure ventilation [IPPV]);
(2) Patients requiring support of two or more organ systems;
(3) Patients with chronic impairment of one or more systems sufficient to restrict daily activities (co-morbidity) and who require support for an acute reversible failure of another system.

(Intensive Care Society, 1997)

Although Ethel has a good pre-morbid state, post-operatively, it is likely that Ethel will require the following:

- Mechanical ventilation
- Circulatory support in the form of vasoactive drugs as well as fluids
- Possible renal support in the form of renal replacement therapy

In view of these, the intensivist as well as the surgical team will need to make a decision whether surgery is the best option, and if so, what the likelihood of her recovering to an acceptable quality of life is. However, from this clinical scenario, it is unlikely that Ethel will survive this episode without surgical and intensive care interventions. Therefore, the decision-making process will need to take into account Ethel's prognosis without surgery as opposed to her likely prognosis following surgery. This requires them to apply ethical principles to guide their decision-making.

Key consideration

What are the ethical issues involved in this situation?

What are ethics?

'Ethics' is a generic term for examining and understanding moral life (Beauchamp and Childress, 2001); health-care dilemmas, however, are usually considered to be 'ethical' rather than 'moral'. The development of 'medical and nursing' ethics implies that practitioners are experts in knowing what is right and wrong in health and care provision (Downie, 1996). This creates an assumption that health-care professionals are authorities in moral dilemmas but they may have no more 'moral' expertise than anyone else who has a caring or compassionate nature. Health-care practitioners do, however, have a specialist knowledge that gives credence to decision-making involving an ethical difficulty (Downie, 1996). Therefore, health-care providers have a social morality as well as professional morality to guide their practice. Within health care, rules exist about the role of practitioners; therefore, although rules of informed consent and confidentiality are based within more general moral codes respecting autonomy and preventing harm, these rules are very pertinent to practitioners and may, in reality, only be relevant to a minority of people outside of health care (Beauchamp and Childress, 2001). Codes of medical and nursing ethics, codes of research ethics and public commission reports all assist to formalise professional morality, and also help to make explicit rules in relation to professional etiquette.

Everyday and technical ethics

Everyday ethics is associated with life situations and dilemmas, and creates tangible links with general moral codes. These are widely shared creating a stable social consensus of behaviours and attitudes. Generally, everyday ethics are associated with norms about right and wrong conduct (Beauchamp and Childress, 2001). Technical ethics are grounded in abstract, logical theory and help avoid the variances of everyday ethics and hence contain principles and notions that complement each other (Seedhouse, 1998). Technical ethics can be subdivided into dramatic/specific ethics, persisting ethics and ethics in a general sense (Seedhouse, 1998), although the boundaries between them are not distinct or clear-cut.

Dramatic ethics, persisting ethics and ethics in a general sense

Dramatic or specific ethics are associated with cognitive processes that are undertaken when a specific ethical problem is encountered and a decision has to be made. Often this involves making the 'tragic choice', with either choice bearing a heavy cost (Seedhouse, 1998).

Underlying these 'tragic choices' and, to some extent, creating their foundation are persisting ethics where fundamental philosophical questions exist in conjunction with moral principles (Seedhouse, 1998). For example, during cessation of life-sustaining interventions, the decision to withdraw treatment would relate to dramatic ethics, whereas the questions of patient benefit and 'doing good' in a futile situation create the persisting ethics. Underpinning persisting ethics are ethics in a general sense which relate to reflecting about how best to conduct one's life in general. From this, alternative courses of action can be identified, which will have different consequences. Depending upon the pathway chosen, one's own life, as well as others, can be enhanced or damaged.

Goodness

In conjunction with these subdivisions of technical ethics are 'aspects' of technical ethics, three of which relate to health care. One of these seeks to understand 'goodness' on the assumption that if goodness is defined, anyone can aim to be good (Seedhouse, 1998). Although 'good' itself can be perceived in different ways, such as good is something that is enjoyable; in health care, 'good' describes a moral concept, with the person wanting to do 'good'. In this respect, the activity that is 'good' affects other people, not just the individual who is carrying out the activity. In critical care, there are links between doing 'good' and the decision-making process because the decision made needs to be sound and right for that person (the decision maker as well as the patient) and the circumstances.

Consequences/Duty

The second aspect of technical ethics that relates to health care is based on either consequences or duties (Seedhouse, 1998). Basing decisions on likely consequences is the cornerstone of a utilitarian approach. For utilitarians, the best actions are those which yield the most favourable balance over good and bad. In view that the outcome is to do good, actions undertaken should achieve that outcome, and therefore, the right action would produce the best consequences. To achieve this, there would have to be an ethical decision as to what the best outcome is and therefore what the best action is. To assist in this, rules are utilised. These are usually associated with beneficence and non-maleficence and therefore giving the ethical decision, a consequentialist justification (Singleton and McLaren, 1995).

Deontology, or duties, is based in the premise that rightness takes priority over the perceived outcomes, with the most important principle being that a person acted according to duty (Seedhouse, 1998). For example, the outcome of telling the truth could be misery rather than happiness but to tell the truth, and therefore act by a preconceived moral duty, is the correct way to act. In the purest form, the consequences of the action are not taken into consideration just so that duties are performed without exception (Seedhouse, 1998). Kant placed duty above consequences and in doing so believed that principles of behaviour could be discovered by any rational person as some principles are so moral in essence that they are cognitively recognised (Singleton and McLaren, 1995). Thus, a moral person does not weigh up rights and wrongs but will know what ought to be done because they know that they must follow moral law. Within health care, conflict between duties may exist, for example, truth telling could result in harm; in situations such as this, Kant's deontological approach is problematic and creates tensions (Singleton and McLaren, 1995). Health-care professionals have a duty of care in the provision of treatment to ensure patient benefit; in futile situations, arguably this duty of care shifts from provision of active treatment to provision of palliative care so that a moral obligation to relieve suffering is fulfilled.

Deliberation

The third and final facet of technical ethics that relates to health care is 'deliberation' (Seedhouse, 1998). There are two key aspects to this: the process of deliberation and the goal. The process is a conscious path in which the person must have an understanding of principles as well as personal maturity (Seedhouse, 1998). The aim of the process is human flourishing, which is considered to be the most fundamental form of morality. Therefore, the essence of deliberative ethics is contemplation of the best ways to develop oneself and others. This corresponds to Aristotle's view because he considered a reflective process as core to identifying the worth of the activity. Rules and principles can be used in this process, but there is recognition that these may be broken to create better human potential. Therefore, rather than the enforcement of an imperfect set of rules or principles, development of these rules and principles are encouraged to further enhance growth (Seedhouse, 1998).

A number of these ethical stances are incorporated into the four principles that make up the biomedical ethical model that is widely used within medicine and nursing.

Biomedical ethical model

Ethical decision-making within critical care is predominately based on Beauchamp and Childress' (2001) model of biomedical ethics. This framework has four main principles: autonomy, non-maleficence, beneficence and justice. The implication of using these principles to guide decision-making is that adequate guidance is provided so that a satisfactory answer is obtained to ethical problems that are encountered (Seedhouse, 1998). This model has gained widespread popularity because of its simplicity and that it is applicable in a wide range of situations. However, this quality may create difficulties if the four principles conflict with personal ethical stance, for example, a utilitarian may not fundamentally agree with the principle that is being utilised (Seedhouse, 1998). Additionally, within the four-principle approach there is no clear indication as to why it should be followed. Therefore, the philosophical theory of the four-principle approach is unclear.

In Ethel's situation, the intensivist and surgical team will be considering her current situation and the consequences of surgical intervention and intensive care admission. Therefore, they will be cognitively 'weighing up' beneficence and non-maleficence to come to a decision about what is the best way forward for Ethel and her rights as an autonomous adult.

Autonomy

Autonomy relates to 'self-rule' and incorporates concepts such as self-governance, freedom of will, liberty rights and individual choice (Beauchamp and Childress, 2001) and is essential to health care. Autonomy can be viewed in two different ways: firstly, as being able to do and secondly, as being able to have one's expressed wants fulfilled (Seedhouse, 1998). Therefore, to exercise autonomy, the person must be able to understand, reason, deliberate and have independent choice (Beauchamp and Childress, 2001). Autonomy is an intrinsic personal quality and autonomous choice is a right of patients – they may or may not choose to exercise it. For example, a patient may wish to be informed about their medical situation, but they may not wish to make their own medical decisions (Schneider and Young, 1998). Therefore, it is imperative that an individual has a right to hold views, to make choices and to take actions on personal values and beliefs. The health-care practitioner must respect these principles and act upon those choices rather than just have a positive attitude towards them (Beauchamp and Childress, 2001).

Autonomy does not mean obedience to patient choice but the health-care professional must facilitate a situation where the patient can exercise reasoned choice. Additionally, autonomy does not mean that doctors have a duty to provide treatment, which they feel is grossly inappropriate (Downie, 1996) as doctors have a professional autonomy, which they must uphold. Within the ICU, many patients are sedated or are unable to participate in decision-making because of their disease process; documents such as advanced directive and living wills can give the medical staff an indication of what the patients' wishes would be if they were able to be involved. The British Medical Association (BMA) (2001) emphasises the need to respect advanced directives; however, as McLean (1996) rightly points out, advanced directives often reflect a quality of existence rather than a clinical condition for which the patient may or may not want to be treated. This can then create tensions between clinical freedom, professional accountability and personal autonomy as quality of life is subjective with differences in perceptions of the meaning of 'quality of life' (Heap and Ridley, 1996).

Non-maleficence

Non-maleficence is the obligation not to inflict harm on others and refers to intentionally refraining from harmful actions (Beauchamp and Childress, 2001). Non-maleficence also concerns an obligation of not imposing harmful risks: to knowingly put people at risk is negligence and actions that do this are outside accepted professional standards (Beauchamp and Childress, 2001). A consequentialist philosophy would support the concept of non-maleficence and beneficence as being the opposite poles of a continuum (Singleton and McLaren, 1995); however, the range of application is different in that, within health care, there is a duty not to harm others but there is not a duty to benefit everyone (Singleton and McLaren, 1995).

Part of the decision to offer a patient intensive care is based on non-maleficence. The decision is considered against the burdens and benefits of the treatment in relation to the patient's rights and welfare (Beauchamp and Childress, 2001). Even so, the application of non-maleficence creates dilemmas as there are concerns in how 'harms' are assessed. Perceptions of what counts as harm may well be different to the view held by the individual who is under review (Singleton and McLaren, 1995). From this, a paternalistic attitude to health-care delivery may be fostered in the evaluation of what is harmful even if autonomy is respected. Therefore, Ethel may be willing to take the risk of 'harmful' interventions if there is any possibility that it will improve her prognosis, even if the medical staff feel that the burdens of the treatment outweigh the benefits.

Beneficence

Beneficence is an action that benefits another with balancing of benefits and drawbacks to ensure the best overall outcome (Beauchamp and Childress, 2001). Generally, the rules of beneficence are related to protecting and defending the rights of others, preventing harm and removing conditions that will cause harm to others. Philosophers have used the term *beneficence* to identify a positive obligation to others, and through an act of charity, fulfil this principle. Thus, if they fail to act with beneficence, they are not morally deficient (Beauchamp and Childress, 2001). However, there is no clarity if/when beneficence is optional rather than obligatory. As opposed to non-maleficence, beneficence requires positive actions, does not have to be followed impartially and rarely provokes legal reprimand if rules are not abided by (Beauchamp and Childress, 2001). Again, concerns exist as to how benefits are assessed as health-care providers may hold different views to the patient as to the benefits. Benefits are subjective and depend on careful evaluation of the situation (Singleton and McLaren, 1995). Medicine's paternalistic nature can cause conflict between beneficence and autonomy although ideally they would positively interface and support each other. In health care, the medical staff have a greater knowledge and insight to determine what is in a patient's best interest and this can be shared to influence the patient's right to autonomy. Should this override a known preference, it can be justified if the goal of benefiting, or avoiding harm, is achieved (Beauchamp and Childress, 2001). This supports the notion of passive paternalism in the face of medical futility. If an intervention is 'non-beneficial' in that it cannot heal, palliate suffering or enable benefits to quality of life, denying an intervention is justified (Beauchamp and Childress, 2001). Therefore, although the intervention will not necessarily harm the patient, it will not, however, produce a benefit. This principle is key when admission to intensive care is being considered: will there actually be an overall benefit to the patient?

Justice

Justice has two main themes, which are formal justice and the material principle of justice. Formal justice supports the notion that equals are treated equally, whereas the material principle of justice specifies the characteristics required for equal treatment. Therefore, 'need' could be identified as a requirement for a service. Within the critical care setting, the material principle of justice thus can be demonstrated by patients who require an ICU bed being offered an ICU bed, irrespective of age, sex, class, underlying condition or prognosis. Therefore, in view of justice, Ethel should be offered full intensive care interventions irrespective of her age, social status and likely prognosis.

This widely used biomedical ethical model forms the basis upon which decisions are made in relation to patient admission, care strategies and, as required, care cessation in the ICU setting. Doctors and nurses would claim to use this ethical model and indeed, it is this model that creates the ethical standard against which doctors make decisions. A distinction between medical and nursing ethics can be made, though, by suggesting that nursing ethics are derived from the nurse–patient relationship rather than models of 'patient good', notions of autonomy or the professional practice contract that exists between doctor and patient (Fry, 1989). From this it can be postulated that doctors view situations, from an ethical perspective, within a 'justice' orientation, whereas nurses view it from a care perspective (Oberle and Hughes, 2001), that is, an approach based on the application of abstract principles of fairness versus an approach based on relationships.

The role of outreach

> **Key consideration**
>
> What is the role of the outreach team in the identification of patients requiring level 2 or level 3 care?

The identification of the critically ill or deteriorating patient is essential in effective critical care. Outreach services, as a multiprofessional collaborative service, have a key role in ensuring that patients receive relevant and timely treatment in an appropriate clinical area (DH, 2000). They can also enable the timely admission to critical care as well as 'stepping up' patients into level 2 or 3 care settings (ICS, 2002). In Ethel's situation, the outreach team has been notified and are offering support to the ward staff prior to Ethel's surgery and admission to a critical care setting; this sharing of skills and expertise helps to educate and reskill ward staff in the recognition of deterioration and initiation of essential patient resuscitation, for example, with fluids and oxygen.

Identification of the patient at risk

The identification of patients who are deteriorating or are at the risk of deteriorating is fundamental to outreach services. Patients who require level 3 care, for example, those requiring advanced respiratory support, are relatively easy to identify; however, it is the patients requiring level 0–1 or level 1–2 care who are more difficult to identify; there is greater overlap in classification and greater quantities of patients. Some patients will deteriorate quickly, others will have more subtle physiological derangements which may be more difficult to quantify. It is the second group of patients who pose the challenge in timely identification and intervention as they may have a gradual deterioration over hours or days. A patient at risk of deterioration may be identified by the following:

(1) Demonstration of abnormal physiological signs
(2) Their condition (e.g. major surgery) or pre-morbid state
(3) Staff intuition of the patient not being 'quite right'

(ICS, 2002)

The National Confidential Enquiry into Patient Outcome and Death (NCEPOD, 2005) highlighted that patients frequently have prolonged periods of physiological instability prior to their admission to intensive care. Systems based on abnormal clinical signs, such as the modified early warning score (MEWS) and track and trigger systems, have been developed and can be used to guide timely 'triggering' of outreach. Tools such as these can enable early detection of the deteriorating patient by ward-based staff so that outreach services can become involved. However, studies have shown that with the introduction of early warning systems, unexpected admissions to ICU have reduced but there has been little impact on mortality (Bristow *et al.*, 2000; Pittard, 2003).

Patient treatment

Early goal-directed treatment has been shown to improve the mortality of patients presenting with sepsis (Rivers *et al.*, 2001). Outreach are in an ideal position to initiate this management strategy, which aims for the following:

(1) Central venous pressure (CVP) 8–12 mmHg (self-ventilating patient)
(2) Mean arterial pressure (MAP) $\geq$65 mmHg
(3) Urine output $\geq$0.5 ml/kg/hr
(4) Central venous or mixed venous oxygenation saturation 70% and 65%, respectively

(Dellinger *et al.*, 2008)

Colloids or crystalloids can be used to fluid resuscitate the patient, although greater quantities of crystalloids will be required, with recommendations that 1000 ml of crystalloids are used as opposed to 300–500 ml of colloids over 30 minutes. Ongoing haemodynamic management with vasoactive support may be required: the use of vasopressors or inotropes will need to be overseen by an experienced practitioner, if this treatment is commenced in the ward setting.

Patient choice

At the moment, it appears that Ethel would benefit from surgery and post-operative intensive care management. However, some patients may not benefit from intensive care interventions because their illness is beyond recovery or their premorbid state is such that treatment would be inappropriate and futile. The outreach team would be in a position to explore and discuss appropriateness of critical care admission with the admitting consultant as well as the patient and his or her family.

Ethel, though, on discussing the surgery and requirement for post-operative intensive care treatment with staff experienced in intensive care, may not want the surgery and admission to the critical care area. This decision would need to be taken with a full understanding of the consequences of not having the surgery or critical care admission. Ethel, at this time, could also discuss with the intensivist any limitations of treatment that she would want, for example, if her quality of life was likely to be poor, then she would prefer that heroic measurements are not taken.

Ongoing patient scenario

Ethel has now been mechanically ventilated on the ICU for 8 days following her surgery, and requires high concentrations of oxygen and positive end-expiratory pressure (PEEP) to achieve a pO_2 of >7 kPa. She requires vasoactive support. She also requires renal replacement therapy. Her lactate is 4. She does not tolerate enteral nutrition. Her family feels that she has had 'enough'.

Futile situations

> **Key consideration**
>
> What are the ethical issues surrounding life-sustaining treatment when the situation may be futile?

The goals of intensive care management are focused on maintaining life and relieving suffering; however, the intensive care team can face the dilemma of having to decide whether it is in the patient's best interest to withhold or withdraw treatment. Ethel's condition has significantly deteriorated and she has developed multiorgan failure. Ethel's family members express their view that she has had enough and therefore treatment should be withdrawn. This is a familiar situation within ICU as advances in nursing expertise, treatments and technology have increased the number of patients within ICU who are being supported and cared for although their prognosis is poor. Contemporary health-care provision within the ICU setting offers life-sustaining treatments and advanced nursing care: in reflection of this, there have been dramatic increases in the occurrence of withdrawal of treatment within ICU as opposed to death despite full active management (Stroud, 2002). Currently, within the United Kingdom, euthanasia is not recognised; however, studies have confirmed the work of Prendergast and Luce (1997) who found that during the period of 1987–1993 within the United States, there had been an increase from 50% to 90% of patients dying in ICU following withdrawal of life support. Within the United Kingdom, a 72.6% mortality rate following withdrawal of treatment has been reported (Mercer *et al.*, 1998). These studies demonstrate that withdrawal of treatment predominately leads to the death of the patient. Therefore, in the group of patients for whom continued treatment is futile, the ICU team have to find an acceptable path through the legal and moral dilemma of treatment cessation.

Withdrawal/withholding of treatment or euthanasia?

In recognition of these difficulties, it is imperative to define legitimate withdrawal or withholding of treatment and to differentiate it from euthanasia. This supports the medical profession from a legal perspective in their obligation to 'treat' (Gilfix and Raffin, 1984). Withdrawal of treatment, on clinical grounds, should only occur when

> *... the treatment will not benefit the patient or the expected benefits are outweighed by the burdens of treatment.*
>
> (Cohen *et al.*, 2003)

Associated with withdrawal of treatment is withholding treatment, which is

> *a process through which various medical interventions are ... not given to patients ... with the expectation that the patients will die from their underlying illnesses.*
>
> (Luce and Alpers, 2000)

However, euthanasia can be defined as

administering medication or performing other interventions with the intention of causing a patient's death.

(Emanuel, 1994)

Although there are clear definitions, concerns exist over philosophical areas of 'greyness', which surround the distinction between euthanasia and withdrawal/withholding treatment (Seymour, 2000). This has been repeatedly described as the distinction between 'killing' and 'letting die' (Rachels, 1975; Johnson, 1993; Cartwright, 1996; Seymour, 2000). Increasingly, efforts have been made to create an obvious separation between withdrawal of treatment and death, thereby ensuring that there is no 'proximate relationship' (Hoyt, 1995, p. 621). Consequently, central to an ability to place situations into distinct realms is predicting whether a particular course of action is prolonging an inevitable death or facilitating the likelihood of a positive outcome (Seymour, 2000). In withholding or withdrawing treatment, Beauchamp and Childress (2001) claim that, in general, health-care professionals are more comfortable with not starting a treatment as opposed to stopping an established intervention as that decision seems more momentous and of more consequence. Even so, withdrawing and withholding treatment are perceived as being the same. Nevertheless, even if there was a clear difference between the two, not starting an intervention or stopping an established intervention must be ethically justified in futile situations. Both can cause a death and both can allow a death to occur.

Despite situations that have, to some extent, clear boundaries and definitions, conflict and disagreement can result irrespective of the relationship with the patient, be that a doctor, nurse or relative (McGee *et al.*, 2000). Questions may be asked of the decision to either discontinue care or not offer care in respect of futility and a definite poor outcome (Phelan, 1995). Often ICU patients are not competent to participate in the decision-making, and are therefore reliant on others to represent them and their views. The Study to Understand Prognoses and Preferences for Outcomes and Risks of Treatment (SUPPORT Principle Investigators, 1995) demonstrated that the ICU patient may receive unwanted life-sustaining treatment or insufficient palliative care within the ICU setting. In this age of consumerism within health-care provision, the historical paternalist attitude of the medical profession is being challenged by assertive patients and/or family members who demand more involvement in decision-making (Baggs and Schmitt, 2000). This may be seen in either patients/relatives insisting on treatment or by patients asserting their right to have choice at the time of their death by, for example, exploring advance directives and living wills. Both situations can cause difficulties in relation to the ethical principles of beneficence and non-maleficence, and have created debate over physician-assisted suicide and euthanasia (Rieth, 1999).

Protocols/guidelines

To aid the decision-making process, the BMA (2001) and the Intensive Care Society (ICS) (Cohen *et al.*, 2003) have released guidelines both recommending that a coherent management plan is made on ICU admission. Within this plan, any treatment limitations should be made explicit and then regularly reviewed (Cohen *et al.*, 2003). Winter and Cohen (1999) recognise that the question whether to withdraw established interventions has become more of an issue recently because of the ability to maintain life for long periods of time without any real hope of recovery, thereby prolonging the dying process. Even so, the BMA makes it overt that treatment should never be withheld if there is any possibility that a treatment will benefit the patient. Although 'percentage' values of the likelihood of recovery can be quantified and may assist in making judgements over futility of treatment, these are limited as patients, with their particular pre-morbid state and combination of factors, have to be assessed on an individual basis (Gunning and Rowan, 1999). However, doctors can have difference of opinions in view of the risk–benefit balance, which can create conflict (Stroud, 2002).

Patient autonomy

Patient autonomy is a factor in the decision to withhold or withdraw treatment. Advanced directives can offer guidance of the patient's views; however, Goodman *et al.* (1998) found that only 5% of patients over the age of 65 years who were admitted to ICU had an advanced directive. Of the 5%, 11% were administered cardiopulmonary resuscitation despite the advanced directive, indicating that the patient did not want this. They also found that the level of care delivered to this group of patients was not significantly different to those who did not have an advanced directive. This suggests that advanced directives may not be complied with and do not necessarily mean care will be different. However, arguably advanced directives can be viewed as an extension of the right to self-determination (McLean, 1996). If there is no indication of what the patient would want, the family's opinion can be sought. The relatives should be informed and involved within decision-making when the situation is futile. However, relatives cannot make that decision on the patient's behalf (Dimond, 1992). Their role is to give an impression of what the patient would have wished for. Ultimately, when the patient is not capable of participating in the decision-making process, it is the consultant in charge of the patient who makes decisions in view of non-maleficence and beneficence.

The process of withdrawing or withholding treatment

The impact of withdrawing or withholding treatment affects the whole of the ICU team and tensions can develop if a strategy to acknowledge and respond to the death is not present (Stroud, 2002). Additionally, the difficulties of caring for the patient and his or her family must be recognised. The SUPPORT Principle Investigators (1995) study identified that many patients receive unwanted life-sustaining interventions and insufficient palliative care, which was mainly orientated towards symptom control. Once the decision has been made, questions arise about the process of treatment cessation so that the dying process is not prolonged and that the patient is pain-free and comfortable (Levin and Sprung, 1999). However, there is a lack of clear protocols for this withdrawal process. Faber-Langendoen (1994) showed that in 84% of deaths following treatment cessation, the life support was removed gradually and sequentially with incremental decisions made on three to four different occasions. These generally followed the steps of first writing a 'Do Not Resuscitate' order usually with a decision about haemofiltration being made at the same time; secondly, limiting parenteral nutrition and then finally restricting mechanical ventilation. Hall and Rocker (2000) found that at the time of death, 59% of patients who had treatment either withdrawn or withheld were not receiving mechanical ventilation (as compared to those who died with active treatment, all of whom were receiving mechanical ventilation). They also found that larger doses of narcotics and anxiolytics were given to the treatment cessation group. It is unclear as to why it is speculated that the palliative care group were perceived to be showing more signs of discomfort (Hall and Rocker, 2000). This may occur as a result of reducing mechanical ventilation, with the increase in opioid analgesia and anxiolytics to counter any signs of dyspnoea. Concerns exist in the administration of these drugs to dying patients who are in respiratory failure that death will be hastened through respiratory depression (Brody *et al.*, 1997). However, patients who have intensive life support withdrawn and are given large doses of opioids for comfort live as long on average as patients who are not given opioids. This suggests that the underlying disease process determines the time of death, not the medication (Brody *et al.*, 1997).

The compassionate and supportive removal of interventions to relieve suffering is an essential part of critical care medicine (McGee *et al.*, 2000). However, although there has been an increase in the practice of the withdrawal of treatment, there are suggestions that medicine is failing to provide compassionate care (SUPPORT Principle Investigators, 1995). A time frame cannot be applied to withdrawal of treatment, as there is unpredictability after treatment has ceased. Nelson and Meier (1999) suggest that a palliative care framework should be applied to these situations, thereby ensuring that an integrated, systematic approach to comfort is employed. This would require a change in philosophical perspective (Nelson and Meier, 1999) but would allow for a change of practice, which currently may be inadequate and inconsistent.

Role of the nurse

Key consideration

What is the role of the nurse in the decision-making process?

Nurses are key in treatment cessation and a number of studies have investigated their role and the effect of nurses' experiences of caring for this patient group. It is largely recognised that the families of patients who die in ICU require ongoing support and bereavement care; however, there has been little to demonstrate that the needs of the staff looking after the patient are understood or provided for (Schneider and Young, 1998; Stroud, 2002).

Treatment cessation creates anxieties and those more experienced in critical care demonstrate less anxiety than those who are newer to the area (Erlen and Sereika, 1997). Experiential knowledge and trusting those who make the decision is likely to contribute to feeling less anxious. A feeling of impotence seems to be experienced by nurses as they are involved within a situation which they have little control over but are instrumental in the delivery of. Nurses have expressed concerns over the legal aspects related to the treatment withdrawal such as competence, family involvement in decision-making and euthanasia. Nurses have also identified a feeling of responsibility as it is the nurse who is the practitioner actually carrying out the reduction in life-sustaining therapies. Therefore, nurses have concerns about whether that makes them legally and/or morally responsible for the death of the patient especially in the eyes of the relatives. All of these contribute to ICU nurses having a negative perception of the situation (Simpson, 1997; Schneider and Young, 1998).

Collaborative decision-making

Collaborative decision-making is essential in deciding whether treatment should be withdrawn or withheld. Doctors and nurses have different perceptions of the ethics of withdrawing or withholding treatment with doctors having the burden of making the decision, whereas nurses have concerns with living with the decisions made by another (Oberle and Hughes, 2001). Bucknall and Thomas (1997) found that nurses were frustrated with a lack of decision-making by the medical staff, feeling that decisions were made too late or that decisions were ambiguous, for example, that a specific intervention should continue but not another. The nurses also expressed dissatisfaction that junior doctors, who were less experienced in ICU, made decisions, which then the nurses had to implement although they disagreed with the decision made. Simpson (1997) recognised that a distrust of nurses towards the medical staff inhibited the family and patient's grieving process. Situations that would create distrust included, for example, a communication failure, ambiguous decision-making, a lack of collaborative decision-making or poor communication with the family (Simpson, 1997). These conflicts could result from a lack of understanding between the medical staff and nurses about each other's role within this process (Viney, 1996). Nurses do not appear to have an active role; whereas, the medical staff seemed to be making decisions in isolation and did not receive support for their decisions. Ultimately doctors question themselves as to whether the right decision is made while nurses question doctors whether the right decision was made leading to moral distress for the nurses and moral dissonance for the medical staff. Both professional groups have the same goal of minimising patient suffering though.

Nurses make little differentiation between withholding treatment and withdrawing treatment. However, discontent among nurses is present in situations when patients were continued to be aggressively treated when the nurses felt the situation was futile (Bucknall and Thomas, 1997). Situations such as this do demonstrate that the medical staff and the nursing staff view these situations differently. Doctors and nurses use the same ethical principles to guide their practice but doctors are more likely to use a utility-based model, whereas nurses base their interpretation of situations on a virtue/relationship model (Robertson, 1996). This suggests that doctors and nurses have a difference in perception of ethical problems in practice, which could cause conflict. This offers an explanation as to why there can be discord in the decision-making process as there may need to be a degree of compromise with doctors and nurses viewing the situation from different vantage points, philosophies and professional orientation.

The transition from a 'curative' role to one that facilitates the dying process can be difficult (Kirchhoff and Beckstrand, 2000). This shift of focus may happen over a very short period of time and requires considerable skill to be able to cope with the changing situation. To facilitate the dying process following withdrawal of treatment, the transition from curative to care needs to be polished and problem-free. This is difficult, though, if there is uncertainty about process management in a time frame that is unpredictable.

Conclusion

Critical care, by its very nature, will involve ethical decision-making. Recommendations have been made that nurses should have formal education in ethical principles and how ethics are applied within the clinical setting (Viney, 1996). Also, nurses, if they are to truly act as patient advocates, must be allowed to practice in an environment that supports their role in ethical decision-making. Collaborative approaches to care provision are encouraged and supports notions of shared clinical governance, thereby ensuring that accountability for decision-making occurs at the point of care rather than being a hierarchical process (O'Grady, 1994). The BMA (2001) guidelines stress the need for a consensus decision-making process and emphasis that good communication is key in both making decisions and in the actual process of withdrawing treatment. Therefore, within the ICU setting, there must be recognition of the value of each other's role so that a consensus decision is made in collaboration with the family.

References

Baggs JG and Schmitt MH (2000) End of life decisions in adult intensive care: current research base and directions for research. *Nursing Outlook* 48 (4) 158–164.

Beauchamp TL and Childress JF (2001) *Principles of Biomedical Ethics.* 5th Edition, Oxford University Press, Oxford.

Bristow PJ, Hillman KM, Chey T, *et al.* (2000) Rates of in-hospital arrests, deaths and intensive care admissions: the effect of a medical emergency team. *Medical Journal of Australia* 173 (5) 236–240.

British Medical Association (2001) *Withholding or Withdrawing Life-Prolonging Medical Treatment.* BMJ Books, London.

Brody H, Campbell ML, Faber-Langendoen K and Ogle KS (1997) Withdrawing intensive life-sustaining treatment – recommendations for compassionate clinical management. *The New England Journal of Medicine* 336 (9) 652–657.

Bucknall T and Thomas S (1997) Nurses' reflections on problems associated with decision making in critical care settings. *Journal of Advanced Nursing* 25 (2) 229–237.

Cartwright W (1996) Killing and letting die: a defensible distinction. *British Medical Bulletin* 52 (2) 354–361.

Cohen SL, Bewley JS, Ridley S, Goldhill D and Members of the ISC Standards Committee (2003) Guidelines for the Limitation of Treatment for Adults Requiring Intensive Care [Online]. Available from: www.ics.ac.uk [Accessed 10th August 2008].

Dellinger RP, Levy MM, Carlet JM, *et al.* International Surviving Sepsis Campaign Guidelines Committee (2008) Surviving sepsis campaign: international guidelines for management of severe sepsis and septic shock. *Critical Care Medicine* 36 (1) 296–327.

Department of Health (2000) *Comprehensive Critical Care: A Review of Adult Intensive Care Services.* The Stationery Office, London.

Dimond B (1992) Not for resuscitative treatment. *The British Journal of Nursing* 1 (2) 93–94.

Downie RS (1996) Introduction to medical ethics. Chapter 1 in Pace NA and McLean SAM (Eds) *Ethics and the Law in Intensive Care.* Oxford University Press, Oxford.

Emanuel EJ (1994) Euthanasia: historical, ethical and empiric perspectives. *Archives of Internal Medicine* 154 (17) 1890–1901.

Erlen JA and Sereika S (1997) Critical care nurses, ethical decision making and stress. *Journal of Advanced Nursing* 26 (5) 953–961.

Faber-Langendoen K (1994) The clinical management of dying patients receiving mechanical ventilation: a survey of physicians' practices. *Chest* 106 (3) 880–888.

Fry S (1989) Toward a theory of nursing ethics. *Advances in Nursing Sciences* 11 (4) 9–22.

Gilfix M and Raffin TA (1984) Withdrawing or withholding extraordinary life support: optimising rights and limiting liability. *Western Journal of Medicine* 14 (3) 387–394.

Goodman MD, Tarnoff M and Slotman GJ (1998) Effect of advance directives on the management of elderly critically ill patients. *Critical Care Medicine* 26 (4) 701–704.

Gunning K and Rowan K (1999) ABC of intensive care: outcome data and scoring systems. *British Medical Journal* 319 (7204) 241–244.

Hall RI and Rocker GM (2000) End-of-life care in the ICU: treatments provided when life support was or was not withdrawn. *Chest* 118 (5) 1424–1430.

Heap M and Ridley SA (1996) Quality of life after intensive care. Chapter 7 in Pace NA and McLean SAM (Eds) *Ethics and the Law in Intensive Care.* Oxford University Press, Oxford.

Hoyt JW (1995) Medical futility. *Critical Care Medicine* 32 (4) 621–622.

Intensive Care Society (1997) *Standards for Intensive Care Units.* Intensive Care Society, London.

Intensive Care Society (2002) *Guidelines for the Introduction of Outreach Services.* Intensive Care Society, London.

Johnson K (1993) A moral dilemma: killing and letting die. *British Journal of Nursing* 2 (12) 635–640.

Kirchhoff KT and Beckstrand RL (2000) Critical care nurses perception of obstacles and helpful behaviours in providing end of life care to dying patients. *American Journal of Critical Care* 9 (2) 96–105.

Levin PD and Sprung CL (1999) End-of-life decisions in intensive care. *Intensive Care Medicine* 25 (9) 893–895.

Luce JM and Alpers A (2000) Legal aspects of withholding and withdrawing life support from critically ill patients in the Unites States and providing palliative care to them. *American Journal of Respiratory and Critical Care Medicine* 162 (6) 2029–2032.

McGee DC, Weiacker AB and Raffin TA (2000) Withdrawing life support from the critically ill. *Chest* 118 (5) 1238–1243.

McLean SAM (1996) Advance directives: legal and ethical considerations. Chapter 5 in Pace NA and McLean SAM (Eds) *Ethics and the Law in Intensive Care.* Oxford University Press, Oxford.

Mercer M, Winter R, Dennis S and Smith C (1998) An audit of treatment withdrawal in one hundred patients on a general ICU. *Nursing in Critical Care* 3 (2) 63–66.

National Confidential Enquiry into Patient Outcome and Death (NCEPOD) (2005) An acute problem? [Online]. Available from: http://www.ncepod.org.uk/2005report/ [Accessed 30th July 2008].

Nelson JE and Meier DE (1999) Palliative care in the intensive care unit: part I and II. *Journal of Intensive Care Medicine* 14 130–139.

Oberle K and Hughes D (2001) Doctors' and nurses' perceptions of ethical problems in end of life decisions. *Journal of Advanced Nursing* 33 (6) 707–715.

O'Grady PT (1994) *Shared Governance for Nursing: A Creative Approach to Professional Account-ability.* Aspen, Rockville.

Phelan D (1995) Hopeless cases in intensive care. *Care of the Critically Ill* 11 (5) 196–197.

Pittard A (2003) Out of our reach? Assessing the impact of introducing a critical care outreach service. *Anaesthesia* 58 (9) 882–885.

Prendergast TJ and Luce JM (1997) Increasing incidence of withdrawal and withholding life support from the critically ill. *American Journal of Respiratory and Critical Care Medicine* 155 (1) 15–20.

Rachels J (1975) Active and passive euthanasia. *New England Medical Journal* 292 (2) 78–80.

Rieth KA (1999) How do we withhold or withdraw life sustaining therapy? *Nursing Management* 30 (10) 20–27.

Rivers E, Nguyen B, Havstad S, *et al.*, for the Early Goal Directed Therapy Collaborative Group (2001) Early goal-directed therapy in the treatment of severe sepsis and septic shock. *New England Journal of Medicine* 345 (19) 1368–1377.

Robertson DW (1996) Ethical theory, ethnography and differences between doctors and nurses in approaches to patient care. *Journal of Medical Ethics* 22 (5) 292–299.

Schneider R and Young C (1998) Treatment-withdrawal decisions made in ICUs and the impact on nurses, with a commentary on the legal issues raised. *Nursing in Critical Care* 3 (1) 17–29.

Seedhouse D (1998) *Ethics: The Heart of Health Care.* 2nd Edition, John Wiley & Sons, Chichester.

Seymour JE (2000) Negotiating natural death in intensive care. *Social Science and Medicine* 51 (8) 1241–1252.

Simpson SH (1997) Reconnecting: the experiences of nursing for hopelessly ill patients in intensive care. *Intensive and Critical Care Nursing* 13 (4) 189–197.

Singleton J and McLaren S (1995) *Ethical Foundations of Health Care: Responsibilities in Decision-making.* Mosby, London.

Stroud R (2002) The withdrawal of life support in adult intensive care: an evaluative review of the literature. *Nursing in Critical Care* 7 (4) 176–184.

SUPPORT Principle Investigators (1995) A controlled trial to improve care for seriously ill hospitalised patients: the study to understand prognoses and preferences for outcomes and risks of treatment. *Journal of American Medical Association* 274 (20) 1591–1598.

Viney C (1996) A phenomenological study of ethical decision making experiences among senior intensive care nurses and doctors concerning withdrawal of treatment. *Nursing in Critical Care* 1 (4) 182–187.

Winter B and Cohen S (1999) Withdrawal of medical treatment. *British Medical Journal* 319 (7205) 306–308.

Index